Psychiatry

CLINICAL CASES UNCOVERED

Peter Byrne
MA, MB, MRCPsych
Consultant Liason Psychiatrist
Newham University Hospital
London

Nicola Byrne
MBChB, BSc, MSc, MRCPsych
Consultant Psychiatrist
Lambeth Adult Mental Health
The Maudsley Hospital
London

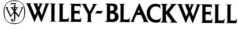
WILEY-BLACKWELL
A John Wiley & Sons, Ltd., Publication

This edition first published 2008, © 2008 by P. Byrne and N. Byrne

Blackwell Publishing was acquired by John Wiley & Sons in February 2007. Blackwell's publishing program has been merged with Wiley's global Scientific, Technical and Medical business to form Wiley-Blackwell.

Registered office: John Wiley & Sons Ltd, The Atrium, Southern Gate, Chichester, West Sussex, PO19 8SQ, UK

Editorial offices: 9600 Garsington Road, Oxford, OX4 2DQ, UK

The Atrium, Southern Gate, Chichester, West Sussex, PO19 8SQ, UK

111 River Street, Hoboken, NJ 07030-5774, USA

For details of our global editorial offices, for customer services and for information about how to apply for permission to reuse the copyright material in this book please see our website at www.wiley.com/wiley-blackwell

Library of Congress Cataloguing-in-Publication Data

Byrne, Peter, MA.
    Psychiatry : clinical cases uncovered / Peter Byrne, Nicola Byrne.
        p. ; cm.
    Includes index.
    ISBN 978-1-4051-5983-8
    1. Psychiatry–Examinations, questions, etc.   2. Psychiatry–Case studies.   I. Byrne, Nicola.   II. Title.
    [DNLM: 1. Mental Disorders–Problems and Exercises. WM 18.2 B995p 2008]
    RC465.B97 2008
    616.890076–dc22

                                                                                    2008009431

ISBN: 978-1-4051-5983-8

A catalogue record for this book is available from the British Library

Set in 9/12pt Minion by SNP Best-set Typesetter Ltd., Hong Kong
Printed in Singapore by COS Printers Pte Ltd

1   2008

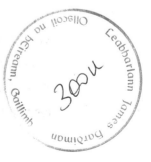

Contents

(**Part 3**) **Self-assessment, 203**

Introduction

Psychiatry is the ultimate clinical speciality. No other branch of medicine relies so much on empathic listening skill and the integration of biological, psychological and sociological theory to unravel a patient's story into a coherent aetiological formulation. Whether you hope to call yourself a psychiatrist or are just passing through, be aware that this is a golden opportunity to acquire competencies that will serve as foundations for your working life (e.g. understanding reactions to illness and adversity, the relationships between physical and mental health, working with 'difficult' patients and relatives, and keeping your cool in unpredictable situations).

The focus throughout the book is on developing your clinical reasoning and core competencies up to a standard of passing undergraduate examinations, workplace-based assessments of your early years as a doctor, and beyond. Part 1 is a guide to psychiatric assessment and introduces the range of treatment options, Part 2 is a collection of case studies covering the range of mental disorders, and Part 3 is for self-assessment. Ultimately, clinical judgement comes from experience, and the more patients you encounter, the more skilled you will become. Some clinical dilemmas have no 'textbook' right answer. Medical professionalism is based on working within our shared ethical framework (Box A); whenever the rights and wrongs of a situation are opaque, it can be helpful to return to these first principles to determine your action.

You will get the most from the case studies by stopping to answer every question posed as the responsible doctor. The cases vary in complexity, beginning with easier ones. An index of cases by diagnosis is provided on p. 223 – useful for revision or if you want to select a case for peer group learning or tutorials. All cases are amalgams of patients and situations we have come across, and none describe identifiable individuals.

In relation to diagnoses, we have used the World Health Organization's categorization of mental disorder, the ICD-10 (International Classification of Diseases).

> ## Box A The duties of a doctor
>
> Patients must be able to trust doctors with their lives and health (General Medical Council: www.gmc-uk.org). To justify that trust you must show respect for human life and you must:
> - Make the care of your patient your first concern
> - Protect and promote the health of patients and the public
> - Provide a good standard of practice and care
> - Keep your professional knowledge and skills up to date
> - Recognize and work within the limits of your competence
> - Work with colleagues in the ways that best serve patients' interests
> - Treat patients as individuals and respect their dignity
> - Treat patients politely and considerately
> - Respect patients' right to confidentiality
> - Work in partnership with patients
> - Listen to patients and respond to their concerns and preferences
> - Give patients the information they want or need in a way they can understand
> - Respect patients' right to reach decisions with you about their treatment and care
> - Support patients in caring for themselves to improve and maintain their health
> - Be honest and open and act with integrity
> - Act without delay if you have good reason to believe that you or a colleague may be putting patients at risk
> - Never discriminate unfairly against patients or colleagues
> - Never abuse your patients' trust in you or the public's trust in the profession
>
> You are personally accountable for your professional practice and must always be prepared to justify your decisions and actions.

The terms here are used to describe disorders, not people: people with borderline personality disorders or schizophrenia are not 'borderlines' or 'schizophrenics'.

Diagnoses do not define identity, and they need to be used sensitively in mental health.

We have both been lucky enough to learn through great clinicians we have been taught by and worked with, and from the generosity of our patients. None of us can fully understand what something is like until we experience it ourselves, and first-hand accounts of mental disorders that we have found valuable are listed in Further reading below. You will not need them to pass exams, but they are worth reading to balance your clinical experience and reading with the realities of mental illness and its consequences.

Peter and Nicola Byrne
2008

Further reading

Sunbathing in the Rain: A Cheerful Book about Depression. Gwyneth Lewis (2007) HarperCollins. The author is a poet, and her experience of a severe depressive episode is charted as her investigation into the mystery of how she came to arrive at the point of psychological collapse. She re-evaluates assumptions about depression as simply a problem, exploring its meaning for her and its potential role as a signal that her life needed to change. Comprising a series of short sections which can be dipped into, she speaks to those involved in caring for depressed people, and those currently depressed themselves and unable to digest long tracts of text.

An Unquiet Mind. Kay Redfield Jamison (1995) Vintage. A psychiatric 'classic', the author is an eminent American professor of psychiatry who describes her experience of bipolar affective disorder. With frequent intersections between the personal and the scientific, it is widely read by professionals and patients.

Smashed: Growing Up a Drunk Girl. Koren Zailckas (2005) Ebury Press, London. A young woman's experience of using alcohol to avoid social anxiety and uncomfortable emotions in the transition into adulthood. Gives a good – albeit retrospective – account of her innate predisposition to becoming addicted, illustrating how some people might powerfully 'take' to a substance after only limited exposure, which can seem bewildering to people with no such inclination. The collateral damage of substance misuse to her close relationships and the striking descriptions of her physical and sexual vulnerability when drunk are complicated by the blank horror of her alcohol-induced amnesia.

Drinking: A Love Story. Caroline Knapp (1999) Quartet Books, London. An account of alcohol addiction from the perspective of a highly functioning journalist from a 'respectable' middle-class background, who goes on to seek help from Alcoholics Anonymous (AA). Provocative reading for those who drink to excess socially or to relieve stress, and for whom the line between harmless and harmful drinking may not always be clear.

Beyond Crazy: Journeys Through Mental Illness. Julia Nunes and Scott Simmie (2002) McClelland and Stewart, Toronto. Compiled by two successful Canadian journalists, the whole range of mental disorders is presented, written in different styles and from many perspectives, but the book ends with clear explanations and useful advice. Almost every account moves logically from setting out painful, real experiences to discovering universalities that promote understanding and recovery.

Speaking Our Minds: An Anthology. Jim Read and Jill Reynolds (1996) MacMillan, London. An anthology of writing from over 50 individuals, from diverse perspectives and backgrounds, who have experienced mental distress and have had various forms of treatment. Useful to understand the nature of their difficulties and what authors did and (frequently) did *not* find useful from mental health services.

Is That Me? My Life With Schizophrenia. Anthony Scott (2002) A. & A. Farmer, Dublin. A deeply personal account of a life punctuated by schizophrenia. Written in an honest and direct style, the author is generous to the people who helped him along the way and reflective about the obstacles to his full recovery.

Born on a Blue Day. Daniel Tammet (2006) Hodder. A unique account of how a man with Asperger's syndrome experiences reality, filtered through his relationship with words and colours. Unusually, he is able to explain the nature of his 'savant' mathematical abilities and to describe the mutual incomprehension between him and those around him growing up. It is also an impressive account of someone transcending their own limitations.

Stuart: A Life Backwards. Alexander Masters (2005) Fourth Estate, London. Strictly speaking a biography, this is a life story traced backwards, starting from Stuart's adult position as a chaotic, homeless, 'personality-disordered' and at times violent drug-user existing in a social underclass. The author is one of his care-workers and (like most doctors) hails from a background of relative advantage and security that is in marked contrast to Stuart's. The book is simultaneously an account of his relationship with Stuart, often characterized by mutual irritation and exasperation. Stuart's behaviour initially appears bewildering, but increasingly makes sense as we are led backwards to its origins. In turns hilarious and terrifying, his story is a challenge to instinctive reactions to reject this type of 'difficult' patient.

Telling is Risky Business: Mental Health Consumers Confront Stigma. Otto Wahl (1999) Rutger's University Press, New Brunswick. This is a catalogue of people's experiences of isolation and misunderstanding by others as a result of their mental illness. Drawing on first-hand accounts of stigma, it demonstrates how negative stereotypes have invaded every aspect of Western culture to make discrimination against 'those people' the norm, not the exception.

How to use this book

Clinical Cases Uncovered (CCU) books are carefully designed to help supplement your clinical experience and assist with refreshing your memory when revising. Each book is divided into three sections: Part 1, Basics; Part 2, Cases; and Part 3, Self-Assessment.

Part 1 gives a precis of history and examination, and key treatments based on best evidence. Part 2 contains many of the clinical presentations you would expect to see on the wards or crop up in exams, with questions and answers leading you through each case. New information, such as test results, is revealed as events unfold and each case concludes with a handy case summary explaining the key points. Part 3 allows you to test your learning with several question styles (MCQs, EMQs and SAQs), each with a strong clinical focus.

Whether reading individually or working as part of a group, we hope you will enjoy using your CCU book. If you have any recommendations on how we could improve the series, please do let us know by contacting us at: medstudentuk@oxon.blackwellpublishing.com.

Disclaimer

CCU patients are designed to reflect real life, with their own reports of symptoms and concerns. Please note that all names used are entirely fictitious and any similarity to patients, alive or dead, is coincidental.

Approach to the patient

Psychiatric histories are complex. The challenge is to cover a wide range of areas in a limited time, often with the patient at a time in their lives where they are least able to give a coherent account of themselves.

This section begins with the content of the assessment – the 'what': **history, mental state examination (MSE), physical examination** and **formulation**. You will come across different versions of the interview schedule in terms of the ordering and grouping of information – find a version that makes most sense to you and stick to it. We outline our preferred version here. The second part of this section looks at the process of conducting interviews, or the 'how'.

History

History-taking has been compared to shining a torch around a dark room. Initially, you need to use a systematic approach to find what you are looking for, using an established framework to structure your history (Table 1), until you know instinctively where to focus your attention. A comprehensive assessment will take about an hour depending on the patient. For example, when interviewing an adult in crisis in accident and emergency (A&E), focus on the presenting problem, role of substance misuse if any, medical and psychiatric history, pertinent current social circumstances and indicators of risk. By contrast, the planned psychiatric outpatient assessment of an adolescent will be a time-intensive process, covering detailed family, personal and developmental history, including collateral information from the parents and, if possible, their family doctor and school.

Table 1 details the content of the history. When presenting a history, verbally or in writing, introduce the case with a brief **background** to put the information that follows in a specific context (i.e. who the patient is; when, where and why you were interviewing them).

The **presenting complaint/history of presenting complaint** should use the patient's own words to describe their problems (e.g. 'I just feel numb') not the technical labels for them. These come later in the MSE ('affect was depressed'). The structure echoes that of any medical history, covering symptom onset, trajectory and relationship to other problems. Differentiate between the patient's report and that of others. *Relevant negative findings* are included as they help signpost towards your differential diagnoses later (e.g. if schizophrenia is the primary problem, list the lack of mood symptoms that exclude bipolar disorder).

Family history explores biological (e.g. genetic) vulnerability to illness as well as formative experiences (e.g. losses and dysfunctional relationships). In the **personal** history you are looking for evidence of developmental problems (normal development is summarized in Table 2), getting a sense of the family atmosphere in which they grew up, and exploring their capacity to form relationships and to direct the course of their lives (school, occupation). **Social circumstances** indicate level of current functioning, and the social network that supports this.

The **substance misuse** history may permeate all the other areas of the history, but needs to be addressed in its own right to clarify all the important information (for the worked example of alcohol see Box 1).

Under **medical**, specifically enquire about a history of epilepsy or head injury. Ask women about their obstetric history (e.g. number of pregnancies, miscarriages, terminations of pregnancy) and older patients about vascular risk factors.

If past **psychiatric** history indicates a relapsing recurring disorder, explore why things were better during periods of relative health.

Any **forensic** history may well link to **premorbid personality** in terms of social habits (e.g. binge drinking), impulse control and capacity for remorse/victim empathy. A history of violence not formerly prosecuted should also be included here: past violence is the best predictor of future violence.

Table 1 The psychiatric history.

Background to assessment
- Basic **demographics**: name, age, gender, ethnic background, marital status, children, type of employment and if currently unemployed, for how long?
- **Current treatment status**: any established diagnosis; nature of current involvement with psychiatric services; if an inpatient, voluntary or involuntary admission
- **Context of your interview**: who referred the patient, where you saw them

Presenting complaint
- In the patients **own words** (e.g. 'There's nothing wrong with me. I've no idea why I'm in hospital')

History of presenting complaint
- **What** is the problem? **When** did it start? **How** did it develop: onset/progress/severity/consequent impairment (e.g. unable to work, end of a relationship)
- What makes it **better** or **worse**; **relationship to other problems**
- **Relevant negative** findings
- **Collateral** history from informants (e.g. friends, family, GP, work colleagues). Note any contradictions

Family history
- **Family structure** describes biological/adoptive/step-parents and siblings: age, state of health or cause and age of death, occupations, quality of relationships. Currently, who supports the patient and who exacerbates their problems?
- **Family history of mental disorder** includes substance misuse, suicide

Personal history
- **Obstetric and birth**: conception planned/unplanned, wanted/unwanted; maternal physical and mental health during pregnancy and postnatally, any prescribed medication or substance misuse; birth full-term/premature, obstetric events and complications, low birth weight, congenital abnormalities, neonatal illness, maternal separation and bonding
- **Development and milestones** (Table 2): delays in interaction with others, speech; motor control, walking, toilet training; sleep difficulties; emotional or behavioural difficulties, hyperactivity; physical illness
- **Family atmosphere and stability**: e.g. warm and caring; abusive; emotionally impoverished or volatile; material circumstances; periods of separation from caregivers (e.g. in hospital due to childhood illness; in foster care due to parental difficulties)
- **Social development**: establishment of friendships, imaginative play, experience of bullying, any juvenile delinquency
- **Educational attainment**: specific learning difficulties, school refusal, age left education and qualifications
- **Occupation**: periods of employment, nature of work/skills
- **Psychosexual**: age of first sexual experience, sexual orientation, number, length and quality of significant relationships, marriage(s), children from all previous relationships

Social circumstances
- **Housing** situation (e.g. renting, numbers of people in the house), **employment, finances, benefits, debts**
- Daily **activities**
- Sources of family and social **support**

Substance misuse history
- **Alcohol** use, amounts (Box 1)
- **Illicit substance** use: type, pattern of use including frequency, dependency; associated problems – occupational, social, relationship, health and criminal activity
- Abuse of any **prescribed** or **over-the-counter** medications

Medical history
- Past and current **physical illness** and **treatment**, allergies
- Current **medication**, including any over-the-counter drugs taken regularly

Table 1 (*Continued*)

Past psychiatric history
- **Age** of onset of symptoms and first contact with services (there is always a time gap); nature and progression of difficulties; **diagnoses**
- **Hospital** admissions: when, length, voluntary or under section
- Past **treatment** – medication, psychological, ECT: what has helped in the past, what has not, medication type, doses prescribed and actual doses taken (i.e. concordance with prescription); history of side-effects

Risk history
- **Risk episodes**: deliberate self-harm (**DSH**) and **suicide attempts**; **self-neglect** and **exploitation** by others (financial, sexual), thoughts of and actual **harm to others**
- **Context** of episodes, **worst harm resulting**

Forensic history
- **Arrests, charges and convictions**: nature of offences, outcome (custodial sentence, community service, probation)
- Include criminal activities where patient was **not arrested, crime not detected**

Premorbid personality
- When did they last – or have they ever – felt 'normal': what is normal for them, how is that different to now?
- General: how would they describe themselves, how would friends/family describe them?
- Specific:
  - **Character** traits (e.g. anxious, sensitive, suspicious, dramatic): 'how would you describe yourself as a person?'
  - **Prevailing mood** and **stability of mood**
  - **Impulse control**
  - **Nature of relationships with others**: partners, friends, colleagues (e.g. close and confiding, casual only)
  - **Leisure** interests (hobbies)
  - **Spirituality** and religious affiliation
  - **Tolerance of stress** and coping style, including use of substances to manage stress, modify mood or facilitate social interaction

ECT, electroconvulsive therapy.

Mental state examination

The MSE describes the *here and now* at interview, analogous to a physical examination. If recent symptoms such as hearing voices or sleeping poorly are not present at interview, they should be mentioned in the presenting complaint rather than here. If current symptoms are discussed in the presenting complaint, do not repeat that detail here: the MSE is the place to summarize and classify. For example, if a presenting complaint describes an account of persecution from neighbours, the MSE would simply state 'evidence of persecutory delusional beliefs regarding neighbours, as described'.

Table 3 details the content of the MSE. **Appearance and behaviour** sketches a portrait of the patient. If you are presenting the patient's details over the telephone, the listener should be able to picture that patient. This description will be your main finding in patients who are unable or choose not to engage with the interview.

Speech can elucidate the more subtle cognitive deficits of schizophrenia or developmental disorders such as autism. If you are unable to access or clarify the subjective **mood**, **thought content** or **perceptual experiences** of a reluctant or incapacitated historian, this is not (hopefully) a failure of your examination, but a finding in itself: when presenting do not stumble over information not obtained, state clearly why that was the case (e.g. 'Unable to access thought content as the patient declined to answer questions' or 'Evidence of some poorly elaborated persecutory delusional thinking regarding staff, but the content of these beliefs unclear due to the degree of their thought disorder as previously described'). An essential part of the mood MSE is to clarify the degree of **suicidal ideation** and **intent** and/or any **thoughts of harming others**.

Cognition is often briefly described in terms of orientation in time, place or person. Asking patients to

Table 2 Normal development and developmental milestones.

Stage	Normal development	Milestones: at approximate ages
Up to 1 year **Infancy**	*Social:* formation of secure relationship with main carer/s *Motor:* balance, sitting, crawling, walking	*Smiling:* 3 weeks; selective smiling 6 months *Speech:* cooing 2 months, babbling 6 months, first words: 40 weeks to 1 year *Walking:* first steps 1 year
Up to 2 years **Year 2**	*Continued social:* keen to please parents, anxious if meets with disapproval	Short-lived temper tantrums: 'the terrible two's' *Speech:* 3-word sentences *Motor:* sphincter control, jumps, laterality
2–5 years **Preschool years**	Rapid language development and curiosity (questions++); learns place in the family, gender role	Tantrums subside, development of fantasy life/imaginative play *Speech:* ↑↑vocabulary, subtle voice tones, end of 'baby talk' *Motor:* full postural control
5–10 years **Middle childhood**	Learns role at school and in wider community/society	*Speech:* inflection, pronunciation and abstract talk. Reading and writing *Motor:* boys better gross motor skills than girls
11 years + **Adolescence**	Puberty 11–13 for girls, and 13–17 for boys; described as a period of emotional turmoil	Increased self-awareness and moves towards autonomy. Complex social interactions: peer groups become more important, intimate relationships begin

---

Box 1 The alcohol history

Screening

In general medicine, a commonly used screen is the **CAGE**: have you ever felt you needed to **C**ut down your drinking; felt **A**nnoyed by others criticizing your drinking; felt **G**uilty about your drinking and/or needed an **E**ye-opener in the morning to steady your nerves. Two or more suggest a significant problem, and merit full enquiry.

Alcohol history
- **Amount consumed weekly** in units: 1 unit = half a pint of regular strength beer, a small glass of wine (125 mL), a small (liqueur) glass of fortified wine (e.g. sherry) or a *single* measure of spirits. One bottle of wine is 7 units; fortified wines are higher. Many popular beers in the UK are stronger and wine is served in larger glasses. One bottle of spirits contains 30 units

- **Pattern of use**: binges, steady intake over the week, throughout the day
- **Features of dependency: compulsion**; **increased salience** of drinking; **difficulties controlling use** despite harm; **tolerance**; physiological **withdrawal** as blood alcohol levels fall. Withdrawal manifests as a range of symptoms:
  - *mild:* tremor, nausea or retching, mood disturbance, sleep disturbance
  - *moderate:* perceptual distortions and hallucinations
  - *severe and potentially life-threatening:* full-blown delirium tremens (confusion, terror, severe tremor, seizures, leading to coma and death)
- **Harm from use: physical, mental, relational, occupational, criminal** (Table 18, p. 62)

Table 3 The mental state examination (MSE).

Appearance and behaviour

General appearance, physical state, abnormal movements, behaviour and rapport
- Style and manner of **dress, hygiene**: self-neglect
- **Physical state**: signs of physical illness, drug/alcohol withdrawal, self-harm scars
- Manner of **engagement** during interview (e.g. suspicious/guarded/relaxed). Quality of **eye contact** (e.g. fixed stare, avoidant). **Distractibility** and preoccupation with internal world (e.g. appearing to respond to auditory hallucinations)
- **Motor** movements: involuntary **tics, chorea, tremor, tardive dyskinesia** (repetitive movements, typically orofacial, due to high-dose antipsychotics) and **akathisia** (external manifestation of internal sense of restlessness, again a side-effect of antipsychotics). **Motor stereotypies** are regular repetitive non-goal directed movements (e.g. rocking). **Mannerisms** are idiosyncratic goal-directed behaviours (e.g. style of walking). **Catatonic** symptoms include 'automatic behaviours' such as *echopraxia* and *echolalia* (imitation of interviewer's movements and speech, respectively), *perseveration* (repetition of a movement, words/syllables or maintenance of a posture once context has passed), *forced* (automatic) *grasping* of objects offered. Catatonia is a rare motor manifestation of schizophrenia or frontal lobe lesions
- **Hyper-/hypoactivity**: relevant in delirium and mood states

Speech

Rate, amount, form and coherence
- Increased/decreased; fast/slow; loud/soft
- **Verbal stereotypy**: repetition of irrelevant words or phrases
- **Formal thought disorder** disruption to the continuity of thought. Answers may be initially appropriate but **circumstantial**, straying far from the topic before returning or **tangential**, where they do not return. The latter represents mild **derailment**, with more severe forms seeing the juxtaposition of completely irrelevant ideas, also known as **loosening of associations**. The most extreme form of thought disorder is known as **word salad** where meaning is indecipherable. **Flight of ideas** in hypomanic/manic states is the rapid transition between topics via internal links (connected words, themes, rhyming, alliteration e.g. 'Black cats scare me, I've a black bag'), or the inclusion of external distractions into the train of thought (e.g. subsequent comments on interviewer's black shoes)
- **Poverty of thought** describes insubstantial speech that conveys little meaning
- **Neologisms**: words or phrases invented or used idiosyncratically to denote new meaning ('I don't like my boss: he's a bosstard')

Mood

Subjective mood, objective affect; thoughts of self-harm and of harming others
- *Subjectively* patient description of their *current* mood: rated out of 10, with 0 lowest; it is useful to rate their 'usual' mood
- *Objectively* interviewer's appraisal of their **affect** (external manifestation of emotional state) and emotional range during interview, **euthymic** (within normal range) and normal reactivity/**incongruous** affect given context/**perplexed/blunted** emotional range
- **Presence or absence of thoughts of self-harm** or **harming others**, state any **plans** and **degree of intent** (e.g. passive death wish, suicidal ideation or suicidal intent)

Thought content

Morbid preoccupations (i.e. ruminations), obsessions, overvalued ideas, delusions
- **Obsessions**: repetitive, intrusive, unwanted, stereotyped thoughts or images
- **Overvalued ideas**: those held with a morbid intensity, but without fulfilling the criteria for a delusion. They are not argued beyond the bounds of reason (e.g. patients with anorexia nervosa are not deluded but have overvalued ideas about their weight)
- A **delusion**: a fixed (usually false) belief held without evidence that is out of keeping with an individual's sociocultural background. Delusions may be primary or secondary. **Primary** (delusional mood, perception and autochthonous delusions) occur out of the blue (i.e. without prior morbid experience). **Delusional mood** is an unpleasant sense that surrounding events refer to oneself. As the mind abhors a vacuum, delusional mood is usually resolved by the formation of an explanatory sudden delusional idea (an '**autochthonous**' delusion): delusional mood is unlikely in a current MSE but may be recalled retrospectively. **Delusional perception** is the sudden attribution of self-referential meaning to a normally perceived object (e.g. 'The position of that cup on the table means I will be famous'). **Secondary** delusions (usually) evolve from pre-existing morbid psychological processes (altered mood, hallucinations, other delusions). They include delusions of **persecution, grandiosity, reference, guilt, poverty, nihilism** (i.e. extreme negation of self or world; e.g. believing part of the body has died). **Passivity** describes the experience that one's mind (thought passivity), emotions, actions, will or body (somatic passivity) is not under one's control. They include **thought insertion, withdrawal** and **thought broadcast** (loss of the sense of barrier between one's mind and external world). Passivity is usually linked with a delusional explanation (e.g. thoughts removed by the government)

Table 3 (*Continued*)

Perception
Sensory distortions, sensory deceptions (illusions, hallucinations)
- **Distortions** are changes in *intensity* or *quality* of real sensory phenomena (e.g. micropsia in a temporal lobe seizure)
- **Deceptions** are either **illusions** (i.e. *misinterpretations of real stimuli*), often in altered mood states or consciousness (e.g. hearing an innocuous noise as a sinister footstep when anxious) or **hallucinations**, which are *internally generated* perceptions in the absence of an external stimulus. **Auditory** hallucinations include noises and voices. **Second person** auditory hallucinations talk to the patient, including giving **commands**. **Third person** auditory hallucinations discuss the patient, sometimes in a **running commentary** on their actions. **Thought echo** is hearing one's thoughts repeated aloud after one thinks them. Other hallucinations include **visual, somatic, olfactory, taste, sexual and touch**. 'Formication' describes hallucinations of touch where small animals/insects are felt to be crawling all over the body, classically seen in organic disorders such as cocaine psychosis. **Reflex** hallucinations are triggered by an external stimulus *in another modality* (e.g. seeing a bus triggering a somatic hallucination of electric shocks). **Functional** hallucinations are triggered by an external stimulus and are experienced at the same time as the stimulus (e.g. auditory hallucinations associated with the sound of running water). **Extracampine** hallucinations are experienced as outside of the sensory field (e.g. voices heard from another country). **Hypnagogic** and **hypnopompic** hallucinations occur with reduced levels of consciousness when drifting off to sleep and on waking, respectively
- **Pseudohallucinations** are experienced as arising from within the patient (e.g. 'voices in my head') rather than the external world, but they are beyond conscious control. In contrast to hallucinations, they are not experienced as having a material reality. They occur in normal grief (seeing or hearing the deceased) as well as a range of disorders including schizophrenia, post-traumatic stress ('flashbacks') and borderline personality disorder

Cognition
Global, dominant and non-dominant hemispheres, frontal lobe function
- **Global: level of consciousness** (if abnormal, use the Glasgow Coma Scale), **orientation** in time, place and person, **attention and concentration** (e.g. test naming months of the year backwards), **memory**: anterograde short-term ('working') memory tested by immediate recall of three given items; long-term tested by their recall 5 minutes later. Retrograde memory includes public (e.g. 'Who is the prime minister?') and personal ('Where were you born?') information, semantic (e.g. how to use a fork) and episodic memory (e.g. 'What happened yesterday?'). Global cognition includes **IQ** (usually estimated rather than formally tested; e.g. 'high', 'low normal')
- **Dominant** hemisphere tests: **language** (naming of objects, repetition of a phrase, comprehension of commands, reading and writing), **calculation** and **praxis** (limb apraxia, e.g. 'Show how you wave goodbye'; finger agnosia, e.g. put pen in their hand with eyes closed – 'what's this?'; conceptual apraxia, e.g. show toothbrush – 'what's this used for?') and awareness of **details**. Draw a clock at 3.45 (see text)
- **Non-dominant** hemisphere tests: **neglect** (hemispatial rather than sensory), **construction** and **visuospatial** ability
- **Frontal lobes** tests: **verbal fluency** (e.g. 'Name as many animals as you can in a minute': tests fluency plus strategy, e.g. listing farm animals first), **similarities and proverb interpretation** (i.e. conceptual thinking, e.g. 'What do a table and chair have in common?'; 'What is the difference between a mistake and a lie?'), **estimates** ('How fast can a leopard run?': frontal lobe lesions typically grossly overestimate) and **alternating sequences** (copying of alternating hand sequence, which tests sequential motor activity dependent on dorsolateral prefrontal cortex function)

Insight
Understanding of illness and its treatment
- Do they think there is anything wrong with them?
- If there is something wrong, do they think it is a physical or psychological problem, or both?
- How do they describe the problem and what caused it?
- Do they think they need treatment, if so what?
- What do they think of treatment offered?

draw a clock at 3.45 is a quick test of neglect (draw both sides?), construction (looks like a clock?) and details (all numbers correct?) as well as frontal lobe function in their strategic approach to the task. Systematic cognitive testing is carried out where there is any index of clinical suspicion regarding cognitive compromise and is performed routinely with older patients (Table 19, p. 68).

Insight is multidimensional and should not be stated as simply being 'present' or 'absent'; delineate insight as described and avoid the presumption that having insight means simply agreeing with your doctor.

Physical examination

Systematic cardiac, respiratory, gastrointestinal and neurological examinations must always be performed for a first psychiatric assessment, and revisited whenever new physical symptoms arise or if there is an unanticipated change in someone's mental state. Physical and mental symptoms are related in complex ways (Box 2).

Physical examination has several aims: it ensures **organic aetiology** is not missed, the **physical impact** of mental disorder is established (e.g. malnutrition in anorexia) and it records **physical side-effects** of current treatment. It also establishes a **physical baseline** before any treatment is started (e.g. antipsychotic medication causing weight gain).

Who performs the physical will depend on context (e.g. it **should** already have been carried out for GP or A&E referrals). On admission to a psychiatric ward, all patients must have a physical repeated by the ward doctor and, if not yet performed, investigations on admission should include a routine blood screen (full blood count

[FBC], urea and electrolytes [U&Es], liver function tests [LFTs], lipids, glucose, thyroid). Whatever the context, it is essential to make sure comprehensive physical assessment has not been missed. If a patient declines to cooperate, it is your responsibility to record that refusal, and flag up the fact it is an outstanding component of their assessment.

Formulation

Structure your formulation as below:

Summary statement

Salient features of the case in a few sentences.

Differential diagnoses

Starting with most likely, give evidence for and against, with each differential. Use the diagnostic hierarchy in Fig. 1 as a prompt for possibilities and a reminder of comorbidity (e.g. 'Depression as the primary diagnosis, comorbid with a secondary diagnosis of anxious-avoidant personality disorder').

Note that classifying mental disorder as 'organic' denotes a presumed or identified gross physical cause (e.g. endocrine disorder or alcohol intoxication). Non-organic mental disorders (i.e. the rest) are sometimes referred to as 'functional'; the disorder arises at the level of the higher mental functions governing cognition, perception, emotion and behaviour. Unlike physical illness, most psychiatric disorders do not therefore map onto measurable material realities; they are best understood as

---

> **Box 2 Types of association between physical and mental illness**
>
> **1** Physical illness presenting with psychological symptoms (i.e. organic psychiatry)
> **2** Physical illness associated with secondary psychological symptoms as a reaction to illness
> **3** Mental illness predisposing to physical illness (e.g. depression as an independent risk factor for coronary heart disease)
> **4** Physical symptoms as the sole presentation of a psychological disorder (e.g. somatization)
> **5** Medication for mental or physical illness causing psychological side-effects (iatrogenic illness)
> **6** Chance association (two disorders occur by coincidence): comorbidity of psychiatric and medical illnesses

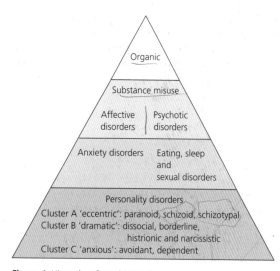

Figure 1 Hierarchy of psychiatric disorders.

end-point presentations of a variety of biopsychosocial processes. Formulate your diagnoses within an aetiological framework (see below), otherwise terms such as 'depression' convey little meaning.

Aetiology

Divide this into **predisposing, precipitating** and **maintaining** factors, further subdivided by **biological, social** and **psychological** type. A 3×3 grid with these headings serves as a framework for collating findings. Avoid rigid iteration of the 'biopsychosocial' model; focus on what is important, give a sense of the relative weight of contributing factors and if, for instance, social factors do not appear relevant, say so. For example, the aetiology of a depressive episode could be described thus: *predisposing* strong family history of depression (bio) compounded by an emotionally (psycho) and materially (social) deprived childhood, this episode *precipitated* by a recent relationship break-up (social) and *maintained* by alcohol abuse (bio) in the context of a personality characterized by limited emotional resources for tolerating stress (psycho).

Aetiological formulation can also be focused along **cognitive, behavioural** or **psychodynamic** lines:

• A **cognitive assessment** would make a current problem list and link these to any associated: (a) *negative dysfunctional beliefs*; (b) *systematic cognitive bias* in information processing about self, others and the world; or (c) *cognitive distortions* (e.g. a tendency to overgeneralize or take an 'all or nothing' view).

• A **behavioural assessment** would consider early faulty learning experience leading to current problematic behaviours, which would then be analysed in terms of how they were currently being rewarded and thereby maintained.

• A **psychodynamic** assessment would look at early childhood experience and the development of psychological defences, associated patterns of interpersonal relating and the relationship of these to current symptoms.

Summary of active risks

Risk to **self**, including **self-harm, suicide, self-neglect**, and risk to **others**, both **general** and to **specific** individuals. State factors likely to increase or decrease risk. For risk to others, note any suggestion that they believe the integrity of their world is under threat (e.g. persecutory delusions and delusions of jealousy may be acted on) and any psychotic experiences that lower their sense of control

(e.g. somatic passivity, command auditory hallucinations), alongside any personality traits such as impulsivity and potentially disinhibiting factors such as alcohol use.

Initial management

Detail your plan for **investigations, treatment** and **risk management**, listing interventions in descending order or priority. Investigations include obtaining physical **tests** (e.g. bloods, electroencephalography [EEG], magnetic resonance imaging [MRI]) as well as **collateral information** and **past records**. Identify treatments (see Mental health treatments) and include specific measures required to reduce risk.

How to conduct a psychiatric interview

Anyone can ask a list of questions. Most patients can talk for an hour. Skilful history taking combines information gathering with a potential therapeutic opportunity. You aim to provide the patient with the relief of being understood and to further develop their own understanding. Where possible, help them to clarify what their thoughts and feelings are, and to make links between their past and current behaviours and their presenting problems. This is an opportunity to reinforce adaptive attitudes and behaviours, encouraging their capacity to manage their situation.

To be effective, clinical interviewing must be like a dance. You are both leading and responding to the patient. Good timing is key: when to let the patient talk, when to interrupt, when to ask something sensitive, when to make a challenging comment or suggestion, and when to stay silent if the patient is not ready to hear it. Throughout this process, you are under observation by the patient, who is gauging what kind of doctor you are, how much to tell you, and whether you are trustworthy. Do not underestimate the importance of first impressions: looking and acting professional reassures people that you are.

If new to psychiatry, start by simply listening to patients as fellow human beings. Be respectful, thanking them for their time in helping you develop your interview skills. They might be bored of being asked the same questions, especially as an inpatient. Stop to **think aloud** about their answers rather than racing on to the next question, and you will both get more out of the process. It is not unusual for students to obtain useful information previously unknown to a busy clinical team, with whom the patient may feel more reserved. Take a systematic approach to one particular area (e.g. taking a careful

MSE or past psychiatric history) before attempting to cover everything.

Throughout the interview be curious and ask yourself – *what would that be like?* Develop your capacity for empathy, which differs from sympathy (pity) as it is an active process. With empathy one accurately identifies with another's situation and is therefore able to have a mirroring emotional response to it that resonates with theirs. Empathy is therefore an essential clinical skill for understanding your patients.

Before starting, clarify

• Why you are seeing the patient – what are the goals of your assessment? What do you need to establish today and what can wait?

• Where you will be seeing the patient? Is there adequate privacy and security? Staff should be nearby for support if needed. Familiarize yourself with the local alarm system (e.g. wall-mounted; 'hand-held'), **and sit nearest the door**.

• How much time do you have? If possible have a clock in view so you can keep track of time, without making the patient feel uncomfortable.

• Who is going to be in the room? If patients are wary of the interview process you might suggest they are joined by a friend or family member, but if possible start an assessment of an adult with them unaccompanied, as others' presence may influence or inhibit their responses. If an adult patient is unquestioningly accompanied by another adult into the interview, ask yourself why. For some families it reflects the fact that the patient became unwell in early life and has never managed to individuate as an independent adult who would normally see a doctor alone. As a rule, encourage patient autonomy where possible – while acknowledging the (possibly central) importance of another person's role and the information they might provide; suggest the patient is seen alone initially, with the other person brought into the interview towards the end.

How do you start?

The interview process starts from when you call the patient's name. Most people feel uncomfortable seeing a psychiatrist, anxious they might be seen as 'crazy'. Put them at ease as you bring them into the room by a comment on the setting or their journey for example: the content is unimportant – you are making a connection with them as a human being rather than as a 'case'. The tone *they* set is often informative.

• Check how they like to be addressed: amongst older people and in some cultures, automatic use of their first name may irritate.

• Explain why you are seeing them, who referred them and why, and orientate them to what to expect. Advise them about confidentiality and what will happen to the information they give you.

• Clarify the time allowed and what you need to achieve in that time (e.g. 'I need to ask you questions about your current situation and past history so we can understand what's been happening and agree a plan about where to go from here'). Warn them there is a considerable amount of information to cover so you may need to interrupt at points to move on, and apologize in advance for having to do so. Suggest there will be future opportunities to return to important topics.

• Start your enquiry with an open question such as 'How are you?' Then listen. A common trap is to interrupt too early. Let them talk in an unhurried way initially as doing so is time well spent. It builds rapport as the patient knows they are being listened to and it orientates you to their perspective. When you move on to specific enquiry, pursue positive responses to their logical conclusion: make sure you have understood what the patient is saying before you move on.

• If the patient is unforthcoming, switch tack to asking why they think they were referred, or why others might be concerned. Consider also whether you need to change your approach (see below).

• As a rule, you need to make notes as there will be too much to remember. Explain this clearly.

How do you clarify the nature of the presenting complaint?

Start **broad** with **open-ended questions** about a topic (e.g. 'What's your mood been like recently?'), gradually refining your understanding with increasingly focused questions, eventually clarifying details by moving to **closed** questions that invite a yes or no answer (e.g. 'So if I've understood right, you only sleep around 4 hours most nights?').

Use **reflective listening** and **summarize** at regular points throughout the interview: this gives the patient feedback of what you have understood in a form that helps them make more sense of it themselves, while also inviting their comment or correction. This technique of active listening is a skill not to be confused with simply repeating what the patient has just said.

Formulate hypotheses to test your assumptions with the patient. Assist the patient to reflect on what the nature of their emotional experience has been, especially if they find this difficult and struggle to make connections between how they feel and how they behave.

If a patient is resistant to a certain line of questioning, move on. Change to a less anxiety-provoking area, and return later taking a different approach: **push where it moves**. For example, if during family history, the patient speaks of hearing his late father's voice, explore this now. Interviewing schedules (Tables 1 and 3) need to be flexible to respond to the patient, not the other way round.

If you are struggling to engage the patient in the interview, try modifying your approach. Everyone has a preferred clinical style depending on personality: the skill is to know when to adapt it, and how. Do not persist with a casual informal approach if that individual might feel more comfortable with a reserved business-like manner. Gain a sense of what is right for that individual at that time.

Once you have established the nature of the presenting problem, stop to consider how it might relate to other perhaps more fundamental difficulties for that individual: how might it function as a solution to these, however maladaptive and unconscious this process may be. This perspective may explain why resolution of the presenting problem has proved impossible to date (e.g. alcohol misuse following bereavement).

How do you ask about delusions and hallucinations?

Advise the patient you need to ask some questions that may sound strange, but they are 'routine questions' everybody gets asked. Introduce each topic with open questions (e.g. for persecutory delusions, ask 'How are other people treating you generally at the moment?'). Depending on the answer, pursue this downstream with more specific closed questions (Box 3).

Box 3 Asking about delusions and hallucinations

Delusions

- *Persecutory:* are you currently under threat from any individuals or organizations?
- *Reference:* are things happening around you that seem to have a special significance just for you? Prompt: like seeing things about yourself on television or in the newspapers or perhaps in songs or being talked about on the radio?
- *Grandiose:* do you have any special powers or mission?
- *Guilty:* do you feel you have committed a terrible crime or sin that deserves punishment?
- *Hypochondriacal:* are strange things happening to your body that you can't explain?
- *Nihilistic:* do you have a sense something terrible is about to happen? Does something feel wrong inside you?
- *Thought passivity:* start broad – are you able to think clearly at the moment? Then, is there any interference with your thoughts? Have you been a victim of telepathy? Once described, clarify:
  - **thought insertion**: are thoughts put into your head that you know are not your own?
  - **thought withdrawal**: do you ever have the experience thoughts are taken out of your head by some external power?
  - **thought broadcast**: do you ever have the experience your thoughts are leaking or being transmitted from your head in some way, so that others can hear them?
  - **thought echo**: do you ever have a thought and then hear it being spoken afterwards?
- *Somatic passivity* (i.e. made actions, body functions, emotions or will): e.g. is your body ever controlled by another force or agency?

When delusions are present, enquire how the patient understands that experience (e.g. by the elaboration of more delusional ideas) and summarize:
(i) **type** e.g. paranoid; (ii) **complexity** e.g. part of a complex delusional system involving many people; (iii) **mood congruity** e.g. none (threatening idea has no impact on patient emotionally) or congruous (a hypochondriacal delusion coincides with low mood); (iv) **influence on behaviour** e.g. none, patient does not act in accordance with his belief that he is the prime minister

Hallucinations

- When on edge or under stress some people hear or see things that are not there: has anything like that happened to you? Have you heard voices, mutterings or noises when there is no-one there or nothing else to explain it? Repeat for visual, etc.

When auditory hallucinations are present, clarify:
(i) **content** (if clear); (ii) from **where** the patient hears them; (iii) **second or third** person quality; (iv) **mood congruity**; (v) **timing** and **frequency**; (vi) **effect on the patient**

How do you cover large amounts of information?

Avoid getting bogged down in detail. You are taking an overview, not a life story. Focus on establishing the **best and worst** of important parameters. For example, with employment, establish their highest level of past functioning in comparison to now, so ask about their most senior past position and their longest time in one job. For their risk history, establish the most serious harm to self or others caused. With multiple hospital admissions, clarify dates of the first and most recent, how long was the longest, and how many were under section?

Where possible, **link topics** (e.g. 'When you have been drinking like that have you ever got in trouble with the police?') When an abrupt change in direction is required, explain this by making **linking statements** (e.g. 'What you're telling me is clearly important and will need to be thought about more. For today, we need to cover some more basic information, so I have to change topic now and ask about medication'). Keep orientating the patient to where you need to take them.

How do you assess someone from a culture unfamiliar to you?

No-one expects you to be an expert on all world cultures, but be aware of your own ignorance and ask questions to avoid making culturally biased assumptions. For example, when a patient hears God, it can sometimes be difficult to differentiate illness from normal religious experience: check with family, friends or church members to confirm what is culturally normative.

Avoid assuming that a patient shares the dominant beliefs and values of their culture. Think of the subcultures within your own culture.

Beyond ethnicity, be sensitive to other factors such as socioeconomic circumstances. Most doctors have backgrounds of reasonable emotional and material security; the impact of adverse events or the difficulty of change will be underestimated if a doctor unthinkingly applies their own emotional, social and financial resources as a benchmark.

How do you ask about sensitive topics?

Normalize the question, again by prefacing it with a statement that it is a routine question you ask everybody. Have a **straightforward manner** that conveys professionalism and makes the patient feel you have asked this question hundreds of times before, and have heard a range of answers. Shame is a powerfully aversive emotion and a patient may avoid disclosure if they fear either feeling stupid or exposed by your reaction to what they say.

Normalize potentially undesirable answers concerning generally or culturally prohibited behaviour (e.g. sex, substance misuse or aggression) by putting the behaviour into context. For example, do not ask 'Do you hit your partner?' but rather 'It sounds like you've been at your wits' end. Have you ever reached the point where you felt you had no option but to hit her to get through to her?' With a patient experiencing persecutory delusions, you might say 'It sounds as if you have serious concerns about your safety. Have you got to the point you feel you need to take matters into your own hands to protect yourself?' These are leading questions, but you have established basic facts first. You are not pretending to condone such behaviour, but demonstrating you can understand it.

Deliberate assumption is sometimes useful, in particular with substance misuse. For example, with young adults, do not ask if they smoke cannabis or use cocaine, ask how much or how often. They will tell you if they do not. With alcohol, most people underestimate how much they drink. If alcohol is or might be a problem, deliberately **overestimate** an amount for that patient (e.g. 'So would you drink a bottle of spirits most days?') Patients usually correct you with a more accurate figure as if freed to do so by an exaggerated one.

Do not avoid topics that make you feel uncomfortable. Asking about suicide, for example, will never make someone suicidal. That said, excessive attention to suicide method is unhelpful. Use stepped questions, becoming more specific (e.g. 'What's been happening sounds very stressful. Have you got to the point where you felt you couldn't go on? Have you got to the stage of thinking about taking your own life? What did you think you might do? Did you make any plans?').

Remember medication may be a **sensitive topic**. Around half of all patients do not take it as prescribed – regardless of type – but may not disclose this to avoid doctors' disapproval or disappointment. Never assume they take it at the prescribed dose and frequency: start by asking how often they manage to take it and at what dose, and take it from there.

It can be useful to revisit the issue of **confidentiality**: patients are often concerned about this, but reluctant to ask.

Be explicit with what it is you are asking, otherwise both you and the patient will be confused as to what they have said yes to.

What is your last assessment question?

'Is there anything else you'd like to tell me?'

Mental health treatments

Core interventions

Mental health interventions are divided into biological (typically, medication and electroconvulsive therapy [ECT]), psychological (psychotherapy) and social (financial advice, vocational interventions). This assumes treatments fit neatly into these boxes, but several (e.g. cognitive–behavioural therapy [CBT] and group therapy) are both psychological *and* social. Our approach presents nine essential treatments (Table 4), listing another 17 options later (Table 5). Two core interventions, assessment and home treatment/admission, are examples of biopsychosocial treatments. No treatment will achieve its full potential if given in isolation or without proper negotiation with the *individual* who receives it. Concordance is a two-way process between an informed patient and a flexible doctor. It is the best way of maximising patients' taking medication regularly (compliance).

A for assessment

During your assessment, it is not enough to set out the sequence of events from no symptoms to symptoms, with indications of symptoms' severity over the time course. You must place these in the context of the person's situation (relationships, job, housing, lifestyle) and *precipitants* (p. 8). A high-quality assessment, where a patient begins to see his/her difficulties in a context amenable to interventions, is in itself therapeutic.

KEY POINT

The first statement of the Hippocratic oath is 'First do no harm'. Stop and think before you rush into interventions, perhaps under pressure to do something, *anything*. Balance any potential benefits with the negative consequences of the treatment.

B for behavioural therapy

A broad definition of mental disorders is that they are abnormalities of thinking, feeling and behaving. We know that disturbances of thinking (confusion, holding paranoid beliefs about strangers) and feeling (low mood, episodes of anxiety) invariably manifest as abnormal behaviours. Consider these in reverse: how we behave impacts on our thoughts and our mood. Identifying unhelpful behaviours (withdrawal, aggression) will guide patients into evaluating the costs (in symptoms and consequences) of continuing to act in a way that makes their life more difficult. A cost–benefit analysis contrasts how things are now with how they could be *if* changes were initiated. Box 4 gives the most common behavioural intervention, a slow breathing exercise to reduce anxiety, especially panics. Analysis of behaviours is complex; it is good to advise someone with dependency traits (Table 31, p. 105) not to volunteer for every new task at work, but telling someone with social phobia (p. 59) to avoid new people would perpetuate their symptoms. A standard behavioural approach is to examine ABCs (Table 4) with the patient. Each of antecedents and consequences will list a mixture of thoughts and feelings, many of which cause distress – but interventions target all three to teach ('condition') the patient new ways of thinking and acting.

Box 4 Behavioural techniques: slow breathing exercise

Teaching a **slow breathing technique** is part of a programme to reduce sudden bursts of anxiety:

- *Stop*, sit down or lean against something
- *Hold* your breath for a slow count to 10: try saying to yourself 'one – one hundred, two – two hundred . . .'
- At the count of 10, breathe out slowly, thinking 'breathe out' or 'slow breaths'
- Then, breathe in over 3 seconds: 'in – two – three'
- Now, breathe out in 5 seconds: 'out – two – three'
- At the end of 1 minute (7 breaths in and 7 out), *hold* your breath again for a slow count to 10

Table 4 Nine core psychiatric treatments: A to I.

Intervention	Outcomes	Other examples
Assessment Full history + mental state exam + investigate For each of biological, social and psychological, what are the **predisposing**, **precipitating** and **maintaining** factors that led *this patient* to present *at this time*?	Give a context and initial approach to understanding symptoms and behaviours; integrate your knowledge of the profile of people who develop a particular disorder (epidemiology) with your clinical findings, supporting diagnosis and indicating severity	Consider extending your assessments: • Blood tests/imaging studies • Neuropsychological testing (IQ, personality) • Would admission clarify symptoms and behaviours?
Behavioural therapy (the B of CBT) Identifies behaviours that trigger or maintain unwanted symptoms; encourages behaviours that will reduce symptoms and break cycles of behaviour → symptoms → behaviour	For each patient, what are the Antecedents, Behaviours and Consequences (ABCs) of distressing symptoms? Even without behavioural analysis of all symptoms, generic behavioural measures will help (Table 6)	Homework: exercises to reduce antecedents and change behaviours; scheduling (planning a diary) to structure activities and reduce boredom; social skills training for the negative symptoms of schizophrenia
Cognitive therapy (the C of CBT) Identifies thoughts that drive symptoms and behaviours. Cognitive therapy changes a patient's mindset – the way he/she sees the world	Mood diary to identify how ways of thinking are associated with periods of low mood; using a formulation to change thoughts and ways of thinking in anxiety, psychosis, etc.	Albert Ellis' three cognitive distortions: 1 'I must do well'; 2 'You must treat me well'; and 3 'The world must be easy'. Change these musts to reduce distress in everyone
Drugs *The* biological treatment, but psychosocial aspects (e.g. concordance with medication, combination with other treatments) have a key role in achieving the best results	See text and individual cases, Box 2 & Tables 2, 5–7. Drug prescription is symptom-based: symptoms, function and side-effects are the main outcome measures	Added to four major groups in this section: anti-Alzheimer's drugs (p. 160), attention deficit disorder (p. 100), and preventing withdrawal of illegal drugs (Table 42)
Electroconvulsive therapy ECT improves low mood quickly in vulnerable patients: older people, severe depression – including postnatal	ECT should not be seen as a treatment of last resort and is therefore included here: risks for these patient groups when severely unwell increases with delay	ECT has a poor evidence base for its routine use in psychosis; for severe depression, it should be administered only in approved centres
Family interventions From contact with family, family as co-therapists to formal therapy	Family intervention reduces both symptoms and relapse rates in psychosis	Essential in treating young people and eating disorders; marital/couples therapy
Groups Psychological therapies delivered in group settings are time and cost effective	Open (e.g. AA) or closed groups (see text). Specific groups for common mental disorders	Psychoeducation usually takes place in groups: for psychosis, bipolar disorder and bulimia
Hospital admission and home treatment These are principally driven by risk assessment, less often by high levels of distress in a patient	Risks (suicide, harm to others) must be shown to be related to symptoms; both interventions provide intensive treatment to people in crisis	Most models of home treatment are assertive community treatment; there are many inpatient settings based on patients' needs
Individual psychotherapy One-to-one psychotherapy: many different approaches	Similar to flying, the greatest dangers of therapy are at the start and at the end (see text)	Psychotherapy is best considered by school (theory) and by problem (e.g. for addictions)

AA, Alcoholics Anonymous; CBT, cognitive–behavioural therapy; ECT, electroconvulsive therapy.

Table 5 The J to Z of other mental health interventions.

Treatment	Details	Who carries out these tasks?
J Job	Facilitating meaningful work; *place then train* (see text)	Vocational rehabilitation worker; careers' advisor
K Kids (children)	Consequences of illness in an adult on children. Paramount principle: the welfare of the child overrides that of the parent	You and your team; social services; child and family and social services; police and other state agencies
L Legal aspects	Any intervention with legal or forensic services' aspects. Confidentiality, conflicts of interest, consent, capacity	Every doctor should be capable of assessing capacity, specialist forensic psychiatric teams, police, lawyers
M Multidisciplinary	Use your team's experience, different approaches and skills: includes interagency working	Nurses, social workers, psychologists, speech and language therapists, support workers, etc. (see J & O)
N Nidotherapy	Environmental manipulation to reduce symptoms/relapses	Varies: general hospital staff, housing agencies, etc.
O Occupational therapy	OT assessments of all support needs. Ward interventions, social outings, treating phobias, pet/art/music therapy	Occupational therapists carry out the assessments working within the MDT and with others
P Prejudice	Stigma as the second illness: to reduce discrimination	This is everyone's job: users, carers and you
Q Quality of life	What gives meaning to patients' lives? Includes relationships, befriending, spirituality, religion, the Arts and more	Social function (GAF) can be measured by any staff member; focus of interventions determined by the patient
R Rehabilitation	Treating enduring disability: severe mood and psychotic disorders	Many treatment settings and staff involved (see text)
S Surgery	Gender reassignment surgery; last resort in treating people with treatment-resistant OCD	Many psychiatrists ensure independent scrutiny of its use; surgeons in designated centres
T TMS	TMS is not (yet) a proven alternative to ECT in treating depression or pain	Specialist centres: will probably become available in the same settings that currently deliver ECT
U User groups	Promoting recovery, resilience, and empowerment	Peer, advocacy, local and national users' groups
V Voluntary sector	Raising awareness of mental health and funding for specific projects (housing, activities, social networks; see text)	Carer groups, charities, Trusts, other non-statutory services, local and voluntary groups.
W Weight loss	Weight changes in anorexia, depression, dementia, psychosis.	Dietitians and physicians: essential, safe advice
X eXercise	Helping patients maximize exercise and lifestyle changes. Anxiety, mood disorders, reversing drug-induced weight gain	Patients, professionals in primary and specialist care settings, staff in sports and other facilities
Y Yoyo	EMDR. A proven adjunctive treatment (with CBT + drugs) of PTSD	Training in EMDR is brief, and any mental health professional can deliver this treatment
Z Z list (e.g. hypnosis)	Hypnosis (some proven efficacy in *physical* illnesses), aromatherapy, yoga, herbs, meditation, reiki, light boxes	All non-medical/alternative/complementary 'therapists': their independence may be problematic

CBT, cognitive–behavioural therapy; ECT, electroconvulsive therapy; EMDR, eye movement desensitization and reprocessing; GAF, Global Assessment of Functioning; MDT, multidisciplinary team; OCD, obsessive–compulsive disorder; OT, occupational therapy; PTSD, post-traumatic stress disorder; TMS, transcranial magnetic stimulation.

Treatment of panic disorder achieves an understanding of triggers and mechanisms before examining how many actions (avoidance and escape behaviours: p. 39) make panic attacks more likely to recur. People with negative symptoms of schizophrenia also benefit from behavioural approaches. The antecedents might be their symptoms (lack of motivation and spontaneity), their thoughts ('if I go out, people will avoid me: why bother') or physical states (excess sedation of antipsychotics, difficulty sleeping because of hearing voices). Their behaviours (staying in bed, day–night inversion, poor personal hygiene, inactive by day) have adverse consequences: inactivity perpetuates more inactivity and they appear to others, especially their parents, as lazy or raise suspicions that they might be on illegal drugs. Coordinating improvements in morning-time sedation with behavioural changes (regular time for getting up, scheduling appointments, goal-setting, improving personal appearance) will have positive consequences – alone and in combination. The *cost* of making these changes is outweighed by the probable *benefits*: feeling better, more social contacts, more independence *and* the elimination of avoidance behaviour.

C for cognitive therapy

Cognitive therapy maps out an individual's thoughts and thought processes (e.g. negative automatic thoughts: activated by events and ending in the same final common pathway of self-defeating affirmations; jumping to conclusions in someone with psychosis) and helps the person to challenge them. Empirical evidence is sought for beliefs using **Socratic questioning** (interlocutors). What do you *think* when X happens? What is your evidence this is true? Could anything contradict your belief? How certain (from 1% to 100%) are you that what you believe is a fact? What alternative explanations are there? These questions challenge dichotomous (black and white either/or) thinking.

Another Greek philosopher, Epictetus, laid the basis for modern cognitive approaches: 'Men are disturbed not by things (that happen to them) but by the views they take of them.' Cognitive interventions challenge (usually negative) thoughts about events. Take the example of stress at work. This is a product of *our perception* of how much work we have to do multiplied by *our perception* of our ability to carry this out. Most people overestimate their amount of work, and frequently add others' to their workload, failing to share or delegate tasks. Parallel to this, we underestimate our own abilities with thought processes such as **selective abstraction** (excessive focus

on the one item done badly out of many), **arbitrary inference** ('If I fail at this, I will always fail at important tasks') and **overgeneralization** ('I am always the one blamed for everything'). The late Albert Ellis identified three cognitive distortions that hold us back in life (Table 4). If each of us could let these three *musts* go, a major source of self-inflicted misery would be removed. Cognitive therapy underpins the logic of behavioural changes (e.g. sleep hygiene; Table 6). When it is applied to psychiatric disorders, formulations identify current pathways and potential ways of breaking cycles (e.g. Fig. 3, p. 63).

D for drugs

It is right to consider medications *after* both a thorough clinical assessment and CBT formulations and interventions. This reduces inappropriate prescribing: most people with anxiety disorders and mild symptoms of depression do not require medication. All treatments have side-effects; with doctors' ability to prescribe comes great responsibility in informing patients about them, monitoring and acting promptly if these occur (Tables 7–9). Before you prescribe, identify:

- Any previous medication use
- Allergy and other sensitivities
- Comorbid medical illness, current medications, and alcohol/substance misuse that could interact with your chosen drug
- That the patient is physically fit. They may need blood tests, weight and BP done at baseline.
- The risk of overdose. This should guide your choice of drug and the quantities dispensed
- The pros and cons of long-term medication. Discuss the possible consequences of discontinuation (e.g. the adverse impact on symptoms, relapse risk, ability to work or relationships) and their likelihood. If there is a strong indication to continue medication, you might use the analogy of a long-term medical treatment such as insulin for diabetes or antihypertensives (i.e. medications that are needed even when you feel well, **to stay well**).

Antidepressants (ADs), the most common psychiatric drugs prescribed, improve low mood and some have limited efficacy in anxiety disorders (Table 7). Some of one group of ADs, the monoamine oxidase inhibitors (MAOIs), were found to be addictive – these are no longer used in standard clinical practice, mostly for safety reasons and the fact that other ADs have equal efficacy. Many ADs (Table 7) have discontinuation symptoms so are withdrawn slowly over months not weeks. Box 5 gives general prescribing advice and Box 6 looks at AD use in

Table 6 Sleep hygiene measures.

Factors making sleep worse	Suggestion
During the day	
Excessive sleep during day	One brief (30 minute) power nap during day
Lack of exercise	Gentle exercise (30 minutes) during day
Loss of routine	Restore routine: regular times for going to bed and getting up; encourage to plan meaningful activities by day – especially mornings – if unemployed or incapacitated
Before sleep	
Stimulants: caffeine, alcohol, substance misuse, computer games/internet use late at night	Avoid these, or institute a 'curfew time' (e.g. no coffee, computer games after 6 pm)
Lack of preparation for sleep	Winding down time, television or radio, reading (not work or stressful reading matter), warm drinks (non-caffeinated)
Excessive expectation of a full or perfect night's sleep	Adjust goals to an expectation of rest. About one-third of people have a bad night's sleep on any given night. It is not a competition to gain the most hours' sleep
During sleep	
Environment prevents sleep	Safe, warm, quiet environment; agree bed time with partner if sharing bed; address external obstacles to sleep: ear plugs for snoring in partner/outside noise
Discomfort: too warm or too cold	Comfortable bed and night attire; consider ways of adapting the environment
'Clock watching': repeated checks to remind person how much sleep they are missing	Hide clocks or place them out of sight: it is important to set the alarm for a reasonable time the following day
'Tossing and turning' – the bed as a torture chamber	Set a reasonable limit for this: if person feels they are not resting, advise to get up for 15 minutes to read a magazine or book in another room. Then return to bed to rest
Somatic anxiety symptoms, hyperarousal or nightmares	Relaxation training (e.g. breathing exercises of Box 4)
Specific intrusive thoughts	Agree cognitive strategy to contain these: a mantra is useful 'I am here to have a rest from those things'. Recollections of positive past events, achievements or people are also useful to displace these
After sleep	
Disappointment (that heightens pressure to sleep the following night)	Encourage to rate the quality of rest achieved, not the total hours 'definitely asleep' – this is always underestimated by people
Early morning wakening: usually accompanied by anxiety	Highly suggestive of depression. Identify it as a short-term treatable symptom, not a new lifelong habit. It is better to rise earlier and do things rather than institute a failed attempt to regain sleep

Table 7 Common antidepressants (ADs). All antidepressants target components of monoamine synthesis. Prescribers should consult Taylor et al. (2007), Rosenbaum et al. (2005), the *British National Formulary* and local guidelines.

Group	Common group S/E	Example First line AD Second line AD	Therapeutic dose (maximum)	Other indications	Individual drug properties and S/E	Lethality in overdose	Discontinuation syndrome
SSRIs	Nausea, GI upset. Flushing, sweating. Anxiety, insomnia. Sexual dysfunction in up to 30% Weight gain (less than TCAs) Sedation is rare	Citalopram	20 mg/day (60 mg)	Panic disorder	Fewer drug interactions	Low	Common
		Fluoxetine	20 mg/day (60 mg)	Bulimia, OCD	Only proven AD in childhood	Low	Rare (long half-life)
		Paroxetine	20 mg/day (50 mg)	Generalized and social anxiety, PTSD, OCD, panic disorder	Most sedating + anticholinergic S/E of all SSRIs. Short half-life	Low	Highest of ADs: as TCAs plus dizziness, shock-like sensations
		Sertraline	50 mg/day (200 mg)	OCD, PTSD in women	No extra benefits at higher doses	Low	Common
Noradrenaline blockers	Sedation, nausea, postural hypotension	Mirtazapine	45 mg/day (60 mg)	Pain disorders	Weight gain but less sexual S/E	Low	Common: as SSRIs
TCAs: variable serotonin and noradrenaline blockade	Sedation, weight gain, anticholinergic effects (Table 8, p. 18), sexual dysfunction, lower seizure threshold, cardiac effects: promote arrhythmias, postural hypotension	Amitriptyline	150 mg/day (200 mg)	Pain disorders	Anti-pain effects at doses of 10 mg	High	Discontinuation symptoms less common than SSRIs: flu-like symptoms (chills, aches, sweating), poor sleep, excessive dreaming
		Clomipramine	150 mg/day (250 mg)	OCD	Used if anxiety levels are high	High	
		Lofepramine	140 mg/day (210 mg)	No other indications	Milder S/E, but constipation	Low	
		Trazodone	150 mg/day (600 mg)	No other indications	Caution with arrhythmia	Moderate	
SNRIs	At lower doses, same as SSRIs: nausea, etc. At higher doses: sweating, palpitations (as TCAs)	Venlafaxine	75 mg/day (375 mg)	Pain disorders, generalized anxiety	Hypertension at higher doses	Moderate	Common
		Duloxetine	40 mg/day (120 mg)	Pain disorders	Lower seizure threshold; less sexual S/E	Low	Rare

GI, gastrointestinal; OCD, obsessive-compulsive disorder; PTSD, post-traumatic stress disorder; S/E, side-effects; SNRI, serotonin and noradrenaline reuptake inhibitor; SSRI, selective serotonin reuptake inhibitor; TCA, tricyclic antidepressant.

Table 8 Common side-effects of antipsychotic (AP) drugs.

Typicals (in alphabetical order)	Side-effect	Mechanism of side-effect	Side-effect	Mechanism of side-effect
Chlorpromazine Fluphenazine Haloperidol Perphenazine Pimozide Sulpiride Trifluoperazine Zuclopenthixol acetate (by injection)	EPSEs: acute dystonic reaction, akathesia, tremor, rigidity and (late) tardive dyskinesia	Dopamine blockade	Anticholinergic effects: dry mouth, tachycardia, blurred vision, constipation, urinary obstruction, delirium (make confusion worse)	Block acetyl choline
	Sexual dysfunction: impotence, ejaculatory failure	Raise prolactin	Sedation (all APs cause this: typicals more than atypicals)	Block histamine
	Women: amenorrhoea, galactorrhoea	Raise prolactin	Raise seizure threshold (all APs: typicals more than atypicals)	CNS depression
	Weight gain	Insulin resistance	Cardiotoxicity: ↑ QTc interval (ECG)	Block cardiac receptors to reduce conduction
	Postural hypotension	Alpha-adrenergic blockage	Contact sensitization (handling the drug), photosensitive rash, cholestatic jaundice	Chlorpromazine only

Atypicals	Sedation (less than typicals)	Weight gain	Hypotension	Glucose intolerance (diabetes)	Sexual dysfunction (↑ prolactin)	Lowers seizure threshold	Unique or potentially fatal side-effects (formulation/common side-effects)
Olanzapine	++	++	+	++	+	++	
Risperidone	+	++	+	+	++	+	
Amisulpride	insomnia	+	–	+	++	+	Rarely activates
Quetiapine	++	++	+	+	+	+	Cardiotoxicity: ↑ QTc (requires b.i.d. dosing)
Aripiprazole	insomnia	–	–	–	–	prob –	Can activate some patients initially: short-term benzodiazepines useful
Ziprazadone	+	–	–	–	+	–	Cardiotoxicity: ↑↑ QTc – unavailable in the UK (requires b.i.d. dosing)
Clozapine	++	+++	hypertension	++	–	+++	↓↓ White blood cells: Box 7, p. 21 (hypersalivation, constipation)

CNS, central nervous system; ECG, electrcardiogram; EPSE, extrapyramidal side-effects.

Table 9 Features of the three most common mood stabilizers (only some drug interactions are listed).

	Lithium	Valproate	Carbamazepine (second line to first two)
History	In clinical use for 60/years; licensed in the USA since 1970, where it is used less often than valproate	Effective anticonvulsant: US approved as a mood stabilizer since 1995	Anticonvulsant: recently approved for mood. Not as effective as lithium in mania, but better in rapid cycling
Forms (parenteral administration not available for any)	Lithium carbonate: single daily dose. Start at 400 mg/day, and increase gradually	Sodium valproate (SV): two doses/day. Valproate semisodium = SV + valproic acid: t.i.d. dosing.	Extended release preparations: two per day. Must be increased slowly by maximum of 200 mg every few days
Mechanism of action (presumed)	Inositol decrease, serotonin increase; regulates adenyl cyclase and glycogen synthase pathways.	Increases GABA: inhibitory neurotransmitter	Opening of voltage-sensitive sodium channels; the drug then blocks these preventing excessive neurone firing
Preparation of patient	History and physical exam Urea & electrolytes, creatinine Thyroid hormones ECG in patients >50, family history Pregnancy test (teratogenic)	History and physical exam Full blood count Urea & electrolytes, creatinine Liver function tests Pregnancy test (teratogenic)	History and physical exam Full blood count Urea & electrolytes, creatinine Thyroid hormones Pregnancy test (teratogenic)
Follow-up tests **minimum 6 monthly**	Physical exam, drug levels Creatinine Thyroid hormones	Physical exam, drug levels Full blood count LFTs	Physical exam, drug levels Full blood count LFTs
Drug interactions: **raise** other drug	Lithium is increased by: NSAIDs, thiazide diuretics, SSRIs and APs (dehydration)	Antidepressants, APs, warfarin, other anticonvulsant drugs	Enhances the effects of other anticonvulsant drugs and alcohol
Drug interactions: **lower** other drug	Lithium is reduced by: theophylline, osmotic diuretics and caffeine (slight)	—	Most APs, benzos, valproate, contraceptive pill (it is teratogenic!)
Target plasma levels	Acute mania: 0.8–1.0 mM/L Prophylaxis: 0.6–1.0 mM/L	Poorer correlation with plasma levels: probably 50–150 μg/mL	Poor correlation. Use anticonvulsant range: 6–10 μg/mL
Common side-effects	GI upset, weight gain+ Thirst, polyuria, fine tremor Hypothyroidism	Nausea, cramps, weight gain++ Hair loss Transient raised LFTs	Nausea, GI upset Sedation, ataxia, dysarthria, diplopia Transient raised LFTs; low white cells
Skin side-effects	Acne, psoriasis, macropapular rash	Drug rash, erythema multiforme (Stevens Johnson'd)	Rashes 3%, exfoliation reported rarely
Toxic/fatal side-effects	Neurotoxicity: initially, coarse tremor, then confusion, coma, death. Renal failure.	Pancytopaenia (Box 7) Pancreatitis, hepatitis	Pancytopaenia: 1 in 150,000 patients Cardiac conduction abnormalities Hepatitis

AP, antipsychotic; ECG, electrocardiogram; GABA, gamma-aminobutyric acid; GI, gastrointestinal; LFT, liver function test; NSAID, non-steroidal anti-inflammatory drug; SSRI, selective serotonin reuptake inhibitor.

Box 5 Prescribing psychoactive drugs

Prescribers should consult Taylor *et al.* (2007), and the *British National Formulary*

- Be aware of your own 'rush to prescribe' – wanting to help people, wanting to be seen to do something, giving a prescription because other treatments (A to Z) are not available that moment, not wanting to let people (patients, relatives, staff) down
- Psychoactive drugs do not cure mental disorders. They provide symptom relief that can act as an impetus to promote recovery
- Elicit the patient's views about medication and illness generally, and their views about taking it themselves for their current symptoms: do they think they need it? What might they be worried about in taking it? Discuss potential barriers to adherence
- Broadly, three difficulties arise about medication: the need to take it, the need to take it regularly and the need to take it long term. Factors exacerbating these three difficulties include a patient's denial of the psychological nature of their problems, stigmatizing attitudes they and those around them may hold towards mental illness and medication, misconceptions about it (e.g. fears of addiction, losing control, changing personality), side-effects and past negative experiences of medication
- Prescribing should be a collaborative process where the patient is involved as an active participant in decisions wherever possible. Give them information about their options. Clarify what the benefits might be of the alternatives. Let them tell you which side-effects they most want to avoid, and any they think they might benefit from (e.g. sedative effects at night). By doing so, you will encourage their sense of self-efficacy in relation to medication (i.e. their sense of agency in taking it). The more a person feels in control of their medication, including side-effects, the more likely they are to persevere taking it

- If a patient has negative attitudes towards taking medication, encourage them to see their beliefs as hypotheses to be tested (e.g. 'medication *may* not take the voices away') rather than irrefutable facts ('medication *will not* take the voices away')
- Before starting treatment, identify treatment goals (including objective symptom measures) that you will monitor over time
- In terms of dose, **start low and go slow** (increase dose at careful intervals). This is essential in patients at the extremes of age and people with learning disabilities. Remember antipsychotic medication and antidepressants can take days to weeks to take effect. It's not uncommon for doses to be prematurely increased because of anxiety that the patient is not getting better quick enough. One of your roles as prescriber is to contain that anxiety, have a clear idea of what to expect and when, and to communicate that to others – patient, carers, staff. Premature increases do not make the patient get better any quicker, they just increase side-effects and thereby the likelihood of the patient stopping medication
- When you review medication, go back to your treatment goals and record the subjective and objective markers of change. If the patient does not volunteer side-effects, make direct enquiry, systematically checking for known possibilities (e.g. Tables 7–9)
- If no or poor response to medication, consider the possibility that the patient is not actually taking it. There is evidence across the literature, regardless of illness/medicine type, that only 40% of medicines are taken as prescribed on a daily basis. Do not accuse the patient of not taking it – enquire instead how often they are managing to do so. Check for difficulties with dose, formulation, administration (tablets, capsules, liquids) that result in people receiving other than the prescribed doses
- Interactions with other drugs (including alcohol) are a common cause of non-response to medication

particular. **Antipsychotics** (Table 8) and **mood stabilizers** (Table 9) are used to lower elevated mood and to prevent further relapses in people with bipolar affective disorder. In common with ADs, their side-effects frequently determine their prescription and their dose rather than their relative efficacy (Box 7). A fourth drug group, **sedative hypnotics**, is sometimes prescribed to promote sleep (or a quiet life for professionals), but they have problems with tolerance and addiction potential after their first 6 weeks' prescription. There are safer ways

to promote good sleep (Table 6). The short-term prescription of benzodiazepines in delirium tremens (alcohol withdrawal) is life-saving.

Beyond these four groups, other medications are described within individual cases. Some 'unconventional' remedies, fish oils and St John's wort, have been shown to be useful in psychosis and depression, respectively. Administration is best carried out under medical supervision; each has a narrow therapeutic window and common side-effects.

Box 6 Prescribing advice for antidepressants

Prescribers should consult Taylor *et al.* (2007) and the *British National Formulary*

- Antidepressant medication is only indicated for moderate to severe depression, *not* mild (where other approaches work better)
- Start at a low dose: monitor at 1–2 weeks at the start of treatment. Watch out for any increase in agitation or thoughts of self-harm, which have been reported at the start of treatment, possibly due to activating effects of some drugs
- Try one type for 4–6 weeks at an adequate dose first before swapping to another, and then choose an alternative from a different group: you gain little in following one SSRI with another. Slowly cross-taper between two antidepressants
- Before you change to a second antidepressant, reassess your patient: are there non-medication factors keeping mood at a low level? Have these got worse since you prescribed? Is there a biological cause of continued low mood, most commonly alcohol misuse? Are they actually taking it, and properly (Box 5)?
- Antidepressants should not routinely be used in combination due to increased risks of serotonin syndrome (Box 7)
- Sexual side-effects are common, but may not be disclosed *unless you ask about them*, and may lead to undisclosed discontinuation of the drug (non-adherence)
- After response, maintain drug at treatment dose for at least 4–6 months; longer with recurrent depression (potentially years)
- Withdraw slowly over 4 weeks, or longer if withdrawal proves to be problematic (switching to liquid preparations where available may help in this case, also consider alternate-day dose reductions)

KEY POINT

Prescribers of any psychoactive medication should consult Taylor *et al.* (2007), Rosenbaum *et al.* (2005) and the most recent *British National Formulary* as well as local prescribing guidelines.

E for electroconvulsive therapy

The majority of students and junior trainees perceive ECT as an 'old' treatment that should be used only as a *last*

Box 7 Medical emergencies caused by psychoactive medications

1 *Acute drug reactions* (not dose-dependent): allergy, anaphylaxis
2 *Overdose:* frequently taken in combination; most commonly, paracetamol
3 *Neurological syndromes:* usually at higher than recommended doses:
   ○ excess sedation, delirium, coma (all psychoactive meds; Table 20)
   ○ neuroleptic malignant syndrome: symptoms precede rise in creatine kinase and WCC
   ○ lithium toxicity (Table 9)
   ○ respiratory arrest (especially benzodiazepines, barbiturates)
   ○ seizures: almost all antidepressants and antipsychotics lower the seizure threshold
   ○ serotinergic crisis: restless, tremor, hypotension, progressively drowsy to coma
   ○ hypertensive crisis caused by interactions of monoamine oxidase inhibitors (MAOIs) with food/drugs: know the interactions, but *never* prescribe MAOIs unless in a specialist centre
4 *Cardiac arrhythmias:* tricyclic antidepressants, typical antipsychotics and some atypical antipsychotics such as quetiapine
5 *Renal failure:* most common psychiatric cause is lithium (Table 9)
6 *Endocrine disorders:* e.g. thyroid hypofunction caused by lithium, even at therapeutic doses
7 Pancytopaenia = **lowered** red cells (RCC), white cells (WCC)* and platelets. Always **stop** the drug (e.g. valproate, clozapine) and consult a physician. Early detection: regular full blood count (FBC), but note that lithium prescription raises WCC. Clinical detection: (patient reports) weakness, pallor (falling RCC); fever, sore throat (falling WCC); easy bruising or bleeding, skin petechiae (falling platelets)
8 *Liver enzymes increases:* antidepressants (Table 7), some antipsychotics (Table 8), mood stabilizers (Table 9) and benzodiazepines
9 *Other biochemical abnormalities:* high amylase (olanzapine and clozapine); low sodium (selective serotonin reuptake inhibitors [SSRIs], tricyclic antidepressants [TCAs], haloperidol, lithium); low potassium (haloperidol, lithium)

---

*Agranulocytosis = ↓↓ WCC: think VCC (Valproate, Carbamazepine and Clozapine)

resort – when ADs and coordinated treatments fail. This is to demote a modern, safe and life-saving intervention to the bottom of the pile – and thereby neglect a severely depressed patient when he/she needs an effective, fast-acting intervention the most.

ECT was the **first effective antidepressant**, introduced in the 1930s, and it remains the most rigorously tested of all psychiatric interventions. Its risks are those of the anaesthetic used to ensure a short pain-free seizure is induced in a patient, and where the manifestations of a generalized seizure are modified by a muscle relaxant so that direct evidence of seizure may be minimal (e.g. twitching of toes). Side-effects, including short-term memory loss (Table 23, p. 84), should be placed in the context of prolonging severe depressive or psychotic symptoms, risking further morbidity (catatonia/stupor, starvation and dehydration) in a vulnerable patient if ECT is withheld.

It is rarely a first line treatment for depression (Table 15, p. 49) *except* where a speedy response is essential to the patient's well-being. ECT is more likely to be applied in older patients where AD non-response is higher and the consequences of prolonged illness are greater. Although it is prescribed very rarely, ECT should be considered in postpartum depression with psychotic features and it is safe in antenatal depression where it does not harm the fetus. The adverse consequences of severe depression and psychosis in a pregnant woman or new mother are far more severe than the risks of ECT. Its negative perceptions among the public and some mental health professionals are also rooted in the realities of poor practice in its application and overprescription up until the 1970s. In Western countries, its use is highly regulated and frequently requires the agreement of an independent professional before it can be applied.

> **KEY POINT**
>
> In the USA, where ECT remains controversial, people with higher incomes and more health insurance and those who are not from ethnic minorities are *more likely* to receive ECT. This reality counters its poor public image as a punishment dealt out to the poor and dispossessed.

F for family interventions

We like to think psychiatry has come a long way from bogus theories that believed parents *caused* psychosis in

their children ('schizophrenogenic mothers, double bind, schism and skew'), but some parent-blaming attitudes still pertain among staff. Guilt is a common parental reaction to any mental health problems in a child. This can manifest as distress, depression, anger (at their child or at you), delayed presentation and/or resistance to treatments. While the causes of illness are complex, it is important to explore where intergenerational patterns of illness (e.g. psychosis) or problematic relationship patterns (e.g. abuse and neglect) have occurred. At the very least, your management of all children and young adults should include regular consultations that involve their families. Confidentiality (see L) becomes an impediment to harmonious working with families when your patient requests you do *not* communicate with them.

Although family intervention (FI) has become a dying art in adult services, it is the core intervention in children and adolescents, and you should not neglect to recommend it for a variety of patient groups (e.g. psychosis and eating disorders). This may mean enquiring about family practitioners in your team and others, but if you do not raise it, patients will not receive it. There are many schools of family therapy – their principal influences are psychoanalytic, systemic and cognitive–behavioural theories. In implementing behavioural measures (see B) for both anxiety and depressive disorders, enlisting a partner or family member as a co-therapist will ensure that advice is carried out and homework is completed. FI ranges from informal meetings, information sharing, generic support, psychoeducation (see G) and specific interventions to more intensive family therapy. Properly conducted, FI has few side-effects and promotes a shared sense of purpose with mental health professionals. Achieving a consensus between the patient, his/her family and the team strengthens relapse prevention planning; you need to agree clear guidelines about when to contact services if difficulties arise. Both anxiety and depression may be precipitated or maintained by dysfunctional relationships within families or in intimate relationships: couples' therapy may be the key intervention that achieves remission of low mood and prevents future relapse (Table 15, p. 49).

G for groups

This heading highlights two important principles:

1 It reminds us that the most remediable factor predicting recovery from illness and preventing relapse is a person's social network. Losing this (e.g. following a pro-

longed admission) will result in more morbidity and poorer outcome

2 As a trainee clinician, you will have learned by now that more effective learning happens in groups than in individual settings. Discussing what you have read and putting it into practice are the best ways of reinforcing learning Similar processes promote psychological learning.

Despite modern advances, the public stereotype of 'talking therapy' remains the psychiatrist's couch with the wise, bearded, bespectacled psychiatrist listening intently, perhaps writing in the background. This is to assume the main benefit of treatment is interpretation, and neglects that therapy primarily offers:

• A regular time and a safe place to disclose and reflect
• Non-judgemental positive regard for the individual
• Anonymity/confidentiality
• Empathy (*not* sympathy) from the therapist
  Therapeutic groups offer additional benefits:
• Shared sense of purpose: group cohesion
• The learning point for an individual that he/she is not alone in their difficulties: universality
• Positive experiences from other group members (e.g. altruism and identification)
• A real world experience of interacting with others – but in a safe environment where people learn that their ways of interacting may be part of the problem
• More intensive groups (e.g. based on Carl Rogers' person-centred model) produce moments of breakthrough, insight or even catharsis

Groups operate at the levels of shared occupations (traumatized soldiers), experiences (bereaved mothers against drunk driving), addictions (Alcoholics Anonymous [AA]; Narcotics Anonymous [NA]) or disorders (singing sessions or reminiscence therapy group for people with dementia). These are examples of *open groups* where people can join in at any time, and only the latter example requires a group leader to structure the sessions. All groups have rules agreed before commencing (e.g. about confidentiality: 'What we say in the room, stays in the room'). A *closed group* has a set beginning time with specific rules for people who arrive late or begin to miss regular sessions, and usually requires a commitment to a lengthy period. Common short-term closed groups include social skills' training, anger management, bulimia, healthy living and solution-focused therapy groups.

Psychoeducation is the term used to disseminate knowledge of someone's disorder, its triggers and protec-tive factors, and their individual relapse prevention plans – to promote self-management. Randomized trials have shown clear benefits of psychoeducation in common mental disorders, psychosis and eating disorders. Staff do not need lengthy high-level training and supervision (unlike group analysts) and, given its interactive learning nature, psychoeducation is best delivered in a group structure. Intensive group therapies vary with the training of the group leader. They usually have a strong psychoanalytic flavour, and detailed assessments are required to achieve referral of suitable members.

> **KEY POINT**
>
> Anticholinesterase inhibitor drugs are widely used in dementia care, but social interventions (e.g. reminiscence and music therapies) achieve comparable improvements in Mini Mental State scores and social function – these groups are cost effective and have fewer side-effects.

H for home treatment and hospital admission

A textbook written 10 years ago would describe only psychiatric hospital admission here. Despite implementing the above strategies, when a patient has not improved, or is overwhelmed by distressing symptoms, either option is the next and safest option. More usually, admission becomes necessary in someone's illness to manage:

• Risks to self (e.g. high suicidality, emaciated anorexia patient, acting on delusional beliefs) and/or
• Risks to others that cannot be managed in the community

Home Treatment Teams (HTTs) operate alongside community teams to intensify treatment (more support, structured interventions, improved medication adherence), working assertively with the patient and their social network. They will visit the patient in their own home up to four times a day. HTTs manage higher levels of risk than community teams, which lack the staff resources to intensify their efforts during a crisis. They work outside office hours, providing night-time assessments and weekend cover. By common agreement, patients are 'admitted' to a HTT, and discharge planning is as rigorous as that from the wards. Both HTTs and admission to hospital are treatments that facilitate other interventions (A to Z), most especially reconsidering the assessment and ensuring that the appropriate interventions have been chosen *and* are being administered.

> ### KEY POINT
>
> The most common indication for readmission in relapsing patients is that they have not been taking prescribed medication.

Because of the shift to HTTs and other assertive community treatments, hospital as a 'last resort' means the proportion of hospital inpatients who are admitted against their wishes (i.e. under section) continues to rise, raising the temperature on inpatient wards. You must operate with your country's laws (see L) and the decision is a balance between removing your patient's liberty, perhaps compromising your therapeutic relationship, and allowing suffering and risk to pertain when community interventions are failing. In hospital, the patient can also access interventions from members of the multidisciplinary team (MDT; see M) who are based in hospitals. A side-effect of admission is that the person can lose their established skills in daily living, managing finances, employment and community links. *Worse again, iatrogenic dependency may result.*

I for individual therapy

Even a regular outpatient clinic setting, where you may see a patient briefly and infrequently, involves a therapeutic relationship. A patient can form a powerful emotional bond with you, the nature of which may sometimes appear bewildering. At the most positive extreme, they may experience themselves as in love with you, or at least what you *represent* to them. Remember the difference. Conversely, you may instantly sense a patient's hostility before you have even had the opportunity to let them down. To every relationship in the present we bring with us expectations of other people, and patterns of relating to them that are based on our past experience. We all carry basic assumptions about others concerning fundamental questions such as 'Can we trust them?' 'Will they care about us?' Habitual emotional attitudes towards others are particularly rigid in patients with personality difficulties and may lead to obvious problems in their care.

Transference and countertransference are terms originally from the psychoanalytic literature that describe this phenomena in therapy. Broadly, transference describes the process by which an emotional attitude towards another from the past is (inappropriately) experienced in the present. Countertransference describes **your** emotional attitudes towards a patient in return. Over the course of someone's contact with mental health services, different members of staff will experience a range of emotional reactions to them based on what is mutually evoked between them and the patient. Unrecognized transference and countertransference reactions are obstacles to effective treatment. When recognized, they are useful tools to understand a patient.

One-to-one therapy should take place in the context of regular review by the MDT, often with medication as adjunctive treatment. Therapy is a means to an end (see Q), not an end in itself. Clear treatment goals will prevent a dysfunctional relationship between patient and therapist, where therapy becomes open-ended and fosters long-term dependency. Boundary violations (inappropriate gifts, friendships, even sexual relationships between therapist and patient) occur when the interpersonal dynamics of a treatment relationship are not attended to: therapists' supervision guards against this. At the time of writing, some disorders have clear guidelines for which therapy to apply and specific recommendations for the duration of therapy (www.nice.org.uk). You must be guided not just by diagnosis, symptoms and previous treatments, but also patients' mode of thinking and individual preferences (Table 45, p. 147).

> ### KEY POINT
>
> The best predictor of success in individual psychotherapy is the therapeutic alliance (between client and therapist), and this is determined early on in therapy.

Other interventions

The reality of modern mental health settings is that patients are offered the nine treatments above, although there is relative neglect of family and group therapies. Of its nature overinclusive, all other interventions are set out here: be familiar with treatment principles rather than detail. The remaining 17 are in no particular order, coded by letter (J–Z; Table 5). Within each heading, there are opportunities to intervene; for example, nidotherapy (see N) can take place in the home, ward, workplace or elsewhere. Some interventions (legal aspects, prejudice) identify external structural obstacles to full recovery – where coordinated actions will achieve improvements in social functioning. You may need to shoehorn treatments not included here into *your list*, but the important point is that you develop a convenient recall of every strategy (which you will remember quickly in clinical settings and exams) so that you never neglect to consider specific treatments in managing patients. Remain open to new treatments as the evidence builds for their use (see T).

J for job

Before early intervention psychosis teams became standard in the UK, the employment rate of people with first episodes of psychosis was only 25% after 1 year of treatment. Among people with long-term severe mental illness in Western countries, rates of employment rarely exceed 18%, although this is higher in Germany and Italy where social programmes dominate. Few people would argue that these 'patients' are incapable of working; only a small proportion have uncontrollable symptoms that make work impossible. We know that work accounts for the largest proportion of our social contacts, that having a meaningful occupation improves self-esteem and that people in paid employment have higher standards of living and increased opportunities. By contrast, unemployment confers a loss of social role on individuals and is a preventable risk factor for suicide (Table 25, p. 92). In the UK, two out of every three suicides of working age are long-term unemployed, and of the age group under 35 years, over 40% had a diagnosis of either schizophrenia or bipolar disorder. The case is as strong in people with other mental disorders that supporting patients in keeping their jobs, returning to work or achieving new employment are highly effective ways of achieving maximum improvements and relapse prevention.

Vocational rehabilitation is a specialist area, quite different from the more familiar role of occupational therapist (see O). Only a minority of jobs are advertised, and a vocational rehabilitation specialist can be proactive in knowing what is available in a particular locality – and what employers are looking for. Allied to this, knowledge of the variety of training and educational opportunities locally (as preliminaries to employment) is beyond the scope of other mental health workers. It is more effective to place someone in employment and to train and/or support him/her in the months that follow than (the traditional) train–place model previously adopted. The vocational specialist is also likely to be free of paternalistic attitudes found among some mental health staff, for example, a competitive interview or a particular job would be 'too much' for a particular patient. The chances of employment success are increased if the employment is both paid and meaningful, although voluntary work may be a necessary compromise in the short term, especially in areas of high unemployment.

K for kids (children)

All assessments across the lifespan must be framed in the context of each patient's childhood experiences (Table 1). The treatment of children and young people is substantially different from adult management. You cannot claim to have completed their assessment without speaking to their parents, and your formulation must integrate the information gathered. Systemic therapists conceptualize the child as a 'symptom carrier' for the family rather than 'sick' in his/her own right; examples are discussed later (Cases 8, 9, 13 and 15).

The final consideration here is the necessity to ask every patient about their own children, and children who are under their care. This acknowledges a wider responsibility to put children's interests first: the paramount principle. When a conflict arises between the rights of a child and those of an adult – even your patient – the child's rights override those of the adult. You must consider:

- The impact of the adult patient's illness on child care
- Does your patient present specific risks (violence, neglect, sexual behaviour)?
- If so, how will you manage these risks? Supervised visits?
- Do you need to communicate information to the child? How will you do this?
- For inpatients, what are the visiting arrangements for children on the ward?

You cannot manage these complex issues on your own and will need to activate discussion and action with your team (see M). If you have worries about the safety of any child you encounter in your professional life (even if you have not met the child), or you have *any* evidence of abuse (physical, emotional, sexual, neglect) of a child, you must activate referral to Social Services – and at the very least, discuss what you know with a social worker from the *Children At Risk* or similar team.

L for legal

Along with public health doctors, psychiatry is unusal in imposing treatment on patients who do not ask or wish for it. Psychiatrists must operate within both legal and ethical frameworks when treating an involuntary patient. The former are set out as legislation and binding codes of practice that include safeguards to protect patients' human rights. In addition to obeying the law, you have ethical considerations:

- *Consent:* you must have this unless lack of capacity

invokes Mental Capacity or Mental Health Act legislation (Cases 5 and 7).

• *Capacity:* a complex area (Cases 5 and 7), where knowledge of the law and case precedents must be backed up by open discussion with colleagues
• *Confidentiality:* you have a duty to preserve this except where you have information that places your patient or others at serious risk, and you break confidentiality in the best interests of your patient or a third party (see K). For example, fitness to drive may be impaired, and if your patient fails to disclose this, you are obliged to do so
• *Conflicts of interest:* these arise frequently in psychiatry (e.g. a therapist is asked to provide a court report whose conclusions would not help their patient's case)
• *Rationing of treatments:* ensuring that every patient has equality of access to interventions (A to Z)

As a psychiatric speciality in the UK, forensic psychiatry (FP) is just 30 years old. Forensic means anything relating to the courts or the law. FP deals with individuals in whom there is a link (sometimes tenuous and possibly coincidental) between their offence behaviour and their (sometimes obscure) mental illness. The 'criminal' demographic (young, male, misusing substances, personality difficulties, non-compliant with medication, lower socioeconomic group, rootless) is also overrepresented among mental health patients. There is high psychological morbidity in prison populations, some of which is related to prison life (e.g. confinement, conditions, substance misuse, low mood and suicidality) rather than causative of the index offence. That said, court diversion programmes prevent the incarceration of people with severe mental illness for minor criminal offences – for which, statistically, they are more likely to give themselves up or be detected with relative ease. In the UK, considerable financial resources have been diverted to FP services to fund many levels of security for the detention of medically disordered offenders. Referral by general psychiatrists for an FP opinion can be a useful exercise, and will lead to specific recommendations, perhaps joint working with FP teams. A community MDT will also receive frequent referrals from FP as part of step-down care (e.g. Case 11).

M for multidisciplinary team

All cases presented in this book are grounded in a biopsychosocial approach, but constructed for doctors. When we define the medical role as central, this intro-duces some imbalance – perhaps to the detriment of psychological and social perspectives. One aim of MDTs is to correct any bias based on professional training. Arguably, these two neglected perspectives have advocates within the MDT, psychologists and social workers, respectively. Your cognitive assessment and dynamic formulation may be inadequate to explain aspects of presentation or poor treatment response – it is reasonable to enlist a psychologist to measure IQ or clarify other aspects of the case. Equally, your social history (Table 1) might be comprehensive enough to pass psychiatric examinations, but lack practical grounding in complex benefits and state support systems. Would you know where to start (without the assistance of a social worker) to help restore social security benefits, schedule debt relief or apply for emergency housing?

Nurses, who contribute to all 26 interventions, have a holistic approach to the care of patients, and plan their interventions on a needs-based approach. A nurse might prioritize poor self-care, inadequate nutrition, family conflict and rising debts in a newly admitted patient we have diagnosed as having 'severe depression'. In traditional mental health settings, it remained true that doctors prescribed the care but nurses provided it – this too is changing, with nurse prescribing, nurse therapists and other innovative ways of working. A trend has emerged in recent years of superspecialization of MDT workers. Child and adolescent teams require a speech and language therapist (Case 9) and some adult services have a team pharmacist. In the community, a variety of support workers assist the MDT. Although not a member of the team, interpreters are essential in many urban centres – and the team should also draw on the resources of community groups (see V) to address transcultural aspects of their patients' care. The MDT often reaches outside of itself for additional expertise.

> **KEY POINT**
>
> The patient's GP is the most important professional in promoting long-term health. He/she is not a member of the MDT but can attend meetings and communicate in other ways. GPs see more cases of depression in their professional lifetimes than psychiatrists. They also have a central role in physical health care.

N for nidotherapy

The term nidotherapy has been coined by Tyrer and Bajaj (2005) to describe a treatment that systematically adjusts the environment to suit the needs of the person. The Greek word *nidus* means 'nest', and the authors' original targets of interventions were people with severe and enduring mental illness – although it is broadened here to include everyone with mental health problems. Consider the setting of a patient in a ward before moving to other settings. Many environmental factors impact on that person's well-being: layout of the ward and that individual's room, lighting and décor, personal items and their security from interference by others, shared spaces, smoking area (if present), exercise opportunities, places for privacy, and the general state of repair and hygiene of facilities. These are central to managing a confused inpatient. The key here is negotiation between patient and MDT: not every change is possible, but acknowledgement of environmental maintaining factors, and staff willingness to improve what they can, is a far better way to proceed than a confrontational approach. Even if the patient has a treatable medical or psychiatric cause – and the best treatment is to treat the cause – the most effective and least toxic intervention here is to change the ward environment (Box 10, p. 70). The same is true for hospital management of psychosis (Box 11, p. 77).

In the community, the main focus for nidotherapy is housing. Poor housing is a strong maintaining factor for mental ill health. This covers achieving the best housing for patients, modifying their housing (e.g. to improve safety, security measures to reduce cues for anxiety, adaptation for physical disabilities), or supporting them to put their own mark upon their environment (decorating, furnishing, removing clutter). The emphasis in nidotherapy in these circumstances is that the individual patient takes control for the programme of change. This will benefit social functioning and self-esteem (see Q). It is possible to achieve immediate changes of housing in some vulnerable patients (victims of domestic violence, children at risk, victims of local violence and intimidation), but in most cases, you cannot influence housing providers and landlords to that degree. This should not stop you from trying.

O for occupational therapy

The use of work and practical activities to ameliorate the effects of mental illness dates back to the development of humane treatments for mental disorder in the 19th century. As a speciality, occupational therapy (OT) has its roots in restoring people with physical disabilities to meaningful work following the First World War. A specialist in OT will:

- Evaluate a patient's physical and social capabilities
- Assess performance skills and obstacles to carrying out activities
- Evaluate home, workplace and other locations to address risk and maximize function
- Recommend adaptations (e.g. equipment, physical changes) to these locations
- Guide individuals, family and MDT members about training and a patient's potential

These activities are a summary of activities within both general (physical) and specialist *mental health* OT. This is a useful way to consider the contribution that OT makes to patient management, given the high degree of comorbidities in people who are referred to OT. Contributions from OT are essential in:

- Rehabilitation teams (see R)
- Treating older people's mental health problems. Many people with dementia retain some activities of daily living (e.g. dressing, self-care) and, with adequate supports (physical and personnel), can continue to live at home longer
- People with learning disability will gain more from comprehensive OT evaluations than, for example, from measuring their individual IQ as a discrete measure divorced from their functional ability

OT assessment and treatments of psychiatric inpatients are a good place to consider these activities. This is frequently too early an opportunity to assess a patient's ultimate potential, and activities with a lower 'work potential' such as art, music and drama therapies are useful in helping to re-engage and establish structure. Music therapy has good efficacy in reducing symptoms in a range of disorders – dementia, psychosis and common mental disorders – with a growing evidence base that it is also effective in childhood and adolescent disorders. It has been of proven use in many physical illnesses, especially pain and cancer conditions. Trials of other art therapies, including the more established drama therapy, should lead to more widespread clinical indications. The activities of community MDT members who have OT training frequently merge with generic team working. Their skills are invaluable in helping phobic patients in practical programmes of graded exposure to overcome specific and generalized phobias.

KEY POINT

Increases in the evidence that 'unscientific' art-based therapies are efficacious and cost effective has been driven by sound medical research in specialities other than psychiatry.

P for prejudice

No other area of medical practice has acquired the extremes of opinion as has mental health. Although many psychiatrists feel devalued and/or under attack from sections of the public, it is people who have mental illness who bear the brunt of public antipathy. A prejudice is an attitude, usually negative and with a strong affective component, that resists evidence to the contrary: the prejudiced person *prejudges* each situation or person. Doctors too may be prejudiced against people (see F) or treatments (see E). Public prejudice against people with mental illness is common in all societies. They are portrayed negatively in the media, within recognizable stereotypes that see them as self-indulgent, lazy or weak, inflicting illness upon themselves (especially people who overdose or have an eating disorder) or as dangerous (addicts and people with psychosis).

Stigma is a prejudice, based on stereotypes, leading to discrimination. Sometimes the discrimination is subtle – a psychiatric patient does not receive full investigation for physical illness, former friends do not visit or an employer passes over someone because of their past – but overt discrimination, although unlawful, continues to occur. Stigma has been described as the 'second illness' and a cause of distress and major disability. The stigma of mental illness predates the profession of psychiatry, but on occasion professionals contribute to it in clumsy language, although meaning well: 'that schizophrenic could never work – it would be too much for him'. Even the buildings of psychiatry (old asylums, group homes in the worst part of town) contribute to stigma. Negative stereotypes can be internalized as self-stigma: a patient with depression may come to believe, even when his/her mood restores to its usual level, that he/she is lazy and worthless, and a burden on society.

So what does all this have to do with your comprehensive management of patients? Your role should include:
- Awareness of your own prejudices
- Consistent challenges to others' stigmatizing beliefs
- Using 'people first' language: there are no 'schizophrenics', just people with schizophrenia
- Challenging patients who have internalized societal stigma
- Helping patients decide in which circumstances they might disclose their mental health problems to others (family, friends, employers)
- Supporting your patients to challenge discrimination on the grounds of mental ill health, a history of illness or merely the label
- Being aware of protective legislation and agencies that will support patients

Q for quality of life

It may seem an easy question to ask a patient to identify those aspects of his/her life that yield the most meaning and fulfilment, but not everyone can answer this question – far less so when in crisis or through the distorted prism of active mental health problems. Meanwhile, those making the assessment often forget to ask people what they want from interventions. As doctors we tend to be trained to have a narrow focus on addressing discrete symptoms (e.g. hearing voices), but these may not be the patient's main problem (it could be housing, poverty, loneliness). Patients soon learn what a particular doctor is interested in hearing about, and much clinical time is unknowingly wasted by medicalized agendas, whereby what really matters to a patient is missed. There are a variety of scales that measure quality of life (QoL), which serve as a useful prompt to remember the various domains: hobbies, sexuality (frequently impaired on psychiatric medications, especially antidepressants; Table 7) and spirituality to name but three.

One approach in a first episode of psychosis might be to focus therapeutic attention on what that person wants to achieve: restoration of previous relationships, getting back to employment or education, or financial independence. Support to pursue some of these domains can fall outside mental health treatments, but MDT support should at the very least remove obstacles to their pursuit. A related concept here is **social functioning**, defined as:
- The ability to cope with tasks with adequate performance and little perceived stress
- Good financial management
- Secure and settled relationships with family, friends and wider society
- Enjoyment of spare time

There are practical measures of this (e.g. Global Assessment of Functioning [GAF] scale of DSM-IV). How a patient's optimum function is achieved is more complex than the elimination of symptoms or even the acquisition of insight into their difficulties. Ernest Hemingway famously commented that his psychiatric treatment had cured the illness, but killed the patient. Recovery from mental disorders has been defined as a process of a way or growing with, or despite, disability. A recovery model highlights hope, shifting emphasis from symptoms and illness to strengths and wellness. It prioritizes an individual's self-esteem and promotes social inclusion, linking interventions with an awareness of societal stigma (see P). Improving QoL and social functioning are focused ways of achieving recovery.

R for rehabilitation

Prevention of all mental disorders occurs on three levels:

1 Primary prevention is **true prevention**: strategies that stop the disorder from happening in the first place. There are universal general measures that help everyone in society (e.g. Table 36, p. 124), and some specific measures aimed at certain (at risk) groups or at an individual level (e.g. Table 37, p. 125)

2 Secondary interventions form the vast majority of 'front end' medical endeavours: this is our main focus in Part 2. This is **treatment** of a disorder as soon as it presents: early intervention and psychiatric A&E teams treat disorders (e.g. psychosis and self-harm) to prevent long-term disability and other negative outcomes (e.g. suicide)

3 Tertiary interventions are directed at those individuals who have developed the disorder and presented too late for effective treatment and/or failed to respond to treatment. Rehabilitation is synonymous with tertiary prevention

Rehabilitation is an organized statutory or voluntary sector (see V) programme designed to improve physical, mental, emotional and social skills to enable a transition back into society and the workplace. There are many settings for rehabilitation teams:

• *Inpatient facilities for intensive MDT working:* to determine the levels of symptoms and medication dosage that facilitate independent living. For young people who became ill in childhood (e.g. onset of psychosis at 15 years), this is about *habilitation* – training them in activities of daily living for the first time

• *Staffed residential units:* for patients who cannot live independently, even with high levels of support. These are the 'new long stay' patients who 40 years ago would have lived indefinitely in an asylum

• *Independent living* (e.g. group homes, hostels, rented accommodation)

• *Day hospitals, day and drop-in centres*

The challenge for rehabilitation teams is to assemble the necessary resources to manage an individual in the least restrictive setting where his/her functioning is maximized (see Q). The specialty is a victim of its own successes in community care: money previously spent in institutions did not follow the patient to the community. Breakdowns of placements are common and increase rehabilitation teams' workload.

KEY POINT

England and Wales lost 110,000 psychiatric hospital beds over 40 years to 1996, but during the same period only 13,000 hostel and home places were created.

S for surgery

Psychosurgery – brain surgery to treat psychiatric illness – has a discredited history. It was introduced on the basis of a poor evidence base in the 1930s, with results falsified to present it in a better light. Patients were coerced into surgery, or gave 'consent' on the basis of false hopes of cure for depression and psychoses. Surgery was even administered in the 'treatment' of antisocial personality disorder, and these abuses have been powerfully represented in Hollywood films such as *Frances* and *One Flew Over the Cuckoo's Nest*. With this appalling pedigree, it is difficult to discuss *any* psychosurgery in a positive light. There is currently only one indication for psychosurgery, and surgical intervention is a treatment of **last resort**. Patients with obsessive-compulsive disorder (OCD) should only be considered for surgery after a range of psychological and social treatments have been implemented over many years – alongside medication use, with assured adherence to all interventions. The procedure here is to break the connections in the subcaudate nucleus (cingulotomy), and case series (there are no randomized trials) have shown mostly positive results.

Psychiatrists are also consulted to screen patients who wish to change their gender (male to female, female to male) by gender reassignment surgery. If indicated, it follows a medically supervised programme of hormone manipulation and a prolonged period where the preoperative individual lives in the role of the destination gender. Assessment rules out psychosis and other psychiatric contraindications to surgery or long-term hormonal manipulation (e.g. treatment-resistant depression). It should also explore sexuality comprehensively. A fetishistic transvestite gains sexual excitement from wearing clothes of the opposite gender, but does not wish to remain permanently in this gender role. Other transvestites are gay people who wear clothes of the opposite gender for pleasure (but not sexual excitement) or to attract same gender partners (e.g. drag queens). Transvestites do not request sex change surgery. Finally, psychiatrists may be consulted by surgeons if unusual or repeated requests for cosmetic surgery are made: these may be driven by insatiable demands for surgery driven by delusional or quasi-delusional/obsessional ideas, such as body dysmorphophobia.

T for transcranial magnetic stimulation

Transcranial magnetic stimulation (TMS) stimulates the brain using intense, pulsed magnetic fields. The technique is non-invasive, applied across the subject's skin, delivering a magnetic pulse to the cerebral cortex from a hand-held device. It is administered to conscious patients without the need for anaesthesia or sedation of any kind. The pulse passes through bone (the skull) and induces an electrical current in brain tissue sufficient to depolarize neurons. Interest in TMS has increased in recent years as a way of inducing central neuronal changes without inducing a full seizure as is the case in ECT (see E). In theory, specific areas of the brain could be targeted, and most research has centred on the use of TMS to treat affective disorders. Other neurostimulation techniques (magnetic seizure therapy, vagus nerve stimulation and deep brain stimulation) are at research stages only.

A multicentre trial randomized patients with severe depression comparing 3 weeks' treatment with TMS with a regular course of ECT. Entry criteria were that clinicians had referred patients for ECT as a result of severe low mood. Their primary outcome measures were ratings of depression (on a recognized scale) during treatment and at 6 months' follow-up. Findings were:
• ECT was more effective than TMS at reducing depression symptoms
• The costs of a course of TMS treatments were not significantly different from the costs of a course of ECT
• Subjective side-effects of ECT (memory loss) correlated with its antidepressant effects
• When global cognition was compared, there were no differences between the TMS and ECT groups before or after treatment

Small trials have shown that TMS may be effective in reducing pain symptoms in chronic pain syndromes.

Positive effects were concluded as independent of the effect of TMS on either patients' mood or anxiety levels. At the time of writing, TMS has not been shown to be an effective treatment for OCD, and research is ongoing into its use in other mental disorders.

U for users

Many psychiatrists are uncomfortable with the term 'service user', as are some people who have mental health problems. Doctors have *patients*, therapists see *clients*, but modern UK psychiatry refers to *users*. In the USA, the equivalent term is *consumers*, although some former psychiatric patients use the more provocative label *survivors*. These individuals have *survived* the psychiatric interventions, rather than the disorder itself. By now, you might consider someone with a mental disorder under your care not as a passive recipient of treatment, but as a service user and a partner in treatment. Empowerment improves self-esteem (see Q) and makes stigma or discrimination less likely (see P). People are more likely to be stigmatized if there is a large power differential between stigmatizer and stigmatized. Power is not just about money: it is also about information. Gone are the days of 'doctor knows best' because they were the only reservoirs of knowledge. Your patients/users will seek out their own sources of knowledge, and you should be proactive in alerting them to reliable independent sources of information (Table 10). Recently, UK government funding of mental health services has become contingent on the degree to which services have consulted users. Ideally, service users should contribute at every level in monitoring how a service spends public money.

Following on from these advances, user-led audit and research are beginning to effect real change in how mental health care is delivered. We know that modern psychiatry is enriched by MDT working, and in a similar way, users are entitled to consult people other than mental health professionals about their care. There are three broad areas where users become involved in treatment:

1 Advocacy is speaking up for others (e.g. people with learning disabilities, dementia or severe mental disorders). Advocates can be professional service users, friends/family appointed by the person (e.g. power of attorney) or professionals (e.g. solicitors)
2 Mentoring is another form of advocacy. One example is a sponsor who helps a new member of an AA group outside of regular meetings. There are less formal examples where peer support empowers users

Table 10 User and carer organizations in the UK and helpful websites for information about mental disorders and their treatment.

User and carer organization	WEB address	Other organizations	WEB address
Rethink	www.rethink.org	Royal College of Psychiatrists	www.rcpsych.ac.uk *Help is At Hand* Leaflets for each disorder
Mind	www.mind.org.uk	BBC Health Site	news.bbc.co.uk/1/hi/health/default.stm
Mental Health Foundation	www.mentalhealth.org.uk	National Health Service NHS Direct	www.nhsdirect.nhs.uk/help
MDF: the Bipolar Organization	www.mdf.org.uk (formerly known as the Manic Depression Fellowship)	National Institute for Mental Health in England	www.nimhe.csip.org.uk
Depression Alliance	www.depressionalliance.org	National Service Framework for Mental Health	www.dh.gov.uk/en/Publicationsandstatistics/Publications/PublicationsPolicyAndGuidance/DH_4009598
Alzheimer's Society	www.alzheimers.org.uk	National Institute for Clinical Excellence	www.nice.org.uk
Beat: beating eating disorders	www.b-eat.co.uk/Home	See Me – Scottish anti-stigma campaign	www.seemescotland.org.uk
User group – psychosis	www.psychosissucks.ca	Early Prevention Psychosis Intervention Centre, Australia	www.eppic.org.au
Alcoholics Anonymous (AA)	www.alcoholics-anonymous.org.uk/geninfo/01contact.shtml	Initiative to Reduce the Impact of Schizophrenia (IRIS)	www.iris-initiative.org.uk
Carers UK	www.carersuk.org/Home	UK Government programme to reduce drug misuse	www.talktofrank.com/home_html.aspx
National Alliance for the Mentally Ill (US organization)	www.nami.org	Chicago Consortium for Stigma Research	www.stigmaresearch.org

3 Several user organizations (Table 10) may communicate with services, or provide part of aftercare (e.g. drop-in centre)

Doctors have nothing to fear from a relative loss of power over their patients: the end of the deference culture does not mean the end of respect for doctors as professionals.

> **KEY POINT**
>
> The move to empower service users is supported by evidence that self-management programmes are effective in improving outcomes of chronic medical disorders. The greater imperative here is that user empowerment is the right thing to do.

V for voluntary organizations

The jargon 'thinking outside the box' might be usefully replaced with 'thinking outside the clinic'. Voluntary organizations (charities, trusts, self-help networks) are non-statutory bodies (or non-governmental organizations [NGOs]) in that they fall outside the control of the state and are separate from the health services. However, they may receive state funding or become paid providers of a particular service. Most are national organizations who have a local presence. You should make it a priority to find out about the range of NGOs that work in your area. Many of the interventions described above are made possible only through interaction with this sector. Examples might include:
• Supporting a patient who is ineligible for council accommodation to rent his/her own accommodation owned by a housing trust (see N)
• Where someone's benefits are not sufficient, suggesting they apply for charitable funds to improve their home or other circumstances (see N)
• Recommending a patient with alcohol problems attends AA (see G)
• Suggesting that patient's relative or partner attends the same organization's supportive wing (e.g. Al-Anon; see F and G)
• Suggesting a patient with debts (someone with mania has overspent or, more common and difficult to prove, some mental disorders may result in inabilities to plan finances) go to a citizen's advice bureau (see N)
• Directing a patient, declined asylum status and who

has exhausted legal process (see L), to a supportive charity
• Linking patients to local community/religious groups (see G and Q)
• Linking patients to a community programme to promote exercise (see X)
• Suggesting a relative or partner attend a local carer organization (see U; Table 10)
• Supporting clinicians and researchers with service and educational grants

Many NGOs and charities work in the mental health arena. Not every one is listed here (Table 10) but their web addresses are a useful starting point for your users and carers to gain useful information, and for you to begin the process of discovering who does what.

W for weight loss

Loss of appetite and weight are common symptoms of depression (Table 13, p. 45), and both symptoms also occur in anxiety disorders (Figure 2, p. 37) and to a lesser extent in people with psychotic illness. When patients have lost weight *before* the onset of mood or anxiety symptoms, this should alert you to the possibility of an organic (physical) cause of their presentation, notably cancer. Weight loss is of itself a cause of low mood, probably through imbalances of the hypothalamic–pituitary axis, and low weight will maintain pervasive low mood and poor sleep. When people lose weight over a period of months, correction of this loss is a priority but not a medical emergency – unless, for example, a depressed patient is refusing to eat or drink.

Urgent action is required in deliberate weight loss: anorexia nervosa has the highest mortality rate of all mental disorders, of which the medical complications are a major component. Your management plan in patients with severe weight loss of presumed psychiatric aetiology includes:
• MDT discussion (include a physician) of the safest setting to manage the patient
• Examination and investigation for an organic cause of weight loss
• Investigation for electrolyte imbalances: potassium, sodium, urea, calcium (in acute weight loss and at the extremes of low weight)
• Investigation for anaemia, vitamin deficiency (all disorders agreed programme of exercise restriction [bed rest] and increased calorie intake)
• Input from dietitian throughout treatment programme

There are two other settings where weight loss may be an indicator of underlying psychological distress and where supportive treatment is required to restore lost weight. Patients who are unlikely to tell you that something is wrong – people with dementia and people with moderate to severe learning disability – may have weight loss as their only symptom of depression. You would need to rule out medical illnesses and confirm other changes in behaviour and/or that changes in their routine may have precipitated a depressive episode. Weight loss is an inevitable symptom in the advanced stages of dementia, but you should have a low threshold in recognizing comorbid treatable depression in this group.

X for eXercise

Medical interventions are frequently represented as things that happen to a person. A man who has a myocardial infarction receives thrombolysis, angioplasty and medication to make him well again but how *he* responds to illness and what *he* does are strong predictors of his outcome – in this example, how much exercise he takes. The same is true for mental health, directly and indirectly. Moderate ('aerobic') exercise is defined as 30 minutes' activity at least three times each week that increases the resting heart rate. This will reduce:
- Obesity
- Risks of developing cardiovascular disease, diabetes and sexual dysfunction
- Mortality rates from cancer
- Depressive symptoms, and relapse rates in people with a history of depression
- Anxiety symptoms
- Cognitive and emotional barriers in people with Down's syndrome

With the exception of eating disorders, where some patients misuse exercise as a method of reducing their body weight, exercise should be recommended as standard in every psychiatric setting. Increasing physical activity may be all that is required to improve anxiety or mild depression – it is a safer treatment than ADs (Table 7) and cheaper. Although weight gain is an uncommon symptom of depression, usually accompanied by excess sleep, the usual context of weight gain is prescription medication (ADs): dietary advice and an agreed exercise programme can achieve significant weight reduction. The worst offenders in unwanted weight gain are the antipsychotics (APs), with olanzapine causing the greatest increase (Table 8). Pretreatment screening

and follow-up are necessary to identify *metabolic syndrome*, defined by three or more of:
- Abdominal obesity: waist circumference of >102 cm in men, >88 cm in women
- Hypertension: blood pressure ≥130/85 mmHg
- Serum triglycerides >1.68 mmol/L
- Fasting plasma glucose >6.1 mmol/L
- High density lipoproteins <1.04 mmol/L in men, <1.29 mmol/L in women

These parameters are not absolute and should be lowered if the patient is at identified risk. Screening should be performed by, or in collaboration with, the patient's GP: the prevention of the long-term consequences of metabolic syndrome (stroke, myocardial infarction) is an absolute priority.

> **KEY POINT**
>
> A history of psychiatric hospital admission reduces average life expectancy by 10 years. One component of this is premature death resulting from suicide and accidental deaths (e.g. anorexia nervosa), but the unhealthy lifestyle of people with severe mental illness and unmonitored effects of medication drive this high mortality.

Y for yoyo

The mnemonic is laboured here but yoyo (as in back-and-forth) is a reliable way of remembering another unclassifiable treatment. Eye movement desensitization and reprocessing (EMDR) treatment was developed by Shapiro (1989) for people with traumatic memories. Unusually for a psychological treatment, it was developed without a pre-existing theoretical framework. Trauma can lead to a number of different anxiety disorders (Table 11, p. 38), but the syndrome most frequently associated with specific traumatic memories is post-traumatic stress disorder (PTSD). Shapiro asked her patients to identify the memory that drives their symptoms (Table 32, p. 108), and to isolate a single visual image of this, describing in detail where the image is located, and what and who is in it. Patients supplied a negative statement that best suited this single image. They also rated their negative feelings associated with visualizing this image into subjective units of distress and constructed an alternative belief statement about how they might feel if the image no longer troubled them (this is cognitive reframing; see C). The technique of EMDR involves the subject:

- Visualizing the traumatic image
- Rehearsing the negative statement
- With his/her head kept in position, letting their eyes follow the therapist's finger 12 inches from their face in sets of 10–20 bidirectional sweeps across from left to right and back
- Following the therapist's finger moves at two sweeps per second, back and forth
- Stopping to reflect on the image's effects on them (rated numerically on an agreed scale). If an alternative, more traumatic memory reveals itself during EMDR, this is analysed as above, and EMDR is repeated for this image
- Once the intensity of the negative response to the image reduces, the positive alternative belief statement is paired with the image

The last step draws on behavioural theory to recondition a previous stimulus–response that paired the memory/image with unpleasant thoughts/negative feelings with a new conditioned response linking the image to a positive (or at least non-negative) statement. EMDR has been show to be effective in treating PTSD – more effective than more established behavioural techniques such as graduated exposure or systematic desensitization. Although a single EMDR session shows benefits at 3 months, six to eight sessions are recommended, and these should take place in conjunction with other CBT and supportive interventions. Guidelines recommend the use of EMDR as more effective and safer than medication (www.nice.org.uk).

Z for Z list of alternative therapies

There are a number of treatments, requested frequently by a minority of patients, that have not made the grade in terms of evidence that they work any better than placebo treatment. Given the ubiquity of mental ill health, it is unsurprising that herbal remedies and homeopathy have been suggested as possible, if unproven, remedies. Some have achieved limited evidence of efficacy: St John's wort and fish oils (see D), but neither achieve 'cure' on their own. On occasion, patients with long-term mental disorders (e.g. treatment-resistant depression, chronic fatigue syndrome) may link their symptoms with toxic metal poisoning or allergy. Conventional toxicology and allergy testing should establish if this is indeed the case, but it is sometimes hard to prove a negative. Where difficulties arise, it is with unproven 'remedies' to this assumed poisoning or allergy.

For the most part, alternative therapies should be approached with the question 'What harm could they do?' Most are indeed harmless (reiki, aromatherapy) and several are recognized as valuable relaxation methods (yoga, meditation, t'ai chi), which rarely result in deteriorations in mental health and are known to promote physical health and well-being. This is not the case for hypnosis, famously abandoned by Freud, where a trance-like state resembling sleep is induced by the hypnotist. The increased suggestibility that characterizes the hypnotic state could precipitate dissociation (Box 28, p. 169), relapse in psychosis or the development of new 'memories' that distress and bring the patient into conflict with others. There are several related and discredited treatments on the extreme fringes of mental health: abreaction, rebirthing and the use of amphetamines to 'open up' someone's mind. Hypnosis in medical settings has been advocated in anxiety disorders and some functional medical illnesses (e.g. irritable bowel syndrome) but only as part of a comprehensive treatment programme that includes CBT, and under close supervision. It has a modest evidence base in reducing pain during surgical procedures and in some chronic pain conditions.

ICD-10 does not specify a separate category for seasonal affective disorder, but this diagnosis has been endorsed by the American Psychiatric Association. The use of light therapy to improve low mood has been backed up by a small number of randomized trials. Its benefits are marginal, but the treatment is expensive – both financially and in terms of the time required to allow exposure to the light box – and it is not without side-effects. Headache and nausea are common in up to 10% of people who use light therapy, and a smaller proportion report jitteriness or an inability to relax. For Z list treatments, best practice is to negotiate with your patient in an open way, and to respect their choices provided they do them no harm.

References

McLoughlin, D.M., Mogg, A., Eranti, S., *et al.* (2007) The clinical effectiveness and cost of repetitive transcranial magnetic stimulation versus electroconvulsive therapy in severe depression: a multicentre pragmatic randomised controlled trial and economic analysis. *Health Technology Assessment* **11** (24).

Passard, A., Attal, N., Benadhira, R., *et al.* (2007) Effects of unilateral repetitive transcranial magnetic stimulation of the motor cortex on chronic widespread pain in fibromyalgia. *Brain* **130**, 2661–2670.

Penedo, F.J. & Dahl, J.R. (2005) Exercise and well-being: a review of the mental and physical health benefits associated with physical activity. *Current Opinions in Psychiatry* **18**, 189–193.

Rosenbaum, J.F., Arana, G.W., Hyman, S.E., Labatte, L.A. & Fava, M. (2005) *Handbook of Psychiatric Drug Therapy*. Lippincott Williams and Williams, Philadelphia.

Shapiro, F. (1989) Efficacy of the eye movement desensitization procedure in the treatment of traumatic memories. *Journal of Traumatic Stress* **22**, 199–223.

Taylor, D., Paton, C. & Kerwin, R. (2007) *Maudsley Prescribing Guidelines*, 9th edn. Informa Healthcare, London.

Tyrer, P. & Bajaj, P. (2005) Nidotherapy: making the environment do the therapeutic work. *Advances in Psychiatric Treatment* **11**, 232–238.

Further reading

Gabbard, G. (1994) *Psychodynamic Psychiatry in Clinical Practice*. American Psychiatric Press, Washington DC.

Gelder, M.G., Lopez-Ibor, J.J. & Andreasen, N.C. (2006) *New Oxford Textbook of Psychiatry*, Vols I and II. Oxford University Press, Oxford.

Sims, A. (1997) *Symptoms in the Mind*, 2nd revised edn. Saunders, London.

World Health Organization (1992) *ICD-10 International Classification of Disease*, 10th edn. *Classification of Mental and Behavioural Disorders*. WHO, Geneva.

Consensus treatment guidelines for most mental disorders discussed here are set out at www.nice.org.uk. The executive summaries are excellent, and they are frequently revised to give the most recent evidence base for treatments.

Case 1 A 20-year-old student who collapses in the supermarket

Ishmail is a 20-year-old student who fell to the ground in the supermarket. He did not lose consciousness. He says he suddenly felt very unwell, as if something terrible was going to happen to him. Then he felt sweaty, he could not breathe properly and his heart began to race as he slumped to the ground. You are seeing him in the Accident and Emergency (A&E) department.

What systems and associated symptoms do you need to cover in taking his history?

Using the hierarchy approach (Fig. 1, p. 7), organic pathology precedes psychiatric:

1 *Cardiovascular:* chest pain, breathlessness, palpitations, syncope, oedema
2 *Neurological:* syncope, seizures/fits/turns, headaches, tremor, weakness, pain, visual and sensory symptoms
3 *Endocrine:* weight loss/gain, thirst, polyuria, sweating, lethargy
4 *Psychiatric:* principally, mood and anxiety symptoms. What was he thinking prior to this episode? Define the sequence of worrying thoughts and physical symptoms. Can you identify changes in his mood or anxiety levels in the weeks before?

What physical disorders in this age group might explain this presentation?

1 *Cardiovascular:* ischaemic heart disease is highly unlikely in this age group; consider cardiomyopathies (especially hypertrophic obstructive cardiomyopathy), arrhythmias, anaemia and vasovagal episodes
2 *Neurology:* epilepsy, migraine, infection (local and systemic), haemorrhage especially subarachnoid, and the rare carotid sinus syndrome. Transient ischaemic attacks and other cerebrovascular accidents are rare in this age group

3 *Endocrine:* hypoglycaemia, hyperthyroidism and Addison's disease. For completeness, two *very rare* disorders: phaeochromocytoma and insulinoma

---

KEY POINT

When considering a case from a psychiatric perspective (in a psychiatric textbook or during a psychiatric assessment), you must exclude physical causes *first*. Otherwise, you will miss treatable physical pathology – with serious consequences.

Ishmail's physical exam is normal.

What physical tests will you order to help reach a diagnosis? Specify what each test rules out

• Full blood count (FBC) to rule out anaemia, infection, (uncommon) polycythaemia
• Urea and electrolytes (U&E) to rule out dehydration, renal impairment, electrolyte imbalances
• Glucose to rule out hypoglycaemic episode
• Electrocardiogram (ECG) to rule out rhythm and conduction abnormalities or cardiomyopathies
• Urine drug screen for legal (benzodiazepines, sedatives) and illegal substances (ecstasy, amphetamines, cannabis, cocaine, opiates)
• Calcium, thyroid and cortisol levels if indicated
• If he has dyspnoea and/or chest pain out of proportion with and/or independent of anxiety symptoms, consider 24-hour ECG and consult a cardiologist

Here, blood gases to measure carbon dioxide (low in hyperventilation syndromes) inflict a painful procedure on anxious patients, and are unnecessary.

Ishmail's physical tests are normal. However, he continues to appear very anxious. He describes several previous similar episodes over the last 9 months.

As a physical cause now appears unlikely, what are the psychological and physical symptoms of anxiety about which you need systematically to enquire?

• *Psychological symptoms:* fear, apprehension, *anguor animi* (a Latin phrase that translates as 'torment of the soul', an intense feeling that one is about to die – Ishmail complained of this on presentation), thoughts racing, restlessness, irritability, inability to relax, increased arousal to stimuli (e.g. sensitivity to noise, poor subjective concentration, difficulty getting to sleep and fatigue)

• *Physical symptoms* (also called 'somatic'): weakness, dizziness (many patients use the colloquial term, *vertigo*, for this), flushing, feeling faint, headaches, muscle tension, choking feeling, difficulty breathing (hyperventilation or dyspnoea), dry mouth, tetany (if hyperventilation), tremor (fine), sweating, tachycardia, chest pains, nausea, abdominal discomfort or 'butterflies', muscle cramps (Fig. 2). Urinary and faecal incontinence are rare in episodes of anxiety, and suggest epilepsy and other neurological disease

KEY POINT

Pathological anxiety is distinguished from normal stress responses by being disproportionate (i.e. out of keeping with the situation), prolonged and severe enough to interfere with normal functioning.

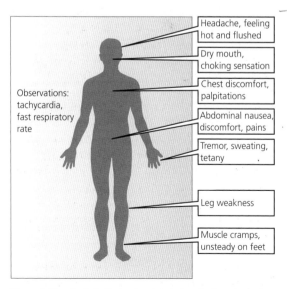

Figure 2 The physical effects of anxiety (adrenaline) on the body.

As Ishmail's history suggests acute anxiety, what positive findings might you find in his mental state examination (MSE)?

• *Appearance and behaviour:* sweating, handshake cold and sweaty; restless, agitated; in extremes of anxiety, patient may 'bolt' from the room to avoid further distress; anxious patients often repeatedly seek reassurance ('Am I going to be alright? It's not serious doctor, is it?')

• *Speech:* repetitive, sometimes loud, fast with mistakes, but with no evidence of thought disorder

• *Mood:* subjectively he may be unable to describe this experience clearly (e.g. 'I don't know, I just feel terrible'), objectively anxious affect; concentration poor subjectively but objectively at a good level. Typically, a highly distractible anxious patient calms down as the interview progresses

• *Suicidality* (thoughts of suicide, suicidal intentions and behaviours): uncommon in anxiety disorders, but people have killed themselves in the context of overwhelming anxiety where the symptoms or ongoing stressors have become intolerable for them

• *Thoughts:* he may perceive his thoughts as 'racing' and there may be evidence of ruminations about specific events or things (phobias), preoccupations about his health and a fear that something bad is going to happen. These ideas will not be delusional (i.e. they will be held on logical grounds, are amenable to challenge and not argued beyond the bounds of reason)

• *Perception:* no hallucinations. Illusions are common in anxious people: mistaking something in the shadows as dangerous (e.g. a potential attacker)

• *Cognition:* no cognitive abnormalities

• *Insight:* frequently very good, but may be poor on first presentation

KEY POINT

When patients are interviewed *after* a panic attack, their MSE may show dysphoria. More usually they have *no* abnormal MSE findings, but the diagnosis is made on history alone (Table 1).

Ishmail has no psychiatric history, with no recent stressful events. He gets about two of these episodes every month – usually in crowded places – but they are unpredictable.

What is the most likely psychiatric diagnosis here?

Panic disorder. Recurrent episodes of sudden onset, severe anxiety symptoms that occur in various (sometimes similar) situations:

• Episodes are random, and not as predictable as a phobia (Table 11)
• Episodes usually terminate within minutes, at most 30 minutes
• Panic disorder is frequently associated with agoraphobia (e.g. a specific fear of crowds, shopping centres, football grounds)

What other related disorders do you need to exclude at this point?

Other anxiety disorders (Table 11) are common in the general public, but mostly undiagnosed and untreated. Like depressive symptoms, anxiety symptoms are likely to be minimized by the person who has them and/or overlooked by clinicians in favour of physical diagnoses.

> ### KEY POINT
>
> You may need to move away from open questions at interview to direct enquiry to distinguish one anxiety disorder from another (Table 12).

Physical complaints (back pain, irritable bowel syndrome and chronic headaches) are common proxy symptoms for anxiety; these have complex interactions with anxiety disorders.

Most patients describe dysphoria (low mood less severe than depression) for minutes, even hours, after a panic attack, but up to two-thirds of people with panics also have comorbid **depression**. Anxiety and depression have a bi-directional aetiological relationship: persistent anxiety makes the development of depressive symptoms *more likely* (perhaps by stimulation of the hypothalamic–pituitary axis and/or the psychological cost of anxiety) and low mood is known to *lower the threshold* for all varieties of anxiety (Table 11).

Table 11 Classification of primary anxiety disorders according to precipitants.

Precipitant	Diagnosis	Course
Stressful life event	Acute stress reaction	Onset immediate, resolves without intervention within hours or days
Stressful life event	Adjustment disorder	Onset within a month, 60% resolve; 20% mild depression; 20% moderate–severe depression
Life-threatening event	Post-traumatic stress disorder	Rarely resolve spontaneously; frequent comorbid depression
Intrusive thoughts	Obsessive-compulsive disorder	Lifelong, with relapses; frequent comorbid depression; can be as disabling as schizophrenia
Specific objects	Specific phobia: animals, heights, flying, etc.	Highly treatable if diagnosed early; many lifelong phobias interfere to a minor degree with social function
Specific situations	1. Crowds = agoraphobia 2. Social situations = social phobia	Chronic course unusual Present late but treatable
Variability of exposures to anxiety: sometimes none	Panic disorder	Treatable but relapse is common (see text)
No immediate precipitant	Generalized anxiety disorder	Usually present by teenage years and run a chronic relapsing course
Health anxieties	Hypochondriasis	Varies: can be trait or state. Always context-dependent

Table 12 The Anxiety and Depression Detector (Means-Christensen *et al.* 2006).

Question: 'In the past 3 months . . .'	Disorder uncovered by question
1. 'Did you ever have a spell or an attack when all of a sudden you felt frightened, anxious or very uneasy?'	Panic disorder
2. 'Would you say that you have been bothered by "nerves" or feeling anxious or on edge?'	Generalized anxiety disorder
3. 'Would you say that being anxious or uncomfortable around other people is a problem for you in your life?'	Social phobia
4. 'Did you have a period of 1 week or more when you lost interest in most things you usually enjoyed?'	Depression
5a. 'Some people have terrible experiences happen to them (give examples of personal trauma, sexual assault or seeing someone badly injured or killed). Has anything like this ever happened to you?' If the answer is yes	Post-traumatic stress disorder
5b. 'Have you had recurrent dreams or nightmares about this experience, or recurrent thoughts or flashbacks?'	

> **KEY POINT**
>
> Primary anxiety disorders are usually signposted by early childhood symptoms or traits. New onset anxiety without this history usually indicates depression – in older adults it may be brain disease, even an early symptom of dementia.

> **KEY POINT**
>
> Lifestyle advice is the safest and most effective way to reduce anxiety symptoms: sensible/no drinking; quit smoking, caffeine, cannabis and other illegal drugs; carry out regular exercise and relaxation training (e.g. yoga); structure days to promote a good work–life balance.

What aspects of Ishmail's lifestyle do you need to consider that might make panic or other anxiety disorders more likely to occur, and make them worse?

- Alcohol or drug misuse
- Sedentary lifestyle
- Social isolation (student, living alone, away from home)
- Excessive cigarette and caffeine consumption
- Poor diet
- Financial problems
- Adverse living conditions (noisy home, location in a rough part of town, overcrowding)
- Stressors unique to that person (exam deadlines, rent arrears, work problems)

What cognitive and behavioural factors are likely to perpetuate these episodes for Ishmail (currently two each month for 9 months)?

- *Anticipatory anxiety:* believes he will become anxious if he goes to that particular supermarket, or similar places. These deeply ingrained cognitions drive the behaviour. Anxiety in these situations becomes a self-fulfilling prophecy
- *Avoidance behaviour:* reduces all activities where panic might occur
- Increase in *illness behaviour:* stops attending lectures and socialising to focus on his symptoms
- *Use of alcohol or other sedatives:* to relieve distress, so-called 'self-medication'
- *Repeatedly seeking medical opinions:* for somatic anxiety symptoms, despite repeated normal investigations and reassurances that the symptoms are psychologically driven. You may be the latest in a long line of doctors who need to find the overlooked physical condition and provide the 'quick fix'
- *Escape behaviour:* when anxiety occurs, or panics begin, the patient bolts ('flight' rather than 'fight' response). This reinforces the cycle of anxiety

What advice do you give to Ishmail on this, his first, presentation?

The key message is that panic disorder is *never* fatal: people only *feel* they will die. If he can identify how his thoughts drive his feelings during an episode, he will be able to limit its severity and duration.

Explain the nature of his physical symptoms, and how his own thoughts are driving them. Avoid phrases like 'all in the mind' as they promote self-blame. **Reassure** him about the benign course of panic disorder; even if he develops depression (a common comorbidity of long duration of panic disorder), both conditions are highly amenable to treatment.

Changing his lifestyle and his behaviour will have immediate benefits for him. **Breathing and relaxation techniques** can be learned from a variety of professionals: nurses, behaviour therapists, psychologists, occupational therapists, even doctors. A programme of **graded exposure** is paired with relaxation exercises and the introduction of cognitive models to understand his panics.

Advise him to attend his GP for **follow-up**. The GP will be able to refer him for psychological treatment in his area. Cognitive–behavioural therapy (CBT) should be offered to all patients, with medication as an adjunct in a minority, to achieve remission. Should panics recur following a panic-free period, the person usually reinstitutes the successful treatment and recovers.

Recommend he **finds out more** about panics and how to overcome them; refer him to leaflets, self-help books and useful internet addresses (Table 10, p. 31).

If you are in a position to carry out CBT under supervision, the paper by Williams and Garland (2002) is an excellent introduction and overview of the area.

In the short term, back in A&E, how might you instruct Ishmail in a slow-breathing technique to manage his panic when it occurs?

First, help him understand that rapid overbreathing is distressing and uncomfortable in itself, and causes many additional physical symptoms (Fig. 2; e.g. chest pain, dry mouth, tingling in his hands). Overbreathing prolongs the panic attacks.

Secondly, outline a slow-breathing technique (Box 4, p. 12) to use when he panics and overbreathes. If he can master this technique, he will be able to take control of subsequent attacks, limit their severity and reduce safety behaviours described above. Most people resolve the distress of their panic, and stop overbreathing within 5 minutes.

> Ishmail has no lifestyle behaviours that contribute to his anxiety. He asks you about medication.

What medications can and should not be used in this condition?

Four classes of prescribed drugs can be used as adjunctive treatment in panic disorder:

1 *Selective serotonin reuptake inhibitors* (SSRIs; Table 7, p. 17): the most common medications prescribed for panic, because of relatively fewer side-effects and a reasonable evidence base. Anxious patients tolerate them better if they are initially prescribed at half the antidepressant dosage then titrated upwards slowly. They take up to 6 weeks to show benefits and should be prescribed for at least 8 months. There is no consensus about when to stop them and this can be negotiated with the patient on an individual basis. If they are the only treatment used (i.e. without any psychological or behavioural treatments), the panics will probably recur after they are discontinued.

2 *Tricyclic antidepressants:* there is limited evidence for the efficacy of imipramine and clomipramine, and they are second line drugs to SSRIs. They show improvement over placebo treatment in the acute phase of panic disorder, but there are no large studies of long-term follow-up. Imipramine is poorly tolerated, and needs to be started at very low dosage (25 mg/day) before increasing. Despite the role of adrenaline in somatic symptoms (Fig. 2), tricyclics that block noradrenaline have no proven role in the disorder.

3 *Buspirone* acts on or close to the benzodiazepine receptor and has weak serotonin agonist properties. It can be sedating and has minimal effects on somatic symptoms. Three of its common side-effects (dizziness, nausea and insomnia) are likely to mimic panic disorder and could reinforce behavioural pathways.

4 *β-Blockers:* these reduce the somatic effects of anxiety (Fig. 2). Even in Ishmail's age group, clinicians should prescribe these with caution. They are contraindicated in people with asthma, heart conduction abnormalities or peripheral vascular disease.

> **KEY POINT**
>
> People with anxiety frequently self-medicate with over-the-counter 'drugs' (herbal remedies, antihistamines); legal drugs (alcohol); prescribed medication (other people's, e.g. benzodiazepines – donated, bought or stolen); as well as illegal drugs (e.g. cannabis). All provide short-term relief only, and most make difficulties worse.

Here is what *not* to prescribe: benzodiazepines. There is no justification to use other sedatives such as barbiturates or (sedating) antipsychotics, because of the other risks these medications incur.

Ishmail tells you he once used some of his mother's prescribed diazepam when he felt in a panic and he found it helpful at the time. He agrees to go and see his GP but asks you to prescribe him some diazepam in the meantime to prevent him having another attack.

How do you respond to Ishmail's request?

Explain:
• Benzodiazepines such as diazepam provide only symptomatic relief of anxiety and should only be used in the short term, because of their highly addictive nature. Patients become tolerant of their effects within 2 weeks
• Their prescription delays other treatment strategies being put in place, and people who take them perform less well in psychological therapy sessions
• Even if patients do not develop addiction to them, they experience withdrawal of their sedating effects and the frequency of panics can *increase*
• In the long term, patients prescribed benzodiazepines as primary treatment have a worse outcome

> **KEY POINT**
>
> Most psychiatric disorders are chronic relapsing conditions. In deciding about drug prescription, you must balance the need for immediate relief with the long-term risks of medication use.

Ishmail acknowledges that his mother has been addicted to diazepam for years and he does not want that to happen to him. He asks you more about psychological treatment and, specifically, which do you think works better – CBT or medication?

What will you advise him?

If he is going to try either medication or CBT alone, generally CBT works better than medication provided it is carried out by a trained professional. It also needs to be of at least 7 hours' duration (spread over multiple sessions) and include self-help strategies.

There is some evidence that medication plus CBT works better for the treatment of anxiety than either treatment by itself. What does Ishmail think he'd prefer?

Patients need to be given general information about what treatments are available, and then guidance interpreting that information in a way that is relevant to their individual circumstances, and takes into account their own preferences.

Ishmail says he is interested in CBT and asks you about it.

How might you describe it?

Following a thorough assessment, a CBT programme might begin with:
• Cognitive reframing of the panic episodes
• Teaching of slow breathing and relaxation techniques
 Once these techniques have been mastered and are being practiced by the patient, 'graded exposure' can begin. This is a collaborative process between patient and therapist that involves the following:
• The patient thinks through the situations that provoke his worst fears, and lists them in a hierarchy – from those causing least distress to maximum distress
• Treatment begins by mastering the easiest situations before graduating to more distressing situations
• Based on the patient's wishes, exposure can be initially *in vitro* or 'interoceptive' (i.e. in the patient's imagination), and is carried out in places of safety (such as an interview room or at home), or it can be *in vivo*, where exposure takes place in real-life distressing settings (e.g. supermarket, crowded cinema)

Ishmail says a friend advised him to see her psychotherapist, but she sees the therapist privately and Ishmail cannot afford this. He asks you if he could get psychotherapy on the NHS and whether it would be better than CBT for his panic disorder?

There is some evidence that a psychodynamic approach can help reduce the symptoms of panic disorder, but the trials have been small. There is a great deal more evidence to support the use of CBT for panic disorder, and at this point this is likely to be the more useful approach for him to try first. This is not to say that a psychodynamic understanding of his panic would not be useful or of interest in the formulation of his difficulties (Box 8).

It is worth noting that psychodynamic therapy is a scarce resource in most health care settings and he is much more likely to be able to access CBT.

In the first instance, you should stress that he needs to see his GP for follow-up and to ascertain what other treatment is available locally. It is also very important that you ensure that a copy of your assessment is sent to Ishmail's GP so he/she is aware of this presentation, your diagnosis and suggested management plan.

KEY POINT

One objective in first presentations of common mental disorders (anxiety and depression) is to prevent the patient from beginning a long 'psychiatric career'. These disorders therefore need prompt identification with appropriate treatment instigated. Psychiatric referral is not always necessary.

Box 8 A psychodynamic formulation of panic disorder

- According to psychodynamic theories, the key drivers of panic are childhood experiences of *loss and deficient coping skills to deal with loss* throughout adolescence and adult life
- *Parental separation* (e.g. through death, marital or other separations, migration) in early childhood is associated with later panic disorder; that association is three times as strong as the (well established) association between parental loss and later life depression
- Evidence shows *maternal loss* as more damaging than the loss of a father
- Linked to separation and loss is a poorly developed sense of 'object constancy'. This concept describes how, normally, an infant learns to cope with their mother's absences by developing an inner sense of their mother. When she leaves their environment they are therefore comforted by being able to imagine her as an internalized 'object' (i.e. they experience their own continuous inner sense of her). Failure of this normal process of early maturation (e.g. when an infant does not form a secure attachment to his/her mother), can lead to acute episodes of anxiety – where the person is overwhelmed by the combination of intense feelings of abandonment, danger and hence panic
- Freud observed two forms of anxiety: the first is driven by biological factors and the second has psychological origins. This second form, which he described as 'signal anxiety', corresponds to *anticipatory anxiety*, which we now know responds poorest to medication
- People with panic disorder may demonstrate abnormal *defence mechanisms*: the settings for panic may have *symbolic* value (e.g. childhood recollections of being lost in a supermarket), or the panics might represent *displacement* of other (less socially acceptable) emotions (e.g. anger)

CASE REVIEW

Interactions between physical and psychological disorders are complex (Box 2, p. 7): it would be unhelpful to begin this assessment convinced that Ishmail's presentation must be 'psychiatric'. Equally, failure to recognize what happens during panics will lead to months of needless A&E visits. The diagnosis of panic disorder was supported by symptoms here, but medical pathology was ruled out first. It has a lifetime prevalence of 2%. Ishmail presents with many typical features of panic disorder and its treatment:

- Sudden, highly somatic presentation in early adult life
- Physical disorders were carefully ruled out to reassure the patient and to avoid unnecessary medical investigations in future presentations
- Patients frequently attempt to reduce anxiety with self-medication *before* presenting for medical help
- First presentations are the best opportunity to counter the dysfunctional beliefs built up about symptoms (p. 13)
- Simple relaxation exercises (Box 4, p. 12) with consistent explanations will bring instant relief, reducing the demand for medication at first diagnosis
- As a rule, the use of medications alone is unhelpful in treating primary anxiety disorders
- CBT can be adapted to individuals' needs to reduce symptoms, with a strong possibility of complete remission – at least in the short term
- A large proportion of patients will continue (on occasion) to experience some anxiety symptoms throughout adult life, but they have excellent social outcomes

Some aspects of his case are *not* typical:

Continued

- His gender: at least twice as many women present with panic disorder
- He did not have comorbid depression, of itself predicting poorer outcome
- Ishmail's lifestyle did not contribute to the onset and severity of anxiety symptoms
- We can usually identify family histories of anxiety and/or childhood symptoms

References

Gabbard, G. (1994) *Psychodynamic Psychiatry in Clinical Practice*. American Psychiatric Press, Washington D.C.

Means-Christensen, A.J., Sherbourne, C.D., Roy-Byrne, P.P., Craske, M.G. & Stein, M.B. (2006) Using five questions to screen for five common mental disorders in primary care: diagnostic accuracy of the Anxiety and Depression Detector. *General Hospital Psychiatry* **28**, 108–118.

Williams, C. & Garland, A. (2002) A cognitive behavioural assessment model for use in everyday practice. *Advances in Psychiatric Treatment* **8**, 172–179.

Further reading

Fava, G.A. (1995) Long-term effects of behavioural treatment for panic disorder with agoraphobia. *British Journal of Psychiatry* **166**, 87–92.

Furukawa, T.A., Watanabe, N. & Churchill, R. (2006) Psychotherapy plus antidepressant for panic disorder with or without agoraphobia: systematic review. *British Journal of Psychiatry* **188**, 305–312.

Milrod, B., Busch, F.N., Leon, A.C., Shapiro, T., Aronson, A., Roiphe, J., *et al.* (2000) Open trial of psychodynamic psychotherapy for panic disorder: a pilot study. *American Journal of Psychiatry* **157**, 1878–1880.

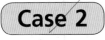 **Case 2** **A 47-year-old woman who lives in fear that God will punish her**

A Nigerian woman, Rebecca, who is a practising Christian, has been talking to her priest about her fears of eternal damnation. He says that she has become 'obsessed' with God's punishment and expresses concern that she has lost weight and does not appear to be sleeping. The priest advises her to see a doctor. When Rebecca comes to see you, she appears low in mood and tells you she is only here because her priest told her to come. Throughout your conversation she thumbs through a well-worn Bible in her hands.

Based on this information, what three groups of psychiatric symptoms do you think you will prioritize in taking her history, and how will you go about exploring them?

1 *Mood symptoms* (Table 13): how does she feel at present?

Begin with Rebecca's current concerns and then focus on systematic exploration of her mood. When and why did she start to feel like this? Open questions (e.g. 'How are you lately? Is something worrying you at the moment? Has anything bad happened to you recently?') should naturally lead you to specific questions about her mood within the context of recent events in her life.

If mood is low, establish if this varies during each day. Diurnal mood variation: is mood worse in the mornings but better as the day goes by? This strongly supports a diagnosis of depression.

The 10 areas of Table 13 are essential to exploring mood. Identify whether or not they are present, and record their duration.

> **KEY POINT**
>
> The assessment of mood is inherently subjective. Ask patients to benchmark their current mood in relation to their usual range of mood (1–10, with 1 worst, 10 best), explaining that most of us would rate our usual mood as 7/10. Chart their current episode of depression: '4/10 last month, but 2/10 today'. This is also a useful marker of progress (or otherwise) when you initiate treatment.

2 *Psychotic symptoms:* what are the nature of her spiritual concerns? Key questions to establish the delusional nature of any such beliefs need to explore *how* she came to believe them, the *certainty* with which she believes them and the *cultural context* of those beliefs (Box 3, p. 10).

Even though it is Rebecca's priest who has expressed concerns, he may be from a different cultural background to her. If possible speak to her partner, siblings or parents to determine whether her views are in keeping with her background and whether they are *out of character* for her.

If she appears to hold delusional beliefs, then systematically explore for *other delusions* and psychotic symptoms.

> **KEY POINT**
>
> If unfamiliar with your patient's religious or cultural background, you need to clarify both what is culturally normative within that community, and what is normal for them as an individual. Family and friends are an ideal starting point.

3 *Obsessional symptoms:* why is Rebecca so preoccupied with God's punishment? The priest described her as 'obsessed' but we do not know if his use of the term describes Rebecca's difficulties with any phenomenological accuracy. You need to establish the quality of this preoccupation:

○ Is Rebecca trying to resist thinking about this topic or is she choosing to dwell on it (i.e. is it 'ego syntonic', under her conscious control)? Remember, with obsessional thinking the individual attempts to resist the thoughts (at least at first) as they are experienced as intrusive and unwanted

○ If her thinking does appear to be obsessional, you need to establish whether there might also be evidence of compulsive behaviour to (temporarily) reduce the associated anxiety. For example, she might visit her church to excess and create her own prayer rituals, leave in a certain way, or wash her hands 12 times each hour (e.g. once for each apostle) to make the obsession go away (Box 36, p. 195).

KEY POINT

The public frequently use 'psychiatric' language to describe how they and others feel (e.g. *depressed, obsessed, paranoid, manic*). These terms do not correspond to precise psychiatric definitions. Do not be misled.

On direct questioning, Rebecca describes 2 months of low mood with loss of energy, lack of interest in things and poor sleep. She tells you she has been thinking a lot about how she is failing to be a good Christian and that she deserves God's punishment. She is not resisting these thoughts. These beliefs do not appear to be held with delusional intensity and she agrees her priest may be right; nevertheless, she has continued to lose sleep worrying about her faith.

Bearing in mind the above discussion about symptoms, if her beliefs about God's punishment are not delusional, how else might you describe these beliefs in your MSE?

1 *Non-pathological preoccupation* with culturally sanctioned ideas in keeping with her subculture. This is often the case with some religious beliefs or core family values. A person's religious beliefs could come under pressure during a crisis and her preoccupation could reflect these doubts. Collateral history will usually clarify this.

2 Depressive or anxious *ruminations*: preoccupation with past events is a cardinal feature of depression and fear of future events indicates anxiety. Her depression may be characterized by acute loss of self-esteem and hopeless-

Table 13 Mood symptoms (ICD-10).

Three major criteria	Depression	Mania and hypomania
Mood	↓ subjectively + objectively	↑ and/or irritable
Energy	↓ with fatigability	↑ subjective excess energy
Interest and pleasure	↓ with loss of emotional reactivity	↑ excessive interests, overtalkative
Seven other symptoms Concentration	↓ subjectively + objectively	↑ but objectively reduced, highly distractible
Appetite	↓ weight loss common	↑ or ↓ (forgets to eat)
Sleep	↓ for most depressed people, with initial insomnia and early morning wakening ↑ in minority of cases	↓ because of a reduction in the person's *subjective* need for sleep
Ideas of self-harm, suicide	Very common	Uncommon but always ask about these
Self-esteem	↓ worthlessness	↑ inflated self-confidence if extreme: grandiosity
Ideas of guilt	Common	Absent. Take more risks than usual for that person
Views of the future	Bleak, hopelessness: strong predictors of suicidality	Unrealistically positive

ness (Table 13), and she may be experiencing excessive ruminations about punishment in this context.

3 A *mood congruent belief* may have developed that her symptoms (low mood, poor sleep, loss of pleasure) are a punishment of some kind. As the belief does not have delusional intensity, she can be persuaded that there are other probable causes for how she feels, specifically, her preoccupations reflect her depression.

4 An *overvalued idea* (i.e. a comprehensible, deeply held idea that dominates an individual's life for long periods). This seems unlikely in Rebecca's case.

5 An *obsession*: again this seems less likely as Rebecca is not resisting these thoughts. However, obsessional thinking can occur in some people who become depressed, and this improves (as do 2–4) once the primary problem of low mood is successfully treated.

There is clearly overlap between these categories. It is helpful to record direct quotations of how she describes her experiences, as well as your own conclusions about her phenomenology. These are likely to change over time and with treatment.

You establish that Rebecca is depressed – what crucial piece of current information about her mental state are you missing?

Suicide risk: has she any suicidal ideas, plans or intent? Has she harmed herself? What has she done or planned?

> **KEY POINT**
>
> *Always* enquire about suicidal ideation. If you have not asked about suicide, you have not interviewed the patient properly.

You are satisfied from the history you have taken that this appears to be the first presentation of depression in a 47-year-old woman, not associated with any immediate risk of self-harm.

What do you need to do now?

Exclude an organic cause of low mood. There are many physical causes of depression (Table 14) and these may have additional physical signs. Look for physical evidence of depression and its possible consequences (weight loss, self-harm, effects of alcohol and substance misuse), as well as comorbid anxiety (Fig. 2, p. 37).

Carry out a **physical examination** in a systematic fashion.

What physical investigations will you recommend to screen for common disorders that could cause or contribute to Rebecca's depression?

Table 14 sets out the common disorders but you need a system to collate these with the common investigations. Start with common tests, easy to carry out and interpret:

• Full blood count (FBC) to rule out anaemia, and a high mean corpuscular volume (MCV) of alcohol misuse, hypothyroidism or folate deficiency
• Urea & electrolytes to rule out dehydration, renal impairment, electrolyte imbalances
• Random glucose may suggest diabetes
• Liver function tests to indicate alcohol misuse (typically, raised gamma glutamate transferase), systemic illness or previously unknown intravenous drug misuse (the vast majority of intravenous drug users are positive for antibodies to hepatitis C)

> **KEY POINT**
>
> Take the time to tell patients the results of the investigations when they are known. This reduces anxiety and prevents excessive preoccupation with physical health. An informed patient is less likely to present to another doctor requesting unnecessary tests in the future.

• Electrocardiogram to rule out ischaemic heart disease in this age group
• Chest X-ray is also useful in patients over 30 years, especially if there are physical findings – in a smoker there may be infection or cancer
• Urine drug screen for legal and illegal drugs
• Calcium and thyroid levels if indicated

| All Rebecca's investigations are normal.

With reference to Table 13, would you define her depression as mild, moderate or severe?

A **mild** depressive episode is diagnosed by two major criteria and two of the others (Table 13) being present for at least 2 weeks; the person usually continues normal social roles and *medication is rarely indicated*.

Table 14 Common organic causes of mood changes.

	Mostly cause depression	Mostly cause elevated mood
Alcohol and substances	Alcohol: the most common legal depressant drug	Alcohol may precipitate or be associated with mania
	Cannabis, cocaine, opioids: heroin, ecstasy	Amphetamines, cocaine, cannabis
Iatrogenic: prescription drugs	Benzodiazepines, sedatives (especially antipsychotics), chemotherapy drugs, β-blockers, digoxin, nifedipine, dopamine agonists, isotretinoin	Steroids, antidepressants, isoniazid, dopamine agonists, amphetamines, antimalarial agents
Neurology	CVA, Parkinson's disease, cerebral haemorrhage, head injury, multiple sclerosis	CVA, acute trauma or bleed affecting frontal lobe, HIV, multiple sclerosis; postpartum psychosis (1/3 organic cause)
Infectious disease	Glandular fever, hepatitis B or C, brucellosis	Malaria
Immunological	Rheumatoid arthritis	Systemic lupus erythematosus
Endocrine	Hypothyroidism, Cushing's syndrome, high calcium: hyperparathyroidism	Hyperthyroidism (also causes depression), Cushing's syndrome,
Cancer	Any cancer: primary or secondary	Unusual
Deficiency states	Pellagra, renal/liver failure	Unusual

CVA, cerebrovascular accident.

A **moderate** depressive episode is defined by at least two major criteria and at least three (preferably four) of the others present for at least 2 weeks. Many of these features will be present to a marked degree and the person has considerable difficulty with social, work and domestic activities.

In a **severe** depressive episode, all three major criteria and four or more out of seven others are present, some of which are of severe intensity. People with severe depression show considerable outward distress, unless psychomotor retardation (sometimes leading to depressive stupor) is a prominent feature. It is highly likely these patients will be actively thinking about suicide and they may even have made plans. If the symptoms are of rapid onset, the diagnosis can be justified before 2 weeks.

You must further classify a **severe** depressive episode as **with or without psychotic features**. By definition, if the low mood preceded delusions or hallucinations (typically both are mood congruent), this is severe depression. The presence of stupor also makes the diagnosis 'severe depressive episode with psychotic features'. Because severe depression tends to present relatively early in Western Society, many of these cases have not yet developed psychotic features.

Most people who develop a first depressive episode will have further episodes. The category **recurrent depressive disorder**, *current episode mild/moderate/severe* describes these. This category is used even if the person has experienced brief elevations of their mood immediately following a depressive episode and/or while taking antidepressant medication.

Rebecca has a moderate depressive episode. She reluctantly agrees with the diagnosis but says there must be a 'cause' of her condition, and knowing this is essential to getting better.

How would you respond to her concerns about what's wrong?

Before giving Rebecca information on depression, first enquire as to whether she has any ideas what has caused her to become depressed. This will help you tailor your answer to address her concerns.

Generally speaking, various factors are known to contribute to vulnerability to depressive illness:

- *Biological:* family history (i.e. genetic inheritance), some medications, current physical illness, alcohol misuse (Table 14)
- *Psychological:* history of loss – especially early parental loss; problems with attachments and relationships; childhood maltreatment
- *Social factors:* such as adverse life events, reduced social networks, poverty

For any individual who has become depressed, relevant factors can be grouped as **predisposing, precipitating** and **maintaining** factors for illness. Note that if any of these factors are present for Rebecca, we cannot be certain that they *caused* her depression: they are associations not causes. There is a complex interplay between someone's temperament, life experience and lack of 'protective factors' such as social support. With recent adverse life events (e.g. Rebecca being in conflict with members of her church), there are strong subjective components to individuals' responses. Was the life event an attack on subjective self-esteem (e.g. Rebecca's sense of her standing in that community)? Did it undermine a core role (e.g. her church activities and sense of purpose there)?

You might discuss a **stress vulnerability model** with her. She had a vulnerability to develop low mood in the context of multiple stressors. Often, a temporary physical illness (e.g. heavy cold, ankle sprain) can act as the 'last straw' in precipitating depression. Social stress also contributes to her difficulties – related anxiety symptoms reinforce her depressive symptoms, and vice versa.

> **KEY POINT**
>
> Depression rarely has a single, simple cause.

Although this is Rebecca's first diagnosed episode of depression, you identify long periods of low mood in her past history.

Does this fit your working diagnosis?

Yes. *Dysthymia* (i.e. persistent low mood that does not fulfil the criteria for moderate or severe depression) can coexist with superimposed periods of clear depressive illness. With dysthymia the person describes long periods over many years (usually beginning in adolescence and continuing throughout adult life) when their mood is below what they perceive it should be, and pleasure is impaired. When someone with dysthymia has a depres-

sive episode, this is sometimes described as 'double depression'.

What is your treatment plan for Rebecca?

Table 15 sets out three broad treatment approaches you need to consider. With the exception of the core principle of avoiding polypharmacy, none are mutually exclusive. The first four of each of biological, psychological and social interventions are commonly prescribed. General and antidepressant specific advice (Boxes 5 and 6, pp. 20 and 21) should be considered prior to choosing a particular medication (Table 7, p. 17).

Given her moderate depression, you refer her for cognitive behavioural therapy and prescribe an antidepressant. Two months later, Rebecca's depressive symptoms are unchanged.

What is most likely to account for this?

Despite current practice there is little evidence to start treatment with both medication and psychotherapy at the same time. Address apparent treatment failure by first revisiting Rebecca's treatment preferences.

Non-concordance with treatment (medication or psychotherapy) is the most common cause of poor treatment response. There may be specific difficulties with medication (e.g. cultural beliefs, fear of becoming addicted, side-effects, drug interactions, cost, inconvenience), or misunderstanding about how she needs to take it (e.g. some patients only take antidepressants on their 'bad days'). You must establish what dose she has been taking, and how often she takes it.

You have referred her to a psychologist – but *has she attended the sessions?* Does she have a problem either with the therapist or the therapy? Cognitive–behavioural therapy (CBT) does not suit everyone. Many patients want the space to speak about their past rather than examine their current difficulties in detail, and may resent the homework that CBT entails. If this is the case here, other psychological approaches to consider include a more focused approach such as problem solving treatment (PST) or psychodynamic (individual psychotherapy, cognitive analytic therapy). Most services have a waiting list for CBT longer than 2 months; PST can be carried out by nurses and doctors in primary care or specialist settings.

Rebecca has complied with treatment but remains depressed.

Table 15 The range of possible treatment approaches in depressive illness.

Biological	Psychological	Social
Improve physical health: exercise, diet, stop alcohol and caffeine, substance misuse	Problem solving treatment (see text)	Provide/improve housing, finances, networks, activities, etc.
Treat medical illness, change/stop depressant medication (Table 14)	CBT (see Cases 7 & 10)	Meet family: empower to use own resources and increase social contacts
Antidepressants: SSRIs, tricyclics, SNRIs as second line (Table 7)	Self-help strategies: see Williams (2001)	Vocational interventions, day hospital referral, occupational therapy
Change antidepressant if no response at 6 weeks	Family/couples therapy if relevant to the patient	Refer to community mental health team; consult Home Treatment Team
Additional strategies to consider if treatment refractory depression		
Lithium augmentation of her antidepressant: lithium at low doses (e.g. 400 mg/day) plus antidepressant	More intensive psychotherapy: interpersonal therapy, cognitive analytic therapy	Nidotherapy: manipulation of patient's environment (Tyrer & Bajaj 2005)
Addition of antipsychotic or thyroid hormone	Group therapy: supportive or psychodynamic	Consider hospital admission
Other specialist medication: see Maudsley Guidelines	Specialist psychoanalytic assessment	Support worker to help structure activities
Electroconvulsive therapy: in severely depressed or psychotic patients, this is *not* a last resort	Consider therapeutic community	Assess for supported accommodation

CBT, cognitive–behavioural therapy; SNRI, serotonin and noradrenaline reuptake inhibitor; SSRI, selective serotonin reuptake inhibitor.

Identify other possible causes for her non-response

1 Comorbidity with *anxiety* symptoms is common. Anxiety symptoms may be overlooked in favour of the more obvious features of depression. The treatment plan must now address these: if they are driving her depressive symptoms they may also have led to maladaptive behaviour obstructing recovery.
2 Cormorbidity with *alcohol* or substance misuse. Do not overlook this in women or in cultures not known for it. Many people use alcohol to alleviate low mood/anxiety in the short term where it can 'block out' problems.
3 Comorbidity with problematic *personality traits* or personality disorder.
4 *Misdiagnosis*: you have only assessed Rebecca once. She may have been guarded and reluctant to elaborate on what were delusional ideas, or obsessional symptoms. You might have missed physical illness.

> **KEY POINT**
>
> The best clinicians are able to challenge diagnoses, including their own.

5 Are there *maintaining factors* for her depression. How are things for Rebecca at home – with relationships, with finances? What is it like for her as a single Nigerian woman to live in the UK? There may be adverse events ongoing that she has not confided in you. Racist abuse and attacks on perceived 'asylum seekers' are very common in Western cities. What are her social supports?
6 *Treatment refractory depression* is usually defined as failure to respond to a therapeutic regimen of an antidepressant (specifically 150 mg of a tricyclic or SSRI equivalent) after 6 weeks. There is currently no agreed approach here. Consider:

○ Alternative approaches to medication (Table 15)

○ Consult prescribing guidelines (e.g. Maudsley Guidelines). There are no guarantees that an alternative antidepressant will improve her symptoms, but it is certainly worth trying this if there has been no response. Choose one from a different class: there is little gain from replacing one SSRI with another

○ Discussion of the case with a colleague may be valuable. Her therapy may need to be modified and made more culturally sensitive. Rebecca coped very well up until now, and is likely to have developed a good coping style of her own in the past. Her therapist should collaborate with her to utilize this to maximum effect

What is Rebecca's 1-year prognosis at this point?

We would have expected some positive responses by now if her depression had a good prognosis. Social factors may be the key here. She may have become isolated and lack meaningful activity in her life. Are there possible environmental changes (nidotherapy, p. 27) that would make a difference here? Her prognosis is guarded, but is likely to be better with the right treatment (Table 15) and if her existing support network improves.

> Rebecca recovers 4 months' later. She expresses a new confidence in herself and has moved in with a close friend whose husband died some years ago. They both had wanted children but it has not been possible. Rebecca has applied to be a foster carer, with her friend, but the authorities raised some concerns about her mental health.

What is Rebecca's 10-year prognosis at this point?

Over two-thirds of people with an episode of moderate depression will experience a recurrence of depression symptoms over the following 10 years. The positive aspects are that they can recognize the problem earlier and will have a strong indication of the measures that improve it. There is good evidence for the role of prophylactic antidepressant use in people with frequent episodes. There is no contraindication in Rebecca's history preventing her from sharing the role of foster parent.

CASE REVIEW

One in four people will become depressed at some stage in their lives. It is the most common psychiatric disorder encountered by the GP. Unless these patients have experienced depression before – in themselves or others – they may not volunteer depressive symptoms (Table 13). Like Rebecca, they present because *something else* happens, usually a change in social functioning. It takes time to tease out the presenting complaints (see the five non-psychotic explanations above). Of all patients with depressive disorders attending GPs, the diagnosis is missed 50% of the time and, of those diagnosed, adequate treatment is initiated in only 50%. Here, the following lessons can be drawn:

- Careful open, then closed questioning (Table 13) confirmed depression
- At the first assessment, four major areas of concern were explored:
  - ○ risks of suicide and self-harm
  - ○ an underlying medical illness that could cause or exacerbate low mood
  - ○ possible psychotic symptoms that would persist with antidepressant treatment alone
  - ○ comorbid psychiatric conditions of anxiety and substance misuse
- Diagnosing low mood as, for example, moderate depression is useful in decision-making about treatments (Table 15) and likely prognosis
- Even a common disorder such as depression represents a challenge when patients or their families ask what 'caused it'. In the same way as we speak about heart disease, it is best to identify a number of 'factors' (family history + childhood experiences + recent stressors) to avoid blaming the individual or others
- Rebecca's presentation raised cultural and religious issues, which required sensitive exploration
- Unusually, her depression did not lift in the first 2 months with the dual prescription of cognitive therapy and antidepressant. Careful follow-up identified treatment nonresponse, and would have uncovered deterioration in mental state. She might have begun to consider suicide

Continued

- Open discussion with collaborative decision-making at the start of the treatment process is the best way to maximize response to treatment. Your patients may dislike the CBT 'here and now' approach and prefer other therapies. Treatment options change over time
- It is best to conceptualize depression as a chronic medical illness. It is calculated that by 2020 it will be the second most common cause of disability worldwide.

A parallel, more positive approach identifies factors that *prevent* depression in a given individual (e.g. their resilience, coping skills, use of social networks, religious beliefs, lifestyle, ability to take breaks/relieve stress). When these are overwhelmed, a pattern of low mood can emerge. If these factors can be improved, any episode of depression will be of shorter duration and less severe.

References

Tyrer, P. & Bajaj, P. (2005) Nidotherapy: making the environment do the therapeutic work. *Advances in Psychiatric Treatment* **11**, 232–238.

Williams, C. (2001) Use of written cognitive–behavioural therapy self-help materials to treat depression. *Advances in Psychiatric Treatment* **7**, 233–240.

Further reading

Mynors-Wallis, L. (2001) Problem solving treatment in general psychiatric practice. *Advances in Psychiatric Treatment* **7**, 417–425.

Mynors-Wallis, L., Gath, D.H., Day, A. & Baker, F. (2006) Randomised controlled trial of problem solving treatment, antidepressant medication and combined treatment for major depression in primary care. *BMJ* **306**, 26–30.

Case 3 An 18-year-old college drop-out gets an eviction order from his parents

Robbie repeated his A-levels to gain a place at a business school. Until the age of 16, he had always been top of his class with lots of other interests but now, aged 18, he struggles at university, attending twice monthly. Quite unlike him, he has made no new friends there and lost touch with former friends. His parents say they never see him; he sleeps by day and spends his nights in his room thrashing about, sometimes laughing or shouting. His 17-year-old brother does not speak to him anymore. His mother has decided she has had enough and she has told him he has to move out or 'get some help'. She brings him to see you, but Robbie tells you everything is fine. He is unshaven and unwashed, wearing dirty clothes.

Before enquiring about specific psychiatric symptoms, how will you approach Robbie?

With an open mind. You might think about his bizarre nocturnal habits, but beware of imposing a diagnosis where there are many non-psychiatric possibilities. Outline what he would like to talk about first, then start with the more neutral topic of university before moving on to address his mother's concerns and any conflict between them.

Explain you would be interested in understanding what has been happening. Try to clarify whether his difficulties at university relate to events there (bullying, relationships, choice of subjects, deadlines, exams) or to factors within Robbie (anger, protest against his parents, medical illness, psychological problems). For example, discuss whether there is anything or anyone that stops him from going. Was it his choice to study business? Why did he lose interest?

Explore relationships with parents and his brother: where does he come in the family? How does he get on with each member of the household? Establish whether there are current difficulties around parental discord or illness, sibling rivalry, financial pressures or other recent

stressors? Ask what he argues about with his parents. Are his rows with his mother different than those with his father? (The details above record that his mother is the one who says she wants him to go.) Why does he think she wants him to leave?

> **KEY POINT**
>
> Establishing family, personal and social history early can confirm a non-psychiatric diagnosis. These details also reveal predisposing, precipitating and maintaining factors in psychiatric conditions.

Robbie gives little detail about his family or university. He makes no spontaneous comments and his answers to your direct questions are brief and uninformative.

What specific psychiatric symptoms will you now look for?
Mood symptoms

When a teenager or adult loses interest in friends/family and studying/work, depression is the most common explanation, so consider this first. Begin with open general questions: 'How have you been feeling?' Move on to specific enquiry (Table 13, p. 45).

Psychotic symptoms

Principally, delusions and hallucinations. Open questions:

- Has anything unusual happened to him lately?
- Is there something different about how people react to him?
- Does he feel something funny is going on?
- Does he think he has any psychological difficulties?

Robbie confirms that he hears people speaking about him when alone in his room at night.

What are the possibilities you need to explore to explain his 'voices'?

Several possibilities arise:

• They are *real*: his room is noisy from inside his home (parents arguing), his neighbours' house or from the street outside. These seem unlikely here

• *Sleep-related hallucinations*: hypnogogic (going to sleep) and hypnopompic (waking up) hallucinations are common in the general population and are *not* associated with psychiatric illness

• *Auditory hallucinations*: if this is the case, he will hear the voices as coming from outside his head, in the absence of any external auditory stimulus (seeing or hearing things when there *is* a stimulus is an illusion). The voices will sound real to him. Hallucinations can be caused by intoxicants, organic states and psychiatric illness. As with all psychiatric diagnoses, you must rule out physical illness before you conclude a patient's hallucinations are a result of functional illness (Table 16).

Robbie says little but confides in you that he is afraid to leave his house for fear 'certain people' will interfere with him. He is orientated in place and time. He denies low mood. His mother confirms he 'has a thing about' MI5.

What do you think?

Several possibilities arise:

• His reasons for staying at home are *realistic*: he lives in an area of high crime, has been bullied, threatened, acquired bad (often drug) debts, etc.

• He has developed a *phobia* – either generalized phobia (agoraphobia) or a social phobia (Table 11, p. 38)

• He has a *persecutory delusion* that people want to do him physical harm and are plotting to do so. Even if there have been assaults locally, he may still argue that he will be attacked by 'you know who' – in an irrational way with faulty reasoning. His delusions may be well-formed (a specific group of people will harm him) or diffuse (he cannot be certain who 'they' are)

Table 16 Physical causes of hallucinations: 'organic hallucinosis'.

Cause/system	Younger adults	Older people
Alcohol and substances	Alcohol common Cannabis, cocaine, ecstasy, amphetamines, illegal benzodiazepines	Alcohol very common: intoxication, withdrawal, Korsakoff's, etc. Ask about illegal drugs
Iatrogenic: prescription drugs	Steroids, antimalarial drugs, aspirin intoxication, isoniazid	Benzodiazepines, anticholinergics, non-steroidal anti-inflammatory drugs, steroids, dopamine agonists, digoxin
Neurological	Epilepsy, especially temporal lobe epilepsy, migraine, head injury, primary tumours, aneurysm, multiple sclerosis, subarachnoid haemorrhage, Huntington's disease, Wilson's disease	Delirium and dementia: cerebrovascular disease, head injury and other traumas, space-occupying lesions: tumours (usually secondaries), abscess, cerebral haemorrhage (especially subdural haematoma), normal pressure hydrocephalus
Infectious disease	HIV, syphilis, encephalitis, mumps, parasites, septicaemia	*Any* infection may precipitate acute confusion/hallucinations in vulnerable older people
Immunological	Systemic lupus erythematosus (SLE)	Temporal arteritis
Endocrine	Thyrotoxicosis, Addison's disease, hyperparathyroidism	Thyrotoxicosis, Cushing's syndrome, hypercalcaemia
Metabolic	Electrolyte abnormalities, porphyria	Electrolytes, malnutrition
Cardiorespiratory	(Unusual in young people) pneumonia, hypoxic encephalopathy	Hypoxia and any cause of acute confusion: cardiac failure, pleural effusion, pulmonary embolism, etc.
Deficiency states	Wernicke's encephalopathy (thiamine deficiency: common in alcoholism)	Wernicke's encephalopathy, B_{12}, folate, nicotinic acid deficiencies, hypothermia

---

KEY POINT

Ask what patients understand about the 'cause' of their psychotic experiences and how they might try to fix that cause. Do they need to obey their voices? Do they have an urge to do something about their beliefs? Risks are increased when patients act on delusions or hallucinations.

You discover Robbie has paranoid persecutory delusions that he is being secretly filmed for reality TV, and he has had auditory hallucinations for several months.

What other psychotic symptoms might he have?

These are positive and negative (Box 9). You cannot rule out negative symptoms without a reliable collateral history.

KEY POINT

The first presentation of psychosis is the best opportunity to establish the extent of symptoms – and document them clearly – before they are treated or partially treated. Patients learn that the more they admit to unusual experiences, the more their medication gets increased.

Robbie becomes suspicious about your questions and is convinced that you are not a doctor but work with the 'others' trying to monitor and harm him. He is shifting around in his seat and looking out the window frequently. He refuses to sit down, and reluctantly agrees to wait outside the room while you continue to talk to his mother. By this point you have established psychotic symptoms but lack his background history.

What additional information could you gain from a collateral history here?

Because he is currently unwell, he may conceal key historical information, be confused about detail or have formed strong beliefs as to what caused his difficulties. His mother could provide information about:
• Birth history: low birth weight (<2.5 kg) is an independent predictor of later life psychosis, and there are weak associations between obstetric complications and schizophrenia
• Family history of any psychiatric illness or suicide
• Developmental history: delayed milestones (Table 2, p. 4) suggest non-psychotic illness

---

Box 9 Diagnosis of schizophrenia (ICD-10)

At least one clear symptom, or two or more 'less clear' positive symptoms, or two or more negative symptoms must be present for at least one month.

Positive psychotic symptoms
'Clear' symptoms
• *Delusions* that are culturally inappropriate and completely impossible, e.g. being able to control the weather
• *Hallucinatory voices* giving a running commentary on the patient's actions or discussing the patient amongst themselves, or voices coming from another part of the body
• *Delusions of reference:* beliefs that random external events in his/her life or wider society (details from a news item, song or television programme) relate in a special way to him/her
• *Delusions of thought interference:* others can hear, read, insert or steal their thoughts
• *Passivity phenomena:* beliefs and/or perceptions that others are able to control their will, limb movements, bodily functions, or feelings
• *Thought echo:* hearing one's own thoughts spoken aloud

'Less clear' symptoms
• *Hallucinations* other than the above, when accompanied by delusions or persistent overvalued ideas. In the paranoid subtype of schizophrenia these are the prominent symptoms
• *Thought disorder:* breaks in the train of thought (thought block), overinclusive and concrete thinking, neologisms
• *Catatonic behaviour* (p. 5)

Negative psychotic symptoms (by definition, these are 'less clear' symptoms)
• *Apathy* (disinterest) manifest as blunted affect
• *Flat affect:* emotional withdrawal
• *Odd or incongruous affect* (e.g. smiles when recounting sad events, and vice versa)
• *Lack of attention* to appearance or personal hygiene
• *Poor rapport:* reduced verbal and non-verbal communication (e.g. eye contact)
• *Lack of spontaneity* and flow of conversation
• Difficulties in *abstract thinking* (e.g. explaining proverbs or common sayings)

- Alcohol and drug use: many teenagers conceal these from parents
- Medical history: this is important for physical causes of his symptoms (Table 16) and to identify potential contraindications (cardiac conditions, diabetes, epilepsy) to antipsychotic medication (Table 8, p. 18)
- Medication use: ask about legal (prescribed), over-the-counter, and illegal drugs
- Evidence for a decline in social functioning (prodrome; see Case 11)
- The sequence of events from age 16 to now. Did paranoid symptoms precede his arguments? Were stressful life events (relationship break-ups, deaths in the family, failures at examinations) a precipitant or an effect of psychotic illness?
- Employment history: has he lost any jobs as a result of his behaviour?
- Is his mother's decision to evict him from the family home final? Would reduction in his distress, alongside improvement in his sleep and behaviour change her decision? Where else could he stay other than hospital or hostel admission?

Using the information you have about Robbie, summarize his mental state examination

- *Appearance and behaviour:* unshaven, shabbily dressed with poor personal hygiene; poor rapport and engagement in the interview; lack of spontaneity; restless and agitated; he appeared distracted by events outside for reasons unknown
- *Speech:* normal rate, tone and volume. His speech is minimal but coherent with no evidence of *thought disorder*
- *Mood: subjectively* he declined to describe his mood; *objectively* he appeared tense and anxious. We have not yet asked about *suicidality*. Suicidality is common in the context of overwhelming psychotic experiences
- *Thoughts:* evidence of systematized persecutory delusions about reality TV and delusions concerning surveillance. These are continuing to evolve and have now included your interview process
- *Perception:* third person auditory hallucinations – people speaking about him when alone in his room
- *Cognition:* orientated in time, place and person. Formal testing not performed
- *Insight:* not assessed as he terminated the interview. However, likely to be poor; he seems convinced that his psychotic experiences are real. He may agree that certain aspects of his presentation might be psychological

> **KEY POINT**
>
> Pseudohallucinations lack a recognized external stimulus. Auditory pseudohallucinations, noises or voices are interpreted as coming from within the person's own head – although some patients become deluded they have an implanted transmitter in their brain. They are a common symptom in psychosis.

You are confident by this point that Robbie's history and mental state examination confirm first episode psychosis, untreated for 7 months.

What risks would you think about here?

- *Suicide and self-harm:* people with psychosis rarely volunteer that they have suicidal thoughts. As their insight increases, they are at a higher risk of suicide. We know that 10% of people with schizophrenia will take their own lives over the course of their psychosis, most doing so in the first 5 years of their illness
- *Self-care and physical health:* Robbie's self-care and personal hygiene is clearly poor. His diet and physical health are also likely to be poor
- *Harm from others:* Robbie is likely to attract attention in public. He is hallucinating, has paranoid delusions and negative symptoms, with little insight. He may be victimized, bullied or assaulted by strangers who meet him and assume he is on drugs. Remember that he has already come into conflict with his family, and we have not explored his brother's grievances with him
- *Exploitation by others:* by strangers, friends, even his family. He may already have accrued debts (e.g. from drug dealers)
- *Harm to others:* the majority of people with psychosis pose risks only to themselves, but explore sensitively this possibility

Robbie cannot tolerate waiting outside the room and comes back in, suspicious about what you have been discussing with his mother. He sits but appears restless.

What will you ask him?

Robbie is unlikely to answer many more questions. Get the most important information you need. Ask him about *immediate risk to self and others*. Do so in a series of stepped questions, becoming more specific about ideas and plans as you go along:

'What's been happening to you sounds very stressful. Have you got to the point where you felt you couldn't cope any more? Have you had any thoughts that you couldn't go on? Have you reached the stage of thinking about taking your own life?' If the answers to these questions are positive, you need to pursue this. What has he thought of doing? Does he know how he would do it? What has stopped him doing it so far, what might stop him now?

'If I've understood you right, Robbie, you believe these people you mentioned want to harm you. It sounds as if you have serious concerns about your safety. Do you know who any of them are? Would you know where to find them? Have you got to the point you feel you need to take matters into your own hands to protect yourself?'

> **KEY POINT**
>
> You must ask about risk. Patients who are psychotic are often guarded and suspicious. Be patient, but follow through this line of questioning if there is any possibility that patients have ideas of harming themselves or (less commonly) others.

Robbie denies any thoughts of self-harm. Although he insists the 'TV people' are involved in a plot against him, he has never actually seen any of these people and does not know exactly who they are. He denies any plans to 'take matters into his own hands'.

What is the most important physical investigation you need to do now?

Urine (or salivary) drug screen. By now, this is unlikely to be simply a drug-induced psychosis, although drugs may have been involved in precipitating the episode. These symptoms are of a duration and severity such that drug misuse has unmasked and augmented them rather than acted as a primary cause. It is common for people with psychotic symptoms to use alcohol and/or cannabis to reduce their anxiety symptoms (i.e. self-medication). Whatever the role of cannabis and other illegal drugs, the challenge is to work with Robbie to reduce and stop their use.

> **KEY POINT**
>
> The only preventable risk factor for schizophrenia is cannabis use. Children who are exposed to cannabis at age 14 or younger are at the highest risk of developing psychotic symptoms in adolescence and early adulthood.

Robbie refuses to give a urine sample. He says he smokes cannabis occasionally. You explain to him and his mother that Robbie is unwell with a psychotic illness and that he needs medication. Robbie's mother understands your explanation, but Robbie repeats over and over that 'he's perfectly alright', and does not appear able to take in the information you are giving him. He suddenly decides he is leaving. You need to formulate a plan.

What are you thinking about at this point?

You have confirmed the diagnosis as *psychosis*, identified some risks and are assessing him in a crisis, when tempers are already running high at home.

It is likely that with poor insight, any continued cannabis use and refusal of treatment, his condition will get worse. The possibility that he will agree to *home or community treatment* appears slim, but you should make these offers. You may wish to discuss his case with an Early Intervention psychosis team.

If he continues to refuse treatment, he will need to be *assessed for compulsory treatment* in hospital under mental health legislation. So far, there are no acute risks identified but you will need to act within days of this first meeting. In England and Wales, he can be placed under Section 2 of the Mental Health Act (1983) for a 28-day period of assessment and/or psychiatric treatment. Two independent medical practitioners and an approved social worker must assess him and agree a course of action. The grounds here are that he is suffering from a mental disorder of a nature and degree that warrants his detention in hospital, and that he be detained in the interests of his own health.

While follow-up and either community treatment or hospital admission under section (more likely here) are being arranged, Robbie and his mother are going back home for the time being. You need to reassure his mother and give her emergency numbers in case matters deteriorate at home. Remind them that if things become intolerable over the next day or so then Robbie can always go (or be taken) to A&E for assessment and admission via psychiatric liaison there.

From what you now know about this presentation, list the possible final diagnoses

1 *Schizophrenia:* he has been hallucinating for some time and has paranoid delusions with negative symptoms (Box 9, p. 54)

2 *Psychotic disorder resulting from substance misuse* (cannabis): this remains a possibility here. There must be a clear temporal relationship between drug misuse and psychotic symptoms, and they must resolve fully between 1 and 6 months following total cessation of substances. Early Intervention psychosis teams take on 'drug-induced' cases for longer term follow-up

3 *Organic delusional disorder:* this may be diagnosed if there is evidence of cerebral disease/dysfunction or systemic physical disease known to be associated with psychosis (Table 16, p. 53)

4 *Schizoaffective disorder* (episodes must show features of mood *and* schizophrenia disorders): less likely given the absence of mood symptoms

Less likely diagnoses for consideration:

1 *Bipolar affective disorder:* presenting with either a manic or depressed episode. Robbie's delusions and third person hallucinations are more common in schizophrenia and a bipolar diagnosis is unlikely without mood symptoms

2 *Schizotypal personality disorder:* rarely made as a primary diagnosis. There must be typical features for at least 2 years of some of the following: eccentric behaviour, odd beliefs or paranoid ideas (*not* delusions), unusual perceptual experiences (*not* hallucinations), vague thinking and odd speech (*not* thought disorder) and short-lived 'quasi-psychotic' experiences

3 *Persistent delusional disorder:* this category comprises patients for whom delusions are prominent (to the exclusion of other psychopathology) and of long duration. Persistent auditory hallucinations (as here), delusions of thought interference/control and organic brain disease (Table 16) are all incompatible with this diagnosis

4 *Acute and transient psychotic disorders:* these are of less than 1 month duration only, and there is usually a stressful precipitant. By definition, the symptoms resolve within 3 months – Robbie has been unwell for too long

5 *Autism and Asperger's syndrome:* unlikely here in the absence of developmental disorder and the presence of a clear change from a 'normal' premorbid outgoing personality to his current presentation

A section assessment is arranged for Robbie but (to your surprise) Robbie engages with community home treatment,

and hospital admission is averted. His psychiatric nurse establishes a good relationship with him and persuades him to take medication to improve his sleep, even if he disagrees he needs it. She also persuades him to stop using cannabis. With daily monitoring of symptoms and medication, and family support, he gradually becomes well over the next 6 weeks, and is given a diagnosis of drug-induced psychosis. Despite abstaining from cannabis and good concordance to medication (Table 8, p. 18), Robbie has a second psychotic episode 10 months later and the diagnosis of schizophrenia is confirmed.

KEY POINT

Psychiatric diagnoses can change with hindsight, over time as an individual's illness evolves and with response to treatment. Here, the initial diagnosis of drug-induced psychosis was not 'wrong' as such: schizophrenia should be diagnosed only when the evidence is clear.

What positive and negative factors would you consider in thinking about Robbie's longer-term prognosis?

These are set out in Table 17. Robbie has at least five favourable and three unfavourable factors.

Even with the best treatments (medication, cognitive–behavioural therapy, family interventions, psychoeducation and vocational interventions), up to two-thirds of people with a first episode of psychosis will have a second. In predicting prognosis following remission, highlight positive factors (Table 17) without giving false hope.

After a first episode of psychosis, the guidance states people who are fully recovered, cannabis-free and lack a family history of psychosis should continue with medication for at least a year *after* they become well. You need to leave the possibility open that the illness could recur and they may need to take medication for longer. This needs to be discussed over time.

Robbie has had a second episode despite favourable factors and changed behaviours. He should stay on medication for longer and other factors (e.g. family, housing, cognitive formulation, vocational rehabilitation, relapse prevention) require closer scrutiny.

Table 17 Factors associated with good and bad outcomes in schizophrenia.

Factor+	Better prognosis	Worse prognosis
Person	Female	Male
	Normal premorbid personality	Poor premorbid adjustment
	High premorbid intelligence	Low premorbid intelligence
Illness onset	Older age of onset: normal personality development	Younger age of onset
	Short illness with precipitant	No precipitant, insidious onset
Family	No family history of psychosis	Family history of psychosis
	Good family support	Poor/no family support
Comorbidity	No substance misuse	Ongoing substance misuse
	Affective component	No affective component
Response to illness	Good response to initial treatment	Poor response to initial treatment
	Takes medication	Refuses medication
	Better insight	Poor insight
Self-harm	No thoughts of self-harm	Suicidal ideation prominent early in the illness

CASE REVIEW

Robbie is far less forthcoming than previous cases. Collateral history was invaluable as an opportunity to obtain core answers.

Schizophrenia has the same prevalence in men and women, about 1%. Men tend to present in the mid to late teens, women slightly later.

Unless the symptoms are intolerable (Box 9), it is the relative, not the patient, who initiates assessment. Robbie's story is a typical tale of delayed presentation with untreated paranoia, established negative symptoms, lost friends and opportunities, lack of insight, treatment refusal and cannabis use. He declined to give a urine sample to establish drug use. If cannabis tests are positive, but denied by the patient, this has negative implications for future adherence and prognosis.

It was a good outcome to engage him with home treatment, removing the need for an emergency mental health act assessment, discussed later. Coercive treatment tends to initiate cycles of poor engagement.

Quick responses to medication tend to attract the (more optimistic) diagnosis of drug-induced psychosis – the assumption is that the cannabis-free patient will remain well. Here, schizophrenia was the more likely diagnosis in that cannabis *at the very least* unmasked an underlying disorder.

Even if he had not relapsed, Robbie should stay under the care of an Early Intervention psychosis team and receive the full range of treatments (p. 57).

Further reading

Byrne, P. (2007) Managing the acute psychotic episode. *BMJ* **334**, 686–692.

Spencer, E., Birchwood, M. & McGovern, D. (2001) Management of first episode psychosis. *Advances in Psychiatric Treatment* **7**, 133–140.

Case 4 An 18-year-old trainee chef who cannot go to work

Jenny, an 18-year-old trainee chef, is brought in by her flatmates. About 2 months ago, following some changes at work, she started to miss work several evenings each week and has now stopped socializing. She tells you she does not wish to be seen in public because she hates people looking at her.

What are the main diagnostic categories you would explore to establish a diagnosis?

Use the hierarchy of psychiatric disorders to structure to your thinking (Fig. 1, p. 7):

Organic illness seems unlikely here but – as with all presentations – its possibility justifies a systemic review. Think too about *substance and alcohol misuse*; both are commonly misused in the context of the late hours and easy access of the entertainment industry (e.g. restaurants, bars, clubs, theatres).

The two major psychiatric categories are *affective* and *psychotic disorders*:

• Psychotic illness must be ruled out first. She may hold pathological beliefs about her appearance either as an *overvalued idea* (non-delusional dysmorphophobia/body dysmorphic disorder) or with *delusional intensity* (i.e. delusional dysmorphophobia). You need to examine the form and content of her beliefs (Box 3, p. 10)

• A depressive episode may have been precipitated by recent 'changes at work' or other stressors; she may have developed an excessive (negative) preoccupation with how people view her in the context of low mood – check for depressive symptoms (Table 13, p. 45). It seems unlikely that these details represent a manic or hypomanic episode

After these, consider the possibility of an *anxiety disorder*. The behaviour appears new and sounds phobic in nature: this is a promising area to explore. Enquire about excessive preoccupation with her appearance related to her weight, and symptoms of food restriction or fear of becoming fat.

In the absence of any support for the above categories, consider the possibility of *personality difficulties*. Specific clusters of personality traits (e.g. anxious avoidant or paranoid) may support a personality disorder diagnosis. These must have been present from an early age, at the very least from puberty, and a collateral history is essential.

Jenny is physically well, not abusing substances and she does not appear to have a depressive illness. There is no evidence of any delusional beliefs or preoccupations with her weight. Before this problem started she seems to have been living an unremarkable life with normal relationships. She tells you her restaurant was redesigned recently to expose the work of kitchen staff to the gaze of its diners. She experiences distress every time she works there: she hates being looked at by strangers while she works. She cannot explain why. Her workmates have tried to reassure her by telling her to ignore it but she says she cannot.

What areas will you ask about in relation to this presenting complaint?

• Explore both *cognitive and somatic anxiety symptoms* (Fig. 2, p. 37), noting in particular how 'serious' she believes them to be. Take a full history of anxiety symptoms prior to this episode. Has she also experienced panic attacks? Screen for other anxiety disorders and recent traumas (Table 12, p. 39). Identify physical symptoms that reinforce her phobia: blushing, tremor, sweating, breathing, etc.

• Establish the relationship between exposure to the stimulus (that kitchen) and her symptoms. Do her symptoms reduce when she leaves?

• What behavioural responses has she developed? She has had these difficulties for 2 months and will have developed (maladaptive) strategies such as avoidance (a 'safety behaviour'), or alcohol use to temporarily reduce her distress

• Has this phobia generalized to other situations? If so, are these episodes driven by the same physical cues? Clarify why she no longer socializes
• Establish which subcategory of phobia she has: specific phobia (i.e. just to this work situation), agoraphobia ('fear of the marketplace') or social phobia

Jenny confirms that her fear of being scrutinized by others extends now to all social situations, explaining her reluctance to leave the house even to socialize.

What three essential diagnostic features are required to make a definitive (ICD-10) diagnosis of a phobia?

1 The psychological, behavioural or autonomic symptoms must be primarily manifestations of anxiety and not secondary to other symptoms such as delusions or obsessional thoughts
2 The anxiety must be restricted to or predominate in particular situations:
  ○ specific phobias ← the presence of the object or situation
  ○ agoraphobia ← crowds, public places
  ○ social phobia ← social situations
3 Avoidance of the stimulus must be a prominent feature

KEY POINT

Some professionals are sceptical about the 'new' diagnosis of social phobia (known also as 'social anxiety disorder') because of concerns that it may be used to medicalize shyness and/or to justify unnecessary prescription of psychoactive drugs.

What findings in Jenny's personal and social history would support the diagnosis of social phobia?

The following factors are relevant to *any* anxiety disorder:
• *Family history* of depression or anxiety disorder. What are her parents and siblings like? Are there familial anxiety traits? A family history of sudden death may also be relevant: as always, ask about familial suicide (as a risk factor for future suicidal behaviour), but enquire too about sudden unexplained death – she may have linked her distressing physical symptoms to a relative's demise

• *Other separations* (Box 8, p. 42). Look for prolonged parental separations in childhood, evidence for childhood anxiety traits, childhood medical illnesses and the way she coped with these. This may also be the time to enquire sensitively about childhood trauma
• *Birth and developmental history:* developmental delay suggests diagnoses other than a primary anxiety disorder
• *School history:* school refusal or delinquency, frequent changes of school, bullying, peer relationships (ease of making friendships, duration, quality)
• *Employment history:* missed training or lost jobs as a result of anxiety or avoidance behaviour
• *Medical history:* organic contributants to symptoms, contraindications to medication (cardiac conditions, pregnancy or risk of pregnancy, epilepsy)
• *Medication use:* legal (prescribed), bought over-the-counter/internet, and illegal drugs
• *Alcohol and substance use:* including caffeine and nicotine
• *Social circumstances and activities:* including exercise (recall Case 1 for lifestyle advice)
• *Relationships:* past and current. Are there links between these and current symptoms? Has she had relationships at work?
• *Premorbid personality:* long-standing traits of avoidance, shyness, self-consciousness. While looking for evidence for the onset of a discrete anxiety disorder (here, social phobia), we also need to consider whether (a) there is evidence of a personality disorder (e.g. an enduring anxious avoidant personality style), and (b) whether this would in itself be sufficient to explain her symptoms and behaviour

Examination of Jenny's premorbid personality did not reveal anxiety traits. You are satisfied she fulfils the criteria for a social phobia.

Would you expect her social phobia to be evident on mental state examination?

Not necessarily. Mental state examination (MSE) is a 'here and now' description at interview. Her symptoms are **situational** and may not be evident in the interview with you now. She might not appear anxious during your discussion: many people with phobias have instituted radical changes in their behaviour (essentially, avoidance of all anxiety-provoking stimuli/situations). They may have eliminated all outward signs of anxiety.

For some people with social phobia, medical scrutiny will be an anxiety-provoking situation and these patients will have objective signs, subjective symptoms and possible cognitive distortions to document in your MSE.

> **KEY POINT**
>
> In phobic anxiety disorders, diagnosis is usually established by history alone.

Jenny finds discussing her problem embarrassing. You need to reassure her you are familiar with this kind of problem and the thought processes that can underline it. She will need some empathic prompting by you to help her disclose her thought processes.

What sort of negative automatic thoughts might you explore with Jenny as possible triggers to her social phobia in the work context?

Fear of negative evaluation that people (customers, colleagues, employers) may see her in the kitchen at work and judge her performance to be inadequate, with her fearing humiliation and embarrassment as a result. You might ask Jenny closed questions 'Do you think things like "I'm no good. I am a useless cook. I will never be a chef"?' She may also have constructed worst case scenarios around failures to perform or potential hazards in the kitchen. 'Customers will see how bad I am. I will be exposed to my boss as no good. I will look totally useless at my job.'

In *social phobia*, automatic thoughts anticipating the negative evaluation of others and the associated shame and humiliation are *worse* when in the presence of *non-peers* – people perceived to be of higher status or importance. In this case, Jenny was coping well with the stressful environment of a busy kitchen, until people other than workmates added to it. Other common performance situations are public speaking ('stage fright'), eating in public and dating.

> Jenny's flatmate confides in you that Jenny collapsed at a party recently, much to her humiliation. Jenny admits that she needs to be drunk at parties and drinks on her own.

Does Jenny's misuse of alcohol surprise you?

It should not. Up to one-quarter of people with social anxiety misuse alcohol, and vice versa. People with any anxiety disorder have twice the prevalence of substance misuse, and the anxiety frequently precedes misuse as 'self-medication'. In Jenny's case, it is not surprising that she turned to a commonly available, cheap and socially acceptable sedative, especially in the context of working late hours in a restaurant. She may have been drinking at and before work. Alcohol is commonly used in preparing for social events – 'Dutch courage' – as it numbs some of the cognitive and somatic manifestations of anxiety. Ironically, for those with social phobia – who overestimate their mistakes and others' negative evaluation when sober – excessive alcohol consumption makes them *less* aware of their errors, and predisposes them to make *more*.

While Jenny may be using alcohol for temporary relief from the symptoms of anxiety, alcohol is likely to be making her anxiety worse overall and partly explains the degree of her current disability. There is evidence that excessive alcohol ingestion interferes with serotonin, noradrenaline and γ-aminobutyric acid (GABA) receptors and these interactions cause increases in both short-term 'rebound' and chronic anxiety.

How will you make links in Jenny's mind between her drinking and her problems?

- Retake her alcohol history carefully (Box 1, p. 4)
- Discuss her alcohol use in comparison to the guidelines for safe maximum weekly consumption – drinking above 16 units will damage her health (Table 18) and health risks are even greater in smokers
- In this case, the duration of alcohol misuse is short (2 months) and she is unlikely to have developed features of dependence. However, you must screen for all complications of alcohol misuse and dependence (Table 18)
- Use evidence of excessive drinking (contradictions in history, physical signs, abnormal investigations and collateral history) to question stated low consumption. The important tactics here are to make sure your patient does not lose face, and not to betray a confidential collateral history without gain
- Remember alcohol is a 'gateway' drug: she may misuse cannabis, cocaine, etc. but only when she has a drink. Explore this.

Table 18 Consequences of alcohol misuse and dependence.

	Category	Examples
Psychiatric	Acute intoxication	Unsafe behaviour, impulsivity
	Harmful use	Problem, binge drinking
	Dependence syndrome	Mood instability (Table 41, p. 137)
	Withdrawal state	Anxiety (Table 42, p. 138)
	Withdrawal state with delirium	Delirium tremens
	Psychotic disorder	Pathological jealousy
	Amnesic syndrome	Memory blackouts
	Residual late-onset psychotic disorder	Hallucinosis when sober
	Other mental and behavioural disorders	Mood and anxiety disorders
		Increases suicidal ideation and behaviour
Medical	Neurological (cerebellar degeneration, central pontine myelinosis, optic atrophy, vitamin deficiencies)	Seizures, dementia, trauma: head injury and haemorrhages, peripheral neuropathy, Korsakov syndrome
	Gastrointestinal (oesophageal varices – end stage of cirrhosis, all GI, liver and mouth cancers are increased)	Oesophagitis, gastritis and ulceration, pancreatitis, *reversible* fatty liver, alcoholic hepatitis, *irreversible* cirrhosis
	Cardiac (cardiomyopathy)	Hypertension and CVA, cardiac arrhythmias
	Respiratory	Aspiration pneumonia, increase all infections – especially tuberculosis
	Haematological	Anaemia: from bleeding and vitamin deficiency
	Metabolic	Hypoglycaemia
	Accidents and trauma	Self-harm, accidental fires, sexually transmitted diseases, hypothermia
	Pregnancy	Unplanned pregnancy, fetal alcohol syndrome
Social	Family problems	Separation, domestic violence, child abuse
	Relationship difficulties	Infidelity, break-up, violence
	Work and financial problems	Poor work record, loss of employment
	Forensic problems	↑ Crime as victim and perpetrator: assaults, drink driving and road traffic accidents

CVA, cerebrovascular accident; GI, gastrointestinal.

> **KEY POINT**
>
> The guidelines for safe maximum weekly alcohol consumption are 16 units for women and 21 for men. Most people minimize their alcohol consumption when talking to health professionals, even those who drink within safe guidelines.

> **KEY POINT**
>
> When a person attempts to remain abstinent from an undesirable behaviour (alcohol or drug misuse, smoking, rituals) but fails, this is a setback not a disaster. Your criticism of this 'failure' will not improve motivation. Reframe this as one less 'attempt' to undergo before they succeed in their goal.

How might you structure a treatment plan for Jenny?

The aim here is to reduce her symptoms and associated social disability. Getting her to link symptoms to her excessive drinking will be the key to her motivation.

> **KEY POINT**
>
> Despite the high prevalence of alcohol misuse and social anxiety, many clinicians take inflexible views about treatment: she must stop drinking *before* psychiatric treatment, or she can only deal with her addiction *after* treatment for her social phobia. Both positions are simplistic, and neither approach will always bring success.

Address alcohol

We know that the most effective time to intervene in alcohol misuse is early in its course, and no future treatment intervention will have as great a chance of success as the first one.

1 Make sure she does not have symptoms of alcohol dependency (if she does, she may require a short course of benzodiazepines; and negotiate a gradual cessation of alcohol use with her
2 Discuss with her if she needs time off work to stop drinking
3 Decide if you need to monitor her alcohol use (to aid her motivation) and if so, how. Blood or salivary tests will detect drinking the previous day.

You need to establish two points early on: cessation of alcohol is a key part of her treatment and, if she cannot remain abstinent, she may need to be referred to a specialist alcohol counsellor.

Address anxiety

Use a cognitive–behavioural therapy (CBT) approach. Begin this by constructing a model of her social phobia. A formulation must be personalized to the patient, and acts as a summary of the information you have gathered so far (Fig. 3). She must understand the range of cognitive and somatic symptoms, and how these are reinforcing her current abnormal behaviour. Treatment will focus on three areas:

1 Challenging her *safety behaviours* (social avoidance, drinking, escaping). The construction of a hierarchy of fears (p. 41) is linked to a corresponding programme of increasingly difficult activities for her to manage without recourse to her escape behaviours. As treatment progresses, use graded self-exposure to feared situations to re-establish her previous functioning
2 Challenging her *negative automatic thoughts* (NATs). This is the cognitive component of CBT. Ask her to write

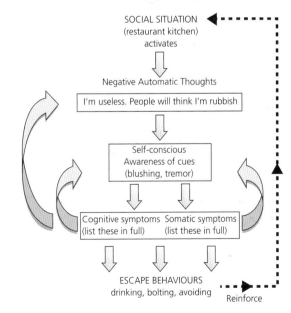

Figure 3 Cognitive–behavioural model of social phobia.

SOCIAL SITUATION
(restaurant kitchen)
activates

Negative Automatic Thoughts

I'm useless. People will think I'm rubbish

Self-conscious
Awareness of cues
(blushing, tremor)

Cognitive symptoms   Somatic symptoms
(list these in full)   (list these in full)

ESCAPE BEHAVIOURS
drinking, bolting, avoiding

Reinforce

down her NATs (e.g. 'People think I can't do my job' (more will be added at subsequent sessions) alongside the evidence that the thought is true. As with obsessions, the thought is intrusive and distressing, but the person does not have to believe it. Challenge her evidence with alternative positive thoughts: 'I got this job over six people at interview. The head chef says I show real promise. I get on with everyone at work. I have been working here for 2 years. People respect me and my work.' One strategy is to pair these thoughts with slow breathing (Box 4, p. 12) or relaxation exercises. These will serve as distraction techniques to reduce NATs and anxiety symptoms.

3 Addressing her feelings of *self-consciousness* is the hardest challenge here. These symptoms are hard to get rid of once they occur. You need to reduce her expectations of cues (Fig. 3) without excessive focus on the cue itself. Blushing is a particular challenge and you may need to consider role play, video sessions or group work to convince her cues are not as 'obvious' to others as they are to her. Group work is an additional treatment for depression (p. 22), but groups for Jenny *early on* could achieve a speedy return to work.

There are a number of instruments that measure social anxiety: these are useful before and during treatment to record her progress.

Consider medication

Recall Box 5 (p. 20) and the discussion of Case 1. As Jenny's drinking may be a continuing problem, use of benzodiazepines, tricyclic antidepressants and/or buspirone will combine with alcohol to cause excess sedation. Sedated patients do not complain, but nor do they socialize or carry out homework. They will miss, or 'switch off' during CBT sessions.

Because her cues may be hard to treat, there is an argument to prescribe β-blockers to reduce adrenergic physical sensations. Their use remains high in performance artists for precisely these reasons, but they are banned in sport.

Selective serotonin reuptake inhibitors (SSRIs; Table 7, p. 17) are now the first line medications used in social anxiety but, if used without other treatments, they have high relapse rates when the medication is discontinued – even after 2 years' medication. Remember that although we perceive SSRIs to have few side-effects, treatment is not risk or side-effect free. Although SSRIs are licensed for social anxiety, there is evidence that people do better with CBT alone.

> **KEY POINT**
>
> For psychological treatments to conquer anxiety, some anxiety needs to be experienced during the treatment. Sedating medication, like alcohol, can interfere with this process by sedating or numbing feelings.

Maximize social treatments

Do not neglect your patient's existing resources. Her flatmates have already shown concern by bringing her to you and are aware of her harmful drinking. They will support her decision not to drink, could stock the kitchen at home with decaffeinated drinks or go to the gym/pool with her to exercise. She may also have a supportive family, a partner or other friends. With her permission, others can act as co-therapists: reading up on social phobia, helping her draw up a fears hierarchy, going out with her, perhaps even attending her CBT sessions.

There may be a downside of recommending a temporary absence from work, making her more avoidant and more phobic (Fig. 3). Part-time work might be the answer. Replace work with other social activities until she is ready to take that step. Encourage hobbies and interests other than solitary ones.

Enlisting the help of a workmate would increase your knowledge of her environment (perhaps others are unhappy with the new kitchen set-up, there are other work pressures or bullying) and provide additional on-site support. It would also help in deciding the best timing for a return to work: this is a balance of when the patient is ready and local factors.

In general, for a return to school or work after an absence with sickness, recommend going back Wednesday or Thursday to increase the chances of success that week, and a full week the following week. In Jenny's case, weekends are the busiest times for restaurants and there may be added demands from shift work. Empower your patient to achieve a phased return to work: most employers welcome the return of a trained, trusted employee, and will be flexible to achieve this.

> **KEY POINT**
>
> The treatment principles for social phobia also apply to the treatment of other phobias. Simple phobias (e.g. fear of spiders) are the easiest phobias to treat.

What is Jenny's likely prognosis?

Her short-term prognosis (6 months) is very good, *provided she stops drinking*. Most studies show major reductions (average 50%) in social anxiety scores, fear of negative evaluation and anxiety symptoms, with parallel improvements in social functioning.

Jenny does not have an anxious premorbid personality, has no current mood symptoms and a short duration of illness. These indicate good prognosis.

Reliance on SSRI medication alone makes further improvements unlikely after 6 months, and increases the probability of relapse thereafter.

The longer term outcome here can cause concern. Even if she responds to treatment, there is evidence that she will carry an increased risk of depression and self-harm in later life. Making the patient and her GP aware of these risks will ensure early diagnosis and treatment of these highly treatable conditions should they occur.

CASE REVIEW

The second most prevalent psychiatric disorder after depression is alcohol misuse and social anxiety combined, with a lifetime prevalence of 22% in Western societies. Social anxiety is common but frequently trivialized as an exaggeration of normal shyness. Untreated, it causes considerable morbidity and comorbidity. Initial diagnosis depended on establishing what she did not have (depression, psychosis), and on teasing out the relationships between symptoms and behaviours (Fig. 3).

Diagnosis is a dynamic process, highly individualized to each patient. Scrutiny of precipitant and maintaining factors allows the clinician to intervene at several points in the cycle:

- Cognitive therapy for NATs
- Psychoeducation to reduce somatic symptoms
- Behavioural measures to extinguish safety/escape behaviours
- Support for alcohol cessation
- Lifestyle changes to increase exercise and reduce caffeine, etc.
- Social networks optimization
- Phased return to work or training

Comprehensive assessment early in a presentation (as here) sets out a clear direction for interventions. In the real world of busy doctors, she might have been referred to a cognitive practitioner, alcohol counsellor, occupational therapist or her GP – with no single professional taking charge of her management. A one-off formulation (Fig. 3 and text) that is shared with all people involved in her care makes speedy recovery and return to work far more likely.

Further reading

Lingford-Hughes, A., Potokar, J. & Nutt, D. (2002) Treating anxiety complicated by substance misuse. *Advances in Psychiatric Treatment* **8**, 107–116.

Stein, M.B., Fuetsch, M., Müller, N., Höfler, M., Lieb, R. & Wittchen, H.U. (2001) Social anxiety disorder and the risk of depression: a prospective community study of adolescents and young adults. *Archives of General Psychiatry* **58**, 251–256.

Tangen Haug, T., Blomhoff, S., Hellstrøm, K., Holme, I., Humble, M., Madsbu, H.P., *et al.* (2003) Exposure therapy and sertraline in social phobia: 1-year follow-up of a randomised controlled trial. *British Journal of Psychiatry* **182**, 312–318.

Veale, D. (2003) Treatment of social phobia. *Advances in Psychiatric Treatment* **9**, 258–264.

Case 5 Sudden deterioration of a 78-year-old woman in a nursing home

Mary has been admitted to a nursing home for 2 weeks' respite while her daughter, her main carer, takes a family holiday. Prior to admission she had mobility difficulties following a failed hip replacement, but still enjoyed concerts and bridge in the evenings with friends. She has no psychiatric history. She became agitated after 2 days at the home, worse at night-time. She now refuses food and fluid. She is confused as to where she is, and wants to go home. She alleges that nursing home staff come into her room to steal from her. You are the local psychiatrist called to assess her.

What are your first thoughts?

Focus on the first category of the diagnostic hierarchy (Fig. 1, p. 7). The details so far suggest _delirium_ (acute confusion) in a previously functioning older woman.

Impaired consciousness is a continuum from delirium through drowsy (inattentiveness, poor response to stimuli), to stuporous (vigorous stimuli are required to elicit a response) and finally to coma. In this case, if she is comatose, you need to rate this on the Glasgow Coma Scale (GCS), and speak immediately to a physician.

Agitation at night-time may reflect 'sundowning' (there is less light to orientate someone visually to their surroundings) and/or that she has an inverted sleep–wake cycle.

> **KEY POINT**
>
> Delirium is a medical emergency – common in general hospitals where organic causes are likely. Normal brain function is impaired by a physical process (or processes) that might be fatal.

Do not allow her allegations of theft (likely to be false) divert you from taking a thorough collateral history from the care home staff. Is she mistaken or deluded? A phone call to her GP will provide invaluable background infor-

mation. At the very least you need her past medical history (we know she has no psychiatric history), medications she is taking (or should be taking) and alcohol use.

> **KEY POINT**
>
> Prescribed medications, from every class, have been implicated as a significant contributor to 40% of cases of delirium.

She presents as alert, responding to questions, but confused. Her GCS is 13/15.

What mental state examination findings would you expect to support a diagnosis of delirium?

- _Impaired consciousness:_ with disorientation and poor concentration. Fluctuating consciousness is the cardinal symptom of delirium
- _Appearance and behaviour:_ psychomotor activity may be increased (agitation) or decreased (hypoactive). This too fluctuates, with more activity by night
- _Mood:_ irritable, perplexed and anxious affects are common
- _Thought content:_ muddled, fleeting, with poorly formed ideas. Delusions are common, usually transient, and easy to understand (i.e. not complex or bizarre)
- _Perceptual ideas:_ hallucinations, also fleeting
- Her accusations about theft may be _delusional, misinterpretations_ (staff will have been checking on her each night when she is more confused) or _visual hallucinations_
- _Cognitions:_ all types of memory are impaired
- Do not be surprised if Mary has _some insight_ – 'I know the trouble I caused last night. I wasn't myself' – it will fluctuate, but insight is absent during delirious states

> **KEY POINT**
>
> Physical examinations are frequently left by psychiatrists for others to perform. This makes missing clinical signs more likely. The more thorough your examination, the more likely you will find a physical cause and improve mental state.

Your history and physical examination identifies a lower respiratory tract infection (LRTI), possibly pneumonia, with some evidence of dehydration. Mary's 'one vice' is smoking and her GP prescribes on average three courses of antibiotics every winter. The nursing home manager tells you he is happy to administer antibiotics and monitor her progress over the next few days.

How will you measure Mary's current cognitive impairment and evaluate the risks of treating her in the current setting?

Complete a cognitive assessment (Table 19).

A standardized assessment of cognitive function, e.g. the Mini Mental State Examination (MMSE) of Folstein *et al.* (1975), is the best way for multiple raters to monitor this over time.

Delirium is a medical emergency: your diagnosis of the cause (LRTI) is only a provisional one, and delirium is frequently of multiple aetiology. Factors to consider are:

• You may have overlooked other pathology causing or contributing to her delirium (Table 20). For example, silent myocardial infarction (infarction without chest pain) is common in this age group, especially in people with diabetes

• There are risks from the delirious state itself resulting from disturbed behaviour: refusing food and fluids, wandering at night, falls, acting on hallucinations, inactivity exacerbating pneumonia or causing bed sores. Does the nursing home have adequate staffing levels (and sufficiently experienced staff) to monitor her progress closely?

• There may be psychiatric comorbidity (depression and anxiety symptoms) requiring monitoring and treatment

• 'Treatments' to control her disturbed behaviour may make her confusion worse, e.g. antipsychotics (Table 8, p. 18) with multiple adverse effects are sometimes prescribed to sedate delirious patients but, like benzodiazepines, frequently make confusion worse.

Should she be admitted to hospital?

Your decision must balance the risks of managing the patient in a low-key setting such as this nursing home with the risks of moving her and initiating a prolonged hospital stay. You recommend that Mary is admitted to the medical ward of the main general hospital.

At this point how do you see your role as a psychiatrist in relation to the medical/nursing team?

Your role is to advise about and treat psychiatric *sequelae* of delirium (principally mood and psychotic states, anxiety and sleep disorders, disinhibited behaviours). It may fall to you to reiterate, as often as necessary, that there are no psychiatric *causes* of her symptoms and she needs medical treatment.

An additional role is to give clear advice about the best environment in which delirious patients can be managed. We have assumed her confusion is caused by her infection, but there were factors at the nursing home that may have made her confusion worse (e.g. absence of her family, sudden social isolation, lack of orientation cues, poor lighting, unfamiliar staff and less of them at night-times).

Just because a disorder has a biological cause, it does not make 'social' treatments redundant. There are basic nursing strategies in the care of patients with delirium that are frequently overlooked (Box 10). There may be other findings in your assessments that help your colleagues manage her illness more effectively (e.g. she has hearing difficulties, lost her spectacles, fears needles).

On discharge, you will need to coordinate an effective care plan for medium-term management and prevention of future episodes of confusion.

> **KEY POINT**
>
> Do not make the delirious patient the subject of a 'turf war' between medicine and psychiatry. The patient frequently needs the best care from both to achieve optimum recovery.

The medical registrar has been trying without success to contact Mary's family and will not agree to his staff administering treatments (intravenous fluids, antibiotics) without her consent. He asks you to 'section' her, that is, admit her against her wishes to a psychiatric hospital. He says she is completely 'crazy' and 'a schizophrenic'.

Table 19 Cognitive assessment component of Mental State Examination.

Parameter	Tests
Consciousness (on a spectrum from full consciousness to clouding, stupor and coma)	Clinical assessment based on patient's best responses. Most Emergency Departments use the Glasgow Coma Scale
Orientation (frequently impaired in delirium)	Remember with confused and some older patients, the questions may be threatening: 'I'm going to ask you some routine questions we ask everybody':
	What is the year, season, date, day, month?
	Time of day?
	Where are we? Country, county/city, town, hospital
Attention and concentration	**Serial 7s**: 'take 7 from 100, and 7 from the next number . . .' (through to 2 if correct). Record number of mistakes and the time it takes to get to the last digit. The normal lower range is two mistakes in 1 minute
	For patients who have poor numerical ability, consider either months of the year backwards (December, November, etc.,) or spelling 'WORLD' backwards. Allow one error for the months until March, and no errors for spelling WORLD backwards
Short-term memory	Testing registration *and* recall at 3 minutes:
	'Repeat after me . . .' three unrelated words (purple, carrot, liberty) or an address (17 North Street, Wandsworth). Make sure the patient repeats the information clearly. Finish other tests and ask for the information back then
Long-term memory	Name five large cities in the country
	Dates of World Wars: 1914–1918 and 1939–1945
	Names of recent UK Prime Ministers/US Presidents
Speech and language	You should be aware of abnormalities at this stage
	Test for dysarthria by asking patient to repeat 'NO ifs ands or buts'
	Dysphasia can be nominal (cannot 'find' some words), perceptive (cannot understand some words) or global (both)
Dyspraxia (parietal lobe dysfunction)	Offer a pen and paper and ask them to draw a CLOCK with all 12 numbers and the time indicated at 3.45
	Keep this in the notes: it is an excellent descriptive snapshot of ability

How would you approach this situation?

There are two issues here:
1 The immediate issue of investigating and treating her physical condition without her consent
2 Who is best placed to manage her care?

Considering these in turn, begin by assessing her capacity to consent to treatment. In England and Wales, the Mental Capacity Act (2005) states: 'A person lacks capacity in relation to a matter if at the material time he is unable to make a decision for himself in relation to the matter because of an impairment of, or disturbance in

Table 20 Causes of delirium (mnemonic from Wise & Trzepacz 1994).

	Category	Subcategory	Examples
I	**I**nfection	Brain-based	Meningitis, encephalitis
		Other organs	Urinary tract infection, respiratory infections, hepatitis, etc.
		Systemic	Viraemia, septicaemia, malaria, subacute bacterial endocarditis
		'Hidden'	Abscesses, dental infection, bed sores, osteomyelitis (possible in this case)
W	**W**ithdrawal	Legal	Alcohol, benzodiazepines, even nicotine withdrawal has been implicated
		Illegal	Any sedating or stimulating illegal substance (Table 42)
A	**A**cute metabolic	Hypoglycaemia	Overdose of insulin (accidental and deliberate), starvation, insulinoma
		The four 'failures'	Cardiac failure, respiratory failure, renal failure and liver failure
		Other glucose, U&Es	Hyperglycaemia (forgotten insulin, infection), *any* electrolyte abnormality
T	**T**rauma	To head	Head injury, four types of intracranial haemorrhage: extradural, subdural, subarachnoid and intracerebral
		To other organs	Burns, heat stroke, hypothermia
C	**C**NS lesions	Structural	Any space-occupying lesion (tumour, haemorrhage, brain abscess, etc.)
		Functional	Epilepsy, paraneoplastic syndrome (non-metastatic malignancy effects)
H	**H**ypoxia	Shock	Cardiogenic shock, haemorrhagic shock, etc.
		Haematological	Altitude sickness, anaemias (causes of low red cells, abnormal haemoglobin)
D	**D**eficiency	General	Starvation: calorie deficiency and/or protein deficiency, cachexia (e.g. cancer)
		Thiamine (vitamin B$_1$)	Korsakoff's syndrome, Wernicke's encephalopathy, cardiac effects (beriberi)
		Nicotinic acid	Pellagra = diarrhoea, 'dementia' (reversible), dermatitis and depression
		Vitamin B$_{12}$ and folate	Tired, weak and breathless (due to anaemia); confusion, other neurological signs
E	**E**ndocrine	Thyroid	Hyperthyroid, hypothyroid
		Parathyroid	Hypercalcaemia
		Adrenal	Cushing's syndrome, Addison's disease
A	**A**cute vascular		Causes of cerebrovascular accident (haemorrhage or embolism), cardiac arrhythmias, hypertensive encephalopathy, post cardiac surgery (insufficient oxygenation or microemboli), etc.
T	**T**oxins		Prescribed drugs (all CNS-acting drugs, especially sedatives) have some role in 40% of delirium cases
H	**H**eavy metals	Lead, mercury	

the functioning of, the mind or the brain.' This covers organic/medical illness and mental illness, whether they are permanent or temporary impairments. People can have capacity for some things (consent to a blood test) but lack it for other matters (consent to surgery); you must carry out separate assessments for each decision. The law assumes a person has capacity, and it is for

you to prove he/she does not. To demonstrate lack of capacity you need to demonstrate one or more of three problem areas in relation to her ability for understanding, retaining and weighing up information to make a decision about treatment (Table 21). Capacity is very important in mental health settings and is discussed again in Case 7.

Box 10 Nursing strategies to manage patients with delirium

1 Frequent observation: 4 hourly or more
2 Efforts by staff to repeatedly orientate the patient to surroundings recognized as a specific part of the management plan
3 Avoid excessive staff changes: special nurse (one to one care) or named, key nurse
4 Patient nursed in a single room
5 Uncluttered nursing environment: beds apart by an adequate distance, and no more than two objects in vicinity that are non-vital or non-orientating
6 Use of individual night light
7 Specific efforts made to minimize noise levels: radio, televisions
8 Relatives of friends specifically requested to visit at regular times, and asked to help with reorientation
9 Observation of sleeping pattern will inform prescription of hypnotic – if this is absolutely necessary

---

Table 21 Assessment of capacity: based on Mental Capacity Act 2005 (England and Wales)

Section 3 (subsection 1):	Section 3 (subsections 2–4):
A person *lacks* capacity if:	A person with capacity:
He is unable to understand the information relevant to the decision	Needs to understand information given in a way appropriate to the circumstances (simple language, visual aids or other means)
or he is unable to retain the information relevant to the decision	Can have capacity (even) if he is able to retain for short periods only
or he is unable to use or weigh the information relevant to the decision as part of the process of making the decision	Needs to understand the information relating to the consequences of choosing one way over another
or he is unable to communicate the decision by talking, sign language, or other means	Is able to communicate his decision with language, visual aids or other means

---

KEY POINT

The assessment of capacity is a core medical skill – all doctors are expected to carry this out without referral to specialists.

Mary is adamant she does not have pneumonia. She denies that her GP has given her antibiotics on many previous occasions. She cannot take in the consequences of refusing fluids and antibiotics.

Does this mean that Mary lacks capacity?

Yes, in relation to the treatment of her pneumonia, she lacks capacity. Her pneumonia should therefore be treated without her consent in her best interests, and under the doctrine of necessity: 'to save life, ensure improvement and prevent deterioration'. The legal framework for this is the Mental Capacity Act 2005.

What about the request to section Mary?

It would be *wrong* to treat her under the Mental Health Act (MHA) as the cause of her impairment is physical and the MHA provides only for psychiatric treatments. Transferring her to a psychiatric hospital under a MHA section might make the medical registrar happy, but would be the *wrong* decision ethically, legally and medically. Reassure the medical registrar that her behaviour may be 'psychiatric' but her illness is not.

As she is seriously medically unwell, she needs to be treated and nursed on a medical ward. Psychiatric wards are not set up to manage physical illness; very few have the facilities or staff to administer intravenous fluids. Psychiatric nurses are not necessarily medically qualified, even to administer intravenous drugs, as many do not have general (i.e. medical) nursing training.

You are asked to prescribe medication to improve her sleep and reduce her shouting on the ward by night. The nurses tell you that the other patients are complaining about her as over the last 4 hours she has been keeping them all awake by repeatedly calling out for her brother (long deceased) and the police.

How do you respond to this request to prescribe?

> **KEY POINT**
>
> In psychiatric presentations, people are sometimes given medication not because they are suffering, but because their behaviour is insufferable.

The best treatment of delirium is to treat its causes (Table 20). All other treatments are symptomatic and have the potential to make confusion worse and may introduce iatrogenic illness (Box 7, p. 21). However, there is a balance of risks here: delirium can lead to falls, fights and many other complications.

Given the above, *if* prescribing some kind of sedating medication is, on balance, in her best interests, you have two choices: antipsychotics or benzodiazepines. The drug of choice here used to be haloperidol, although this is now known to be unsuitable for many patients. Haloperidol has the advantage that it can be administered intravenously (intramuscular injection is known to have variable absorption): 2 mg oral haloperidol corresponds to 1 mg intravenous drug. Its effects on blood pressure, pulse rate and respirations are less than the effects of benzodiazepines. This said, haloperidol causes cardiac conduction delays and can precipitate cardiac arrest in cardiocompromised patients.

Most centres have a local protocol for its use for disturbed behaviour in delirium and it would be wise to refer to these where possible – make sure the guidelines you are reading are for delirium and not for acute agitation or aggression, where higher doses are indicated for more disturbed, younger, bigger, active men.

Many protocols combine haloperidol with lorazepam. This is a short-acting benzodiazepine without the anticholinergic effects of haloperidol (e.g. confusion, hallucinations, urinary retention, glaucoma, dry mouth). One of the few advantages of using benzodiazepines is that if excessive use causes respiratory depression (in susceptible patients such as Mary who has pneumonia), it can be reversed with the drug flumazenil.

If you suspect dementia, and that dementia may be subcortical or associated with Parkinson's disease, do *not* use antipsychotics such as haloperidol. The use of typical antipsychotics (haloperidol) has given way to atypicals such as risperidone and olanzapine. So far, only case reports have recommended the routine use of atypicals

in delirium, and randomized controlled trails have failed to show additional benefits when compared with haloperidol. Prescribing trends will change over time as the evidence base develops.

Document that your decision to prescribe is on the basis of her behaviour and factors such as her sleep–wake cycle, hallucinations or paranoid ideation that are amenable to specific medications. If you fail to document these, you could be accused of treating the staff's anxiety rather than your patient's, and future medication reviews will increase the doses without clear outcome measures.

Remember, you have been called about this request at night, so it may be worth returning to the issue of how she is being nursed by the night shift (Box 10). Is she in a room with sufficient lighting to orientate her?

> **KEY POINT**
>
> If you are writing up as required (p.r.n.) medication, specify the maximum 24-hour dose and record a stop date to ensure review and that the patient does not stay on these, or end up going home on sedatives.

How will you would monitor her mental state from day to day?

As her pneumonia is treated, you would hope that her confusion lifts. Regular Mini Mental State Examinations (MMSEs), perhaps weekly, carried out by *any* health care professional, give a reliable indication about progress or deterioration.

Carry out a good quality MMSE relatively early in your assessments to avoid false positive results from interviewing tired or agitated patients. MMSE are particularly useful in patients where an episode of confusion (delirium) occurs in a patient who has pre-existing chronic confusion (dementia). After an episode of delirium they may well not return to their previous level of cognitive functioning. For many patients, delirium will be a first presentation that 'unmasks' underlying dementia.

Good nursing care and two night's medication achieves some improvements in her condition, and her pneumonia appears to be responding. Mary's daughter returns from holiday and is furious about her mother's treatment. She asks to see you, as the doctor who 'forced' her to go to hospital, 'drugged her to the eyeballs' and wants a separate meeting with the medical doctor treating her mother.

What approach will you take here?

• Suggest you and the medical registrar meet her at the same time. Include any family members and friends she nominates. It is better to face complaints quickly rather than allow them to fester

• Be aware of your own anxieties: this is the 'daughter from California' syndrome – an articulate, informed, close relative who arrives late in the day and challenges medical decisions. In a neutral way, find out what she is angry about

• Many decisions have preceded the current situation:
  ○ her decision to put her mother into respite care
  ○ communication of her mother's known medical conditions at admission
  ○ her choice of nursing home
  ○ the care at that nursing home
  ○ the timing of help seeking: too early or too late – relatives may complain about either decision, sometimes both
  ○ the quality of your initial assessment
  ○ your decision to consult the general hospital
  ○ the shared decision to admit her
  ○ the choice of ward and her location in it
  ○ your assessment of capacity
  ○ medical investigations
  ○ medical and nursing decisions about treatment
  ○ the choice of psychoactive medication or none

• Try and establish a non-defensive atmosphere when you meet her. Perhaps Mary's care has been less than ideal at some stages. Her anger is probably driven by understandable anxiety about her mother's welfare. It's not unusual for people to have an adversarial or aggressively assertive approach to 'authorities' (such as staff in the health care system) out of the (mistaken) belief that otherwise they will not be taken seriously, and their relative will suffer as a result

• Talk through your motivations to help her mother. At some points you had little room for manoeuvre. You would have been wrong to leave her in the nursing home, wrong to take her directly, or later on section, to a psychiatric hospital, and wrong to allow her to die of a treatable infection

• She might blame herself for some decisions (four of the 13 decisions above were hers) but anger is more easily expressed than guilt and may be 'projected' on to health professionals. Support her by active listening. Be transparent. It is best to avoid judgement on others' failings at this point: you will usually be wrong and will be quoted by her from here on

The Mental Capacity Act (2005) allows for the appointment of independent mental capacity advocates (IMCAs) where alternative options or second opinions are sought. If there are unanswered questions, or she remains angry, set a date for a second meeting with you. Prior to that second meeting, convene a case review to identify areas of good and poor practice. You will need to consult with colleagues and your medical director if you think things are getting out of hand.

> **KEY POINT**
>
> The vast majority of complaints, correctly handled at an early stage, do not end up in court. Early, open, non-defensive meetings are the best strategy.

Mary's pneumonia responds and her confusion lifts, as does her daughter's anger.

What follow-up will you arrange?

• Delirium has a high short-term mortality in the context of its causes and additional risks of prolonged hospital stay: hospital-acquired infection, iatrogenic illness, complications of immobility, and loss of social functioning and networks

• Medical colleagues should decide medical follow-up. Infections are rarely 'bad luck' in this age group, even in a smoker. What are her living conditions? Is her nutrition adequate? Does she have regular GP reviews?

• Decide about specialist psychiatric follow-up on the basis of serial MMSEs and psychiatric symptoms. If her score recovered and stayed in the high 20s, follow-up is probably unnecessary. Write to her GP outlining her course, and recommend referral to psychiatry of older adults if there is any deterioration in the MMSE or clinical state

• If she fails to regain her previous good cognitive function, refer her to a memory clinic or a psychiatrist for older people

Could Mary's delirium have been prevented?

Probably not. There are no current randomized controlled trials that identify specific measures to prevent delirium in vulnerable populations. Some medical causes are amenable to prevention (Table 20) and her environment at the nursing home (Box 10) could benefit from scrutiny.

CASE REVIEW

Early on in this case, the issue of capacity in an elderly patient with multiple interacting problems came to the fore. Later, older people's sensitivity to medication and the intervention of a younger carer became problematic. While the diagnosis of delirium is easy to make (acute deterioration in mental state with fluctuating consciousness), its causes are not always apparent. Careful history taking and examination established a chest infection here as one likely cause. You would have been taking a chance had you recommended she stayed in the nursing home: that you had not missed other pathology (her failed hip operation could have led to osteomyelitis; Table 20) and that her LRTI would respond to antibiotics. There is not always one simple cause, and many patients leave hospital without identification of causative factors. Delirium has a significant mortality – 10% at 12 months – and this of itself justifies thorough assessment of every case, and referral onwards where necessary. Despite biological aetiology, many social measures help these patients (Box 10) and psychiatric medication only has a limited role.

Once admitted to a general hospital, you provided a valuable opinion on treating her in the absence of capacity:

- Urging caution in medication
- Helping short and longer term management, with judicious use of MMSEs
- Doing everything right here but entailing conflict with the medical registrar, general hospital nurses and then Mary's daughter
- Facing criticisms quickly and directly. This was in everyone's interests: your patient's, her daughter's, your colleagues' and yours

Your actions here are easy to defend, but this would not be the case if you had done nothing for Mary, or admitted her to a psychiatric ward. Not all presentations are as clear-cut, and delirium can have a subacute onset. Finally, and this applies outside the psychiatric arena, do not see delirium as an 'elderly' condition: children are far more susceptible to delirium (Table 20) than adults.

Reference

Department of Health. (2005) *Mental Capacity Act*. Stationery Office, London. www.dh.gov.uk/en/socialcare/deliveringadultsocialcare/mentalcapacity/MentalCapacityAct2005/

Folstein, M.F. *et al.* (1975) Mini-mental state: a practical method for grading the cognitive state of patients for the clinician. *Journal Psychiatric Research* **12**, 189–198.

Wise, M.G. & Trzepacz, P. (1994) Delirium. In Rundell, J.R. & Wise, M.G. (eds.) *Textbook of Consultation Liaison Psychiatry*. American Psychiatric Press, Washington D.C.

Further reading

Brown, T.M. & Boyle, M.F. (2002) ABC of psychological medicine – delirium. *British Medical Journal* **325**, 644–647.

Leentjens, A.F.G. & van der Mast, R.C. (2005). Delirium in elderly patients: an update. *Current Opinions in Psychiatry* **18**, 325–330.

Meagher, D., *et al.* (1996) The use of environmental strategies and psychotrophic medication in the management of delirium. *British Journal of Psychiatry* **168**, 512–515.

Case 6 A 72-year-old woman with antisocial behaviour

The Housing Department contact the Mental Health of Older Adults' team to refer a 72-year-old woman, Rose, who lives in council accommodation. They have started eviction proceedings because she is in rent arrears and they have had complaints from the neighbours about her antisocial behaviour. She has been seen throwing clothes and personal items into the communal areas outside her flat. She has also called the police several times to her neighbour's flat, accusing them of running a brothel.

What broad differential diagnoses occur to you as you read this referral?
• *Physical illness with neuropsychiatric complications:* any acute physical illness, including delirium, manifesting as disturbed behaviour
• *Dementia:* presenting as disturbed behaviour resulting from cognitive impairment
• *Psychotic illness:* either first onset or an acute exacerbation of previous illness
• There is currently little evidence of an *antisocial personality disorder*

What do you need to establish at this stage?
• Can the Housing Department give you any further information?
• Can you speak with her GP?
• Is Rose known to have any physical health problems?
• Has Rose a known history of psychiatric illness?
• Can you obtain any collateral history (e.g. Rose's family or neighbours)?
• Will Rose agree to a visit from a psychiatrist?

Local mental health services confirm that Rose has no history of previous contact. The Housing Department can give you no other information other than their proposed eviction date: 2 weeks' time. You cannot establish who her GP is, and you have no contact details for her family.

How might you proceed?
A home visit with another colleague from your team. Home visits are usually carried out in pairs in the community for safety reasons (patients' and yours).

The history suggests a deteriorating situation, and Rose is facing eviction so there is a degree of urgency to establish what is happening.

You visit Rose's home, on the third floor of a block of flats. There are old magazines, her smashed television and a pile of clothes outside the door. Rose does not answer the door but you can hear her voice from inside.

Standing outside Rose's door, what might you do next?
• Approach her neighbours to see if you can get any further information
• Put a note through Rose's door to explain who you are, with your contact details

You knock on a neighbour's door and they answer. You show them your ID and explain your visit. Rose's neighbour tells you that she has lived next door to Rose for many years, and she has always 'kept herself to herself'. Over the last 6 months, Rose has been banging on the walls and shouting abuse, and on a couple of occasions when they have passed each other Rose called her a 'whore'. The neighbour says that Rose has gone 'crazy' and 'someone has to do something'.

What else might you ask the neighbour?
It is worth asking if she knows contact details for Rose's family or her GP.

The neighbour has Rose's daughter's number. Her daughter Irene used to visit regularly but stopped a few months ago. Irene tells you by phone that she fell out with her mother months ago because her mother accused her of abusing her. They have not spoken since. Irene is shocked by recent events. She tells you her mother has never been mentally unwell, and her only physical problem is poor hearing. She agrees to meet you at the flat the next day with keys. Irene remembers Rose's GP and you contact him: he confirms her medical and psychiatric history as unremarkable. The next day Irene lets you into the flat. There is rubbish all over the floor. Rose appears from the cluttered kitchen and looks physically well but her clothes are unwashed. She eyes you both suspiciously while Irene introduces you.

How will you proceed?

Before attempting to take a history here you should 'set the scene' for your (surprise) visit by explaining that the Housing Department contacted your team as they were concerned about her eviction.

Remember you are in her home, and she is likely to find your presence intrusive (if not threatening), so ask where she would like you to sit and whether she minds you asking her some questions. It might be useful to say that you will help her in her difficulties with the council.

Rose says she is perfectly well and denies any problems with her physical health. After prompting she tells you her main problem is her neighbours running a brothel. They keep breaking into her flat while she is out and moving things around, and soiling her possessions. She cannot identify evidence for this. When you ask why she has thrown out her television, she says it contained a camera that was monitoring her, and there were programmes on it that were discussing her. She appears distracted, repeatedly looking out the window. She abruptly walks out of the room saying she refuses to answer any more 'stupid questions' and she tells you both to leave. You have established that Rose is mentally unwell, but you are clearly unable to investigate the cause and instigate treatment at this point as she is uncooperative.

What should you try to do before leaving?

• Tell her you are concerned about her health, ask if she would consider coming to hospital, and advise her you will be coming to see her again
• If you have an opportunity, look in the kitchen – are there health and safety issues here or evidence of cognitive impairment? Examples include rotting food and dangerous use of electrical appliances such the electric kettle on a gas hob

• Check for any clues as to a cause for her presentation – evidence of excess alcohol consumption

Summarize your findings thus far in her MSE

• *Appearance and behaviour:* a woman in her seventies who looks physically well but shows self-neglect, wearing dirty clothes. She may be responding to internal stimuli (hallucinations) given her distracted appearance. She is guarded and suspicious and it is not possible to establish a rapport with her
• *Speech:* normal tone but loud (she has hearing difficulties). Often fast. No thought disorder
• *Mood:* objectively appeared irritable, subjectively could not be assessed as she declined to answer the question. Not possible to establish thoughts of self-harm or harming others
• *Thoughts:* evidence of paranoid persecutory delusions regarding her neighbours stealing from her, probable delusions of reference (Box 3, p. 10) Acted on these.
• *Perception:* declined to answer, but behaviour suggests hallucinations
• *Cognition:* no gross cognitive abnormalities, but not formally assessed because of non-cooperation
• *Insight:* none. She does not believe there is anything wrong with her and sees no justification for further assessment, investigation or treatment

What are your working differential diagnoses at this point?

• *Schizophrenia:* she meets the criteria for late onset (Box 9, p. 54)
• *Mood disorder with psychosis:* abnormalities of mood (mood elevation or depression) can be associated with poor self-care and, when severe, psychosis and cognitive disorganization. There is self-neglect but this is more likely the result of her delusions of persecution. Her irritability is not surprising, especially given your surprise visit, which she views as unnecessary and intrusive
• *Schizoaffective disorder:* these patients present with mood symptoms (low or high, p. 57), but the degree and chronicity of their psychotic symptoms excludes a primary mood diagnosis. Most, but not all, experience both groups of symptoms during the same episode. The disorder is best seen on a continuum between mood and psychotic disorders
• *Psychosis associated with cognitive disorders:* people with dementia may present with psychosis (commonly, late in their illness), but Rose's cognitive function appears normal

- *Psychosis caused by a physical condition:* it is possible that an underlying medical disorder (Table 16, p. 53) could present with psychosis and functional decline and this cannot be ruled out here. We know from the GP that physical pathology seems unlikely
- *Substance-induced psychotic disorder:* consider this in everyone. Her disordered behaviour and functional decline may be a result of alcohol intoxication, alcohol-related dementia or alcoholic hallucinosis
- *Delusional disorder:* delusional disorders are encapsulated delusional systems that can be understood as having their own internal logic. They are not associated with hallucinations or a decline in functioning. This is unlikely here and can be discarded as Rose's delusions are widespread, she appears to be hallucinating and there is evidence of functional decline

> After the visit Irene suggests Rose might be tricked into going to hospital straight away if you pretend to take them both in your car to visit her brother Chris.

How do you respond to Irene's suggestion?

Explain to Irene that her mother needs to be assessed for a section of the Mental Health Act. This is the legal framework for admitting people to hospital for investigation and treatment for suspected mental illness without their consent. Although Rose needs admission as soon as possible, this is a situation that has been gradually worsening for months. There is no indication that her immediate safety (or that of others) is in danger; it would be wrong to take her to hospital under false pretences.

You refer Rose for a section assessment, which is arranged for a couple of days later by a social worker and also involves Rose's GP.

> Rose is much the same and refuses to come to hospital. The necessity for formal hospital admission is agreed by the professionals involved. The police are required to help the ambulance crew take Rose to hospital when she becomes physically hostile, screaming 'murderers and rapists'. She calms when the police arrive, although she asks the police to arrest her neighbours. She is taken to hospital without incident and on admission is orientated to the ward by nursing staff, who inform her of her legal right to appeal against her section.

As the doctor on the admitting psychiatric ward, what would you want to prioritize on the day of her admission?

- Take a full history and mental state examination
- Conduct a full physical examination and order appropriate physical investigations
- Decide whether she needs any medication prescribed in the short term
- Decide what level of nursing observation is required

Rose is likely to be angry about her admission, not surprisingly given what she believes. Being brought into hospital against one's will is a frightening experience. She may resist your efforts to examine her, but it is essential you attempt this, and as thoroughly as possible (e.g. she may refuse blood tests, but allow her pulse and blood pressure to be taken). You need to establish if she requires urgent medical review. If any tests or aspects of her examination remain outstanding because of her non-cooperation, this must be clearly documented so they can be completed when she is more cooperative.

Irene asks you what you think is wrong with her mother. Make clear Rose has been admitted to hospital under section for assessment and it is too early at this stage to give a definitive diagnosis. She is experiencing a *psychotic illness* but you do not yet know the exact nature or its cause.

KEY POINT

Although you may strongly suspect someone has schizophrenia, do not underestimate the emotional impact of this diagnostic label and carefully consider the context in which you share this information with both the individual and their family.

> Rose agrees to a physical examination and blood tests.

What investigations will you request for Rose?

- Routine blood tests in this first presentation of psychosis in an older person: full blood count (FBC), urea and electrolytes (U&Es), glucose, liver function tests (LFTs), thyroid function tests (TFTs) plus dementia screen (B$_{12}$ and folate, calcium, phosphate, syphilis serology)
- Further system, i.e. investigation only if indicated on examination (or from abnormal blood results)

Will you start regular psychotropic medication straight away?

This depends on both the degree of Rose's disturbance and how amenable she is to taking it. You may wish to hold-off starting regular medication until she has been further assessed and observed on the ward for a few days and reviewed by the consultant, by which time you will have the results of blood tests.

Rose's physical examination is unremarkable and the blood test results are normal (thyroid results will take a few days). Meanwhile, she has become very distressed, pacing back and forth and shouting that the nurses are trying to poison her. She has refused the food she has been offered.

How might you proceed at this stage?

• You could ask the nurses to try and involve Rose's daughter in trying to reassure Rose that she is safe and to persuade her to eat and drink on the ward. She may trust food·brought in by her daughter

• Given Rose's presentation and degree of distress, it will be necessary to start her on a low-dose atypical antipsychotic (Table 8, p. 18)

• If Rose remains very agitated and disturbed she may need to have additional medication. A low-dose benzodiazepine would be preferable to quickly increasing doses of an antipsychotic because of the potential side-effects of the latter. Benzodiazepines such as diazepam have active metabolites and therefore accumulate in the system, so prescribe cautiously

• The issue of her poor food and fluid intake on the ward is of particular concern. You will need to advise the nurses to start a fluid intake chart to monitor this carefully. If her intake remains poor, take regular U&Es

• Rose is new to the ward, and her behaviour at this stage is unpredictable. You may therefore wish to advise nurses to keep her under close observation (i.e. within eyesight at all times by an allocated nurse) to continue to offer her reassurance, and to ensure she remains safe

KEY POINT

Older people require much lower doses of psychotropic medication to treat psychosis and they are more susceptible to extrapyramidal side-effects, excessive sedation and anticholinergic toxicity (Table 8, p. 18).

Box 11 Management principles in acute psychosis

Byrne (2007)

• Identify and change environmental factors that perpetuate psychotic symptoms

• For manic patients use benzodiazepines with antipsychotics as adjuncts; for patients with schizophrenia use antipsychotics with benzodiazepines as adjuncts

• Consider a dispersible preparation of an antipsychotic, which dissolves quickly on the tongue. This is better than injections or tablets that have uncertain adherence

• Document frequency of nursing observations (blood pressure, temperature, pulse rate)

• Monitor fluid balance (input/output) and body weight (up to daily) in acutely ill patients

• When (not *if*) new symptoms occur, consider unwanted drug effects (Table 9, p. 19)

• Physical exam is an essential part of regular clinical review

• Test for, and persuade/intervene against, persistent substance misuse

• Evidence supports starting psychosocial interventions at the earliest opportunity

Rose settles with medication and sleeps well. Over the next week she eats and drinks. There is no evidence of any cognitive impairment, but she continues to maintain that her neighbours have been persecuting her and the nurses observe her talking in an animated manner when alone, seemingly responding to voices. Her son Chris calls you to say he cannot believe his mother is in a psychiatric hospital because she has never been mentally ill in her life. He says he disagrees with his sister Irene and thinks Rose should be discharged immediately because the hospital is 'driving her mad'.

How might you approach this situation?

• It seems likely that Chris was out of touch with his mother and unaware of her decline before admission

• Acknowledge Chris's concerns while outlining how unwell Rose has been

• Invite Chris and his sister Irene to a ward round so your team can have an open discussion with them. This might be an opportunity to discuss her diagnosis, which now you are confident is *late-onset schizophrenia* (Table 22). As often happens, family members have conflicting views and are communicating these separately to staff.

Table 22 Later onset versus earlier onset schizophrenia.

	Schizophrenia before 40 years	Late-onset schizophrenia
Prevalence (1 year)	0.45% – higher if substance misuse, migration and other social deprivation factors	Probably higher: 10% of non-demented people over 85 years have psychotic symptoms
Of known cases	70% before 40 years old	30% after 40 years old
		Of admissions to an older persons' ward, 10% are for late-onset schizophrenia
Gender ratio	Men ≥ women (close to equal)	Women > men (up to four times)
Aetiology	Mostly unknown Cannabis use	Unknown but some associations with sensory impairments (in Rose's case, deafness) and social isolation (also a factor here)
Family history	Usually negative	More often positive
Premorbid personality	Normal – unless psychosis occurs in early adolescence	Abnormal: paranoid and schizoid traits common
Course	One or more episodes	May run a chronic course
Symptoms	Thought disorder, somatic passivity, negative symptoms – especially disorganization. Mostly *auditory* hallucinations	Paranoia and hallucinations: simple hallucinations common; auditory more than visual (visual impairment common)
Cognitive function	Rarely impaired	Intact unless dementia
Response to medications	Variable	Good: at about 50% of adult doses. Very late onset require even lower doses
Concordance	Variable	Sensory/cognitive impairments, lack of insight and isolation make this even worse
Side-effects	Variable	Higher (e.g. fivefold increase in tardive dyskinesia)

Attempt to reach a consensus by face-to-face meetings with everyone concerned
• Invite their questions about any aspect of her treatment
• Explain your team has a duty of care to treat Rose's illness, even if she disagrees, and this is why she is under a section – but she/they can appeal this
• This is a good time to discuss 'plan B' if she refuses medication (e.g. spits out the tablets). If that happens, consider injected/depot antipsychotic

Chris reluctantly agrees Rose needs treatment and they both persuade Rose to start to take her tablets. Over the following weeks she gradually improves and her persecutory ideas lessen in intensity, and she no longer appears to be hearing voices.

What other aspects of her care do you need to consider before her discharge?

• *Referral to a psychologist:* this is an ideal time to engage in psychological work to challenge her delusional beliefs, reflect on how the illness has impacted on her life and to consider the role medication has played in her recovery
• *Her social situation:* Rose is in rent arrears and facing eviction. She needs to be allocated a key-worker from your community team who will liaise with the Housing Department and inform them of the situation (i.e. Rose failed to pay her rent because she became unwell), so that eviction proceedings are halted. The Housing Department are likely to be sympathetic to a repayment plan once she is out of hospital. Rose may also need more general help with her finances and sorting out any unpaid bills. Before she is discharged, a home visit should be

arranged to ascertain the state of the flat so any repairs can be initiated
• *Long-term follow-up:* Rose needs follow-up by the community team

Rose continues to improve and takes leave from the ward, which is uneventful, and agrees to pay her rent arrears. She no longer believes people are persecuting her and she is free from hallucinations. However, she does not agree she has been ill, and still feels admission was unjustified. She will not see a psychologist. She explains her experiences by saying that she had been under stress and was just not sleeping. Irene and Chris are worried about the plans to discharge Rose and ask you three questions:

1 'Why not keep her in hospital until she really understands what has happened?'
2 'When can she stop taking the tablets?'
3 'Will she become ill again?'

How will you answer?
Insight
It is possible that Rose will never gain any further insight into what has happened, but given how well she is now, there is no longer any justification for keeping her in hospital. There may be several reasons why people cannot recall how unwell they have been:
• From a biological standpoint, during periods of psychosis, the brain often fails to form new or coherent memories in the usual way. Memories of psychotic symptoms may therefore be fragmentary
• Taking a psychological standpoint, it can be upsetting and anxiety-provoking (even humiliating) to recall what one has believed, how frightening it was and how one behaved during a psychotic episode. Understandably, people want to 'seal over' these experiences, and focus on the future

Medication
Under current legislation, Rose cannot be compelled to take medication once she is off section. You advise Rose to stay on the current dose of the medication that has

made her well for at least 1 year as this is a high-risk period for relapse.

After a year, if Rose remains well then discuss slowly reducing and stopping medication. She still has a risk of relapse.

Prognosis
Often, as here, we cannot be definitive: illness course varies between individuals in an unpredictable way. A minority remain well, while most patients will experience relapse. This will depend in part on continuing with medication.

You can say that generally there are some positive prognostic factors in Rose's case as she is: (i) female; (ii) her illness onset was in late life; (iii) her symptoms were of the paranoid type; (iv) she had good premorbid functioning; and (v) she did not have any negative symptoms (Table 17, p. 58).

CASE REVIEW

You have now seen psychosis in a hostile patient, the previous presentation (Case 3) being merely uncommunicative. Rose has many of the typical features of late-onset schizophrenia: no history of psychosis but established social isolation, hearing difficulties, delusions and hallucinations but no thought disorder. She does not have the abnormal, eccentric personality described in classic cases. There are a number of differences between her presentation and Case 3:
• The time frame between being well and unwell was better defined: no prodrome
• As with many assessments of older people, a home visit was pivotal
• Poor hearing may have been a factor in the development of hallucinations
• The patient became **worse** following initial (involuntary, hospital-based) interventions
• Physical examination and investigations were essential to making the diagnosis and monitoring for side-effects of treatment
• Family (in this case, the patient's children) became central to safe management
• Although Rose did not use illegal drugs, there were other obstacles to smooth management of symptoms (e.g. she refused a psychologist, denied being unwell)

Reference

Byrne, P. (2007) Managing the acute psychotic episode. *BMJ* **334**, 686–692.

Further reading

Karim, S. & Byrne, E.J. (2005) Treatment of psychosis in an elderly person. *Advances in Psychiatric Treatment* **11**, 286–296.

Picchioni, M.M. & Murray, R.M. (2007) Schizophrenia. *BMJ* **335**, 91–95.

Schultz, S.K., Ho, B. & Andreasen, N.C. (2000) Clinical features characterizing young-onset and intermediate-onset schizophrenia. *Journal of Neuropsychiatry and Clinical Neurosciences* **12**, 502–505.

A 64-year-old retired teacher's depression is getting worse

Sajida is a 64-year-old mother of four who has lived alone since being widowed 2 years ago. Her GP, Dr Taylor, started her on selective serotonin reuptake inhibitor (SSRI) antidepressants 6 months ago when she presented complaining of poor sleep and lack of appetite. She did not respond and a psychiatrist started her on venlafaxine 3 months later. Her family have now contacted Dr Taylor and requested a home visit, concerned that Sajida's depression is worse and she has taken to her bed. Dr Taylor finds Sajida upstairs in bed, wishing to be 'left alone to die'. On examination, she is pale, tachycardic (pulse 112 beats/min, weak and thready), blood pressure 110/70 mmHg; postural drop 70/40 mmHg. Dr Taylor called an ambulance but Sajida says she does not want to go to hospital.

You are the on-call psychiatrist and Dr Taylor calls you from Sajida's house to ask your advice about an urgent assessment under the Mental Health Act. What do you advise Dr Taylor?

From her presentation, it is clear that whatever the cause, Sajida is physically unwell and needs urgent medical review.

It seems unlikely from what you know so far that Sajida has the **capacity** to make this decision about accepting or refusing medical treatment; Dr Taylor needs to make this decision for her. You might discuss with Dr Taylor how to assess her capacity in this regard (Box 12, Table 21, p. 70).

Dr Taylor confirms that Sajida does not have capacity to refuse treatment, and decides that treating her against her expressed wish (i.e. to be left to die) is in her best interests.

What do you advise?

Sajida must be brought to hospital for urgent medical treatment under the Mental Capacity Act, not the Mental Health Act (as Case 5).

Actions taken must be documented alongside the evidence for her failing any tests of capacity.

KEY POINT

The Mental Capacity Act 2005 protects people who lack capacity. It's principles are (i) capacity is assumed until proven otherwise, (ii) decision-making ability must be optimized, (iii) people are entitled to make unwise decisions, i.e., it is the decision making process not the decision that determines capacity, (iv) decisions made for people without capacity must be in their best interests, and (v) entail the least restrictive option(s).

Sajida is admitted to a medical ward for intravenous fluids and physical monitoring. Her urea and electrolytes (U&Es) are abnormal, and she is found to be borderline hypothyroid. While on the medical ward you are asked to review her, and in particular whether they should continue prescribing the serotonin and noradrenaline reuptake inhibitor (SNRI) antidepressant venlafaxine.

What is your advice about antidepressant treatment?

Hypothyroidism may have precipitated and/or complicated depression, and must be treated. As for venlafaxine – either this was not working or she was not taking it. It is known to cause high blood pressure in some individuals (Table 7, p. 17), but is unlikely to be the cause of her physical difficulties. She should continue this for now.

Her computed tomography (CT) head scan is unremarkable and her electrolyte balance is corrected. The medical team declares her physically fit for discharge from their care. You discuss admission to a psychiatric ward with Sajida but she refuses, again insisting she should be left to die.

Box 12 Capacity – what every doctor needs to know

The test for capacity is outlined in Table 21, p. 70.

1   Medicolegally, capacity is *assumed* until proven otherwise
2   In testing capacity it is not enough to ask a patient if they understand or remember what you have said. You must *demonstrate* that they do. Patients will often say 'yes' to doctors, out of embarrassment, confusion or politeness. You must also give them an opportunity to ask questions
3   To demonstrate a patient has understood and *retained* information you can ask them to repeat what you have said after you have said it (e.g. 'It's important that I know whether you've understood the advice I've given you. Please could you repeat back to me in your own words what you've understood of what I've just said about this treatment.')
4   To know whether they can *recall* the information, you need to leave 5 minutes or so before asking them again, by which point the brain needs to have 'laid down' the information in their *long-term memory*
5   A patient does not need to agree with the doctor to achieve capacity, but they must demonstrate the ability to *weigh up* information – even if they do not come to the same conclusions as their doctors
6   Capacity is *situation specific*. An individual may therefore have the capacity to make one decision but not another, depending on the nature of that decision and what is required to make it. For example, someone unwell with schizophrenia might not be able to weigh up information relating to treatment for their psychosis (perhaps due to delusional beliefs), but may retain capacity to make an informed choice about surgery offered for a physical illness

7   If someone lacks capacity with regards to a specific issue, then you, their doctor, need to take a view as to what – on balance – is in their *best interests*. This will involve identifying all possible outcomes from the various choices involved
8   It is good practice to obtain a *second opinion* from another doctor (as here)
9   *Advanced directives* document an individual's treatment preferences at a time when they have capacity to state what these are. They therefore stand as a record of an individual's decisions made in advance of a hypothesized situation in future when that decision will need to be made. For example, someone may make an advanced directive that they do or do not wish to have ECT if they become severely unwell. Clinicians are obliged to take advanced directives into account. However, they are not legally binding and can be overridden if circumstances (e.g. available treatments) have changed in a way that could not be or were not anticipated by the patient at the time of writing the directive. They can also be overridden if the Mental Health Act has been invoked, or the directive directs the clinician to do something they do not consider to be in the individual's best interests, or even illegal (e.g. euthanasia). In these situations, seek legal advice
10   Doctors should not make capacity decisions in isolation: involve other health professionals (ward nurses, psychologists and occupational therapists) in documented multidisciplinary team discussions, as well as the patient's family.

How might you proceed?

Sajida needs admission to a psychiatric ward but as she is refusing she needs to be assessed for admission under a section of the Mental Health Act (MHA 1983). Collateral history from Sajida's family and Dr Taylor would be helpful at this point.

Dr Taylor tells you Sajida has a history of past depression recorded on the computer system. Her thyroid function was normal when she presented with low mood 6 months ago. Dr Taylor notes that Sajida did not attend the surgery to pick up a repeat prescription for venlafaxine, which was only given in 2 weeks' supply, 3 months ago. Sajida did not attend for a follow-up appointment as suggested by him. You manage to contact Sajida's daughter, Sophie, by telephone. She has limited time to talk.

What might you prioritize enquiring about during this first conversation with Sophie?

• What does Sophie know about recent events?
• Does she know when, how or why Sajida started to deteriorate?
• What made her depression (documented by Dr Taylor) better before?
• Does Sajida have any past history of suicidal behaviour?

KEY POINT

For many patients, collateral history early on can prevent needless repetition of questions, investigations and treatments – for some, it will be life-saving.

Sophie tells you as far as she knows her mother had a 'serious break-down' after the birth of her last child, Sophie's sister Louise, 20 years ago. Sajida tried to kill herself at the time by taking an overdose, and was in hospital for months subsequently. During this time, she received 'shock treatment' and medication. Sajida has not seen a psychiatrist or had other psychological treatment since then, but Sophie says there have been several periods when Sajida has been 'down' and the family worried about her. Sajida is transferred to your psychiatric ward under Section 2 of the MHA. She is still choosing to stay in bed and says she wants to die.

What do you prioritize in her management on her first day on your ward?

• Your priority is to establish her *physical baseline* on arrival to the ward – pulse, BP, U&Es – and to monitor her closely. She will need daily physical observations, weekly weights and U&Es, as well as regular thyroid checks
• Her *oral intake* of food and fluids is likely to remain poor. Advise nursing staff to monitor this using an intake/out-take chart. She may also need to be supervised while eating, and to be encouraged to eat and drink by nurses. Weigh her twice weekly to exclude dehydration or monitor for heart failure (she will retain fluid)
• You need to decide on her level of *nursing observations*. This is determined by her clinical need, including level of risk to herself and/or other people. Initially at least she will require close (eyesight) observations. While there is no evidence she poses a risk to others, her suicide risk cannot yet be established. The degree of her depression, her stated wish to die and her history of overdose are of serious concern and indicate her risk needs to be closely monitored
• *Medication:* either she did not take venlafaxine (for whatever reason – but nausea and headache are common side-effects) or it did not work. In the context of poor sleep and appetite, you might prescribe the SNRI mirtazapine
• Given how unwell she is, Sajida should **not** have any *freedom to leave the ward* at the current time. Although she is not yet requesting to go anywhere, if this changes, pre-empt this in her notes and document your refusal of leave
• Discuss your management plan above with the nurse in charge of the shift and ensure your *documentation* in the notes is clear and unambiguous.

Over the next 2 days Sajida remains uncommunicative. One of the nurses establishes some communication with her, and Sajida confides that she has committed a terrible crime and deserves to die. The nurse asked her why she feels like that, and Sajida replied she could hear people telling her so. The nurses also tell you that Sajida is sleeping very poorly and eating little. Sajida has now had 3 days' treatment of mirtazapine.

Should you increase her mirtazapine?

It is too early for a response to the antidepressant, and increasing it at this stage is unlikely to speed her recovery. There is no evidence that increasing an antidepressant dose *during the first 4 weeks* of treatment is helpful. The evidence for benefit from increases after that point is equivocal.

KEY POINT

Increases in psychiatric medication are sometimes made prematurely because of professionals' anxiety over the length of time patients take to respond. If someone needs temporary relief (e.g. from severe insomnia), then short-term medications such as hypnotics can be prescribed specifically for this purpose.

From what you now know, Sajida has severe depression with psychotic features and therefore it may be helpful to add an antipsychotic to her antidepressant treatment. As she has no history of treatment (successful or otherwise) with antipsychotics, your choice should be determined by side-effect profile. Again, it might be helpful to prescribe a medication that can sometimes stimulate weight gain and promote sleep (e.g. olanzapine).

A week later, the nurses express their concern to you that Sajida is no better and her oral intake remains minimal. Her cardiovascular observations are stable but her U&Es have started to deteriorate.

How might you proceed?

Antidepressants and antipsychotics can take some weeks to work; however, one hopes for some (albeit possibly marginal) improvement over the first week of treatment. Check whether nurses are confident she is actually swallowing the medication.

The nurses inform you they are confident Sajida is swallowing the tablets.

Table 23 Electroconvulsive therapy (ECT) – what patients and relatives need to know.

	Information	Possible questions
Evidence	ECT is the single most tested psychiatric treatment in independent randomized controlled trials	How does it work? Probably by changing neurotransmitter activity through inducing a controlled seizure
Work-up	Two psychiatrists, anaesthetist, nursing staff document patients' physical and mental state	Safeguards? All units must meet minimum safety standards before ECT is allowed on the premises
Preparation	General anaesthetic plus muscle relaxant are administered in a fasting patient	Safety? Anaesthetist assesses patient beforehand and monitors vital signs throughout
Procedure	Electrodes applied to forehead, laterally. EEG records seizure activity during the procedure	Which type? Bilateral more efficacious but unilateral has less memory effects
Dose of ECT	The lowest possible dose of electricity is applied	How strong? The seizure threshold falls after each application, allowing a lowering of the electrical dose with subsequent treatments
What we see	Controlled seizure: no gross limb movements because of muscle relaxant	Drugs ensure physical damage (bruises to limbs, tongue biting) is unlikely with the procedure. ECT does not cause epilepsy
How often?	Twice per week for between 6 and 12 treatments	ECT does not cause structural brain changes
Medication	Usually continues during treatments	Some medications are stopped as they make it harder to induce a seizure: benzodiazepines, anticonvulsants.
Side-effects	Side-effects of anaesthesia, headache, short-term memory effects. Physical injury rare	Mortality is 2 per 100,000 treatments – equal to that for general anaesthesia
Outcome	ECT is more effective than antidepressants	Failure to respond is uncommon and individual contingency plans need to be formulated

At this point you need to initiate a discussion about electroconvulsive therapy (ECT; Table 23). If possible, establish Sajida's views of her previous ECT, her family's views and the views of the nurses and other colleagues. There is much misinformation around ECT, *including amongst health professionals*, so it is important that any misunderstandings can be addressed and people have an opportunity to air their concerns.

How do you respond to family concerns about ECT in a way that makes sense to them?

You need to explain how ECT works and why it is not like the procedure seen in films. While outlining the positive evidence for its use, you must also be trans-parent about the risks and potential for side-effects. You will need therefore to cover the following points:

• ECT has been known as a useful treatment for severe depression since the 1930s, but there are many public misconceptions about its effects (Table 23)

• She has at least two of three predictors of good response to ECT in depression: psychomotor retardation, delusions and a history of good response to ECT

• Usually, any memory difficulties brought about by ECT are transient but some patients experience longer-term difficulties with their memory that they attribute to the treatment. An assessment of cognitive function (e.g. MMSE, Case 5) is completed before the start of treatment and reviewed as treatment progresses and at the end of treatment

KEY POINT

The potential benefit of ECT needs to be balanced against potential risk of that patient having a general anaesthetic and possible memory problems. In a severely unwell patient (as here), the risk of *not* giving ECT must also be considered. NB

ELDERLY → EGFR↓ → ECT AVOIDS
EXCESS STRESS on RENAL SYSTEM (MEOW)

You discuss with Sajida and her family that the risk of ECT for her must be balanced against the risk of continuing with the current situation, which is deteriorating; there is a significant risk here that Sajida may die if things continue as they are.

Should ECT be given against her will?

As Sajida is currently too unwell to give informed consent to having ECT (i.e. she lacks the capacity to do so), she needs to be assessed as to whether she needs to have it under the MHA.

ECT can only be given with the patient's informed consent *or* following a second opinion from an independent psychiatrist appointed by the Mental Health Act Commission. The psychiatrist giving the second opinion usually attends within a few days.

KEY POINT

If ECT is urgent (i.e. the patient is life-threateningly unwell) and in the consultant's view ECT cannot wait for a second opinion to be provided before starting, then up to two ECT treatments can be given as emergency treatment.

Sajida is seen by a second opinion psychiatrist who agrees the proposed ECT is indicated and signs the documentation for up to 12 treatments. Sajida subsequently receives her first treatment of ECT, after which her daughter Sophie contacts you to say she is worried Sajida seemed drowsy and confused immediately after the treatment and now seems no better.

What will you advise Sophie?

Sajida was likely to be drowsy and confused after the treatment because of the general anaesthetic. You reassure her that this wears off.

It is too early to assess her response to ECT after one treatment; people need to have several treatments before

they start to improve. You will be reviewing Sajida before each ECT to monitor her mental state, her response and any side-effects of the treatment.

Sajida continues to receive ECT on a twice weekly basis for 3 weeks. Nurses first report a very small improvement after the third treatment. She then gradually starts to eat more, becomes much more communicative and is no longer hearing any voices. She is also sleeping a little better. Although improved, she still appears depressed. She requests that the ECT be stopped because she does not like having the anaesthetic.

What do you advise Sajida?

ECT should only be continued as long as there is a continued indication to do so. The potential benefit of continuing treatment needs to be balanced against the risks (Box 12).

Although Sajida is far from recovered, she is no longer severely unwell. Given her preference to now stop ECT and the evidence that a treatment response has occurred, it should be stopped. She will continue to require close monitoring on the ward while she remains on medication and her progress continues.

Given Sajida's progress, one of your colleagues decided to reduce Sajida's level of nursing observation so she is on intermittent, as opposed to continuous nursing observation. The next afternoon nurses notice that she has been in the bathroom for a prolonged period and is not opening the door. They unlock the door from the outside – ward door locks are designed for this purpose – with their ward key and find Sajida sitting on the toilet with a ligature around her neck that she has made from a knotted bed sheet.

KEY POINT

In the short-term management of depressed and psychotic patients, attend to **intolerable symptoms** (e.g. agitation, hopelessness and/or guilt, command hallucinations, recurrent obsessions, extreme anxiety).

What do you do?

It appears Sajida was attempting to hang herself so she needs to be physically examined to ensure she has not had any respiratory compromise or harmed herself in any way. Once this is established (assuming that she does not need urgent medical review to assess the effects of possible asphyxia), Sajida will need to be seen by you and an experienced nurse on the ward to discuss what happened, and to offer her emotional support.

This incident does not mean ECT should restart for Sajida, it simply means she needs close continuous nursing observations for the time being to ensure her safety as well as regular medical review of her treatment (biological and psychological). Risk of suicide is not static during an illness episode: it needs to be regularly monitored throughout the treatment process.

The incident should be reported to the appropriate health and safety authority in the hospital as a serious clinical incident: potentially, it could have resulted in Sajida's death. All wards should have been safety checked to ensure that they do not have ligature points from which patients can hang themselves, and in this case it appears that she was indeed unable to find one.

The circumstances in which the decision to take her off close observations was made need to be reviewed. With hindsight, this was an error, and needs to be reviewed in case it should have been preventable or anticipated. This does not mean blaming individuals but does merit examination of the systems used to make important decisions.

Support your ward colleagues. The experience of a patient's suicide, or a 'near miss', is a dreadful one for everyone. Staff can feel blamed or take on the guilt. Explore who else was involved in the incident. Remember, other patients can experience mixed feelings about a failed suicide on the ward.

KEY POINT

Severely depressed patients can be at their highest risk of suicide when they begin to improve. Patients who are severely depressed often lack the cognitive organization or energy (mental or physical) to be able to formulate a plan and act on it. Treatment can improve their ability to do so before their depressed mood improves. The early stages of improvement are therefore a high-risk period.

Sajida makes slow but steady progress over the next 6 weeks. Her affect has become more reactive, she starts to talk of the future, and makes plans for going home. She becomes more involved in ward activities, including occupational therapy. She also interacts far more with staff and other patients, and starts leaving the ward regularly for trips home to see her grandchildren.

What aftercare will you arrange?

Sajida's diagnosis is that of *recurrent depressive disorder* (remember her past history) and this episode has been a **severe** one *with psychotic features* (p. 47). She is at high risk of further episodes.

Advise that to reduce risk of relapse, people who have experienced *one* depressive episode need to continue with medication for *at least 6 months* after they recover. Given Sajida's history of previous episodes, the psychosis component, its severity and slow recovery, her risk is far higher. You recommend she continues with treatment for a year, and remains in contact with her community mental health team for regular reviews. After a year she could make a decision about ongoing treatment with her psychiatrist. Although people are often keen to stop tablets, the risk of doing so needs to be weighed up carefully with her at that point.

Follow-up appointments will determine if her mood stays at this current level. If it does not, one option might be lithium augmentation (Table 15, p. 49), that is, lithium in addition to her current antidepressant.

Now that Sajida has improved, she can consider whether she would be interested in receiving psychological treatment such as cognitive–behavioural therapy (CBT), which she could receive in the community after discharge. CBT will identify relapse prevention strategies – ideally involving her wider family.

KEY POINT

Talking therapies (e.g. individual, CBT, groups) also work for older people.

On the negative side, studies have identified subsequent higher rates of dementia and higher mortality rates (not from suicide, but cardiovascular causes) in older people who develop depression.

Risk factors for suicide will be considered again in the next case and Table 25, p. 92.

CASE REVIEW

Despite the best efforts of her GP (early recognition and treatment, prompt specialist referral leading to a second line antidepressant, follow-up to monitor response to medications, and carrying out thyroid screening at first presentation), Sajida deteriorated to a life-threatening state of severe depression with (initially and then laterally) hidden psychotic features. Admission to hospital and a range of appropriate treatments is no guarantee that patients will improve. Many psychiatric interventions are, or should be, about **negotiation**:

- Advice about capacity supported Dr Taylor's decision to admit her
- The medical team's discharge facilitated the beginning of your interventions
- MHA assessments included open discussion with colleagues
- Examination of her clinical details agreed observation levels with the nurses
- Open discussions of Sajida's treatment with her and both her children
- Once Sajida had improved, she negotiated ECT cessation with you

- You spoke with everyone (patient, relatives, other patients and ward staff) following Sajida's attempted suicide on the ward

When her physical and mental state changed, her suicidal ideas also changed. Cases such as these are always easier to understand with hindsight, but the lesson here is for *at least* daily assessment of suicidality in at-risk patients. She has only two protective factors against suicide: female gender and her children, now grown up. Sajida's risk factors for completed suicide are:

- History of previous suicide attempt – also directly related to low mood
- Older age
- Widowed
- Current severe depression
- Intolerable symptoms: guilt, delusions of being poisoned
- Current medical illness
- Incapacity to change her environment: prisoners have the highest suicide rate of any single group

Further reading

Baldwin, R. & Wild, R. (2004) Management of depression in later life. *Advances in Psychiatric Treatment* **10**, 24–30.

Bellhouse, J., Holland, A., Clare, I. & Gunn, M. (2001) Decision-making capacity in adults: assessment in clinical practice. *Advances in Psychiatric Treatment* **7**, 294–301.

Ottosson, J. & Fink, M. (2004) *Ethics in Electroconvulsive Therapy*. Brenner-Routledge, New York.

Porter, R., Linsley, K. & Ferrier, N. (2001) Treatment of severe depression: non-pharmacological aspects. *Advances in Psychiatric Treatment* **7**, 117–124.

PART 2: CASES

Case 8 | A 17-year-old man has been cutting his arms

Tony is brought to the A&E department one night by his mother. He has no psychiatric history, but has been attending a dermatologist for 2 years. He has psoriasis. Last night his mother noticed blood on his shirtsleeves. She says there are scars on his arms and fresh blood from recent cuts. You are the duty psychiatrist called to assess him.

What are your first thoughts?

The most likely explanation here is deliberate self-harm (DSH). His mother's account of old scars on his arms and new cuts makes it unlikely he will be able to deny that he has been cutting himself, but you will need to establish a good rapport with him to find out – in a non-judgemental way – why he has been doing this.

Less likely causes are that:
• His psoriasis has been itching to an extent that he has scratched these lesions with his fingernails, or
• Someone else has been cutting him. This might occur in a dysfunctional relationship (overly close with bizarre shared beliefs, use of cult internet sites or even a suicide pact) or an abusive one (bullying, extortion). Open questions followed up by clarification (closed) ones, combined with inspection of his arms, will decide on the cause of his cuts

KEY POINT

DSH is defined as a non-fatal act in which an individual deliberately causes self-injury (e.g. cutting or ingesting a substance in excess of prescribed doses).

The A&E Matron is grateful you have come to assess him but has no available room and wants him assessed quickly in the cubicle where he is.

What is your response?

Be polite. Anyone can do a speedy psychiatric assessment in any environment and come up with the wrong diag-

nosis, missing important psychopathology or jumping to the wrong conclusions.

There is clear guidance about this from the National Institute for Health and Clinical Excellence (www.nice.org.uk): 'If a person who has self-harmed has to wait for treatment, he or she should be offered an environment that is safe, supportive and minimises any distress . . . with regular contact with a named member of staff.' A&E units have signed up to this at a national level. He has been managed in an adequate environment until now, and you should acknowledge this to the Matron. You need access to a private, safe and secure room to carry out a comprehensive psychosocial assessment.

Tony's mother is upset. She says he never trusts or confides in anyone, and will lie his way out of A&E. She accuses him of manipulation and insists that she should sit in on your interview. Tony wants the security guards to remove her from the hospital.

What will you do?

Be very polite. DSH is difficult to understand – people who self-harm are often confused as to their own motives. To family and friends, their behaviour can appear to be stupid, provocative, even manipulative. Never use terms like 'manipulative' even if there appears to have been a planned attempt to make others suffer as a result of their self-harm.

It is not just parents who get angry: A&E staff can regard these clients as an unwelcome distraction from 'real patients', and mental health professionals may have similar attitudes. Make it clear to her that you understand why she is upset, but that your priority is to find out why Tony has been doing this, and negotiate the best way forward to prevent more cutting, or worse.

Your first assessment needs to be one-to-one and, at 17 years old, he has a right to privacy. However, you might tell his mother that you will attempt to persuade him to allow her to attend the second part of the interview. Make it clear that her concerns will be addressed, while respecting his privacy.

The possibility of suspiciousness and reluctance to trust anyone might suggest paranoid personality traits (Table 24). More likely explanations are that Tony is a normal, disaffected teenager or that there are difficulties in his relationship with his mother.

> **KEY POINT**
>
> It is unwise to diagnose a personality disorder (Box 13) at one meeting, much less during an emergency assessment or crisis. It takes time to gather evidence that people are not functioning across multiple domains in the ways they think, feel, behave and in relationships.

Tony does not have paranoid traits (Table 24). In fact, he does not meet any criteria for personality disorder (Box 13). His mother accepts your advice but wants a 'quick word' with you before you see him. Tony gives his permission for this.

What will you discuss?

Begin by asking her what her concerns are. The suicide of their child is a parent's worst fear, and many parents are convinced DSH is the beginning of a long psychiatric 'career' for their children. With these concerns come many misconceptions about mental illness and its treatment. Take time to explore these – Tony may share her beliefs and experiences.

> **Box 13 Criteria to establish the diagnosis of personality disorder**
>
> ICD-10 diagnosis of *any* personality disorder requires that:
> * The individual has enduring problematic patterns of *cognition, inner experience, behaviour* and *ways of relating to others*
> * Traits must have been present in adolescence and persisted unchanged until adulthood
> * There must be severe disturbances in character and behaviour, involving several different areas (affect, impulse control, relationships)
> * The combination of traits must lead to 'considerable personal and social disruption'
> * Patterns must be pervasive, and not context-specific
> * Traits must fall outside cultural norms

Give broad contextual advice. DSH is common (5% lifetime prevalence) and for most people where there are clear precipitants, it will be a one-off event. If you can work with Tony to identify these precipitants and help him improve his coping skills and resilience, DSH is less likely to recur.

A proportion of DSH patients have treatable psychiatric illness. It is in Tony's best interests to have this treated, and this will reduce further DSH.

With all 'first episode' DSH patients, further DSH is a definite possibility and there are risks of future suicide; this is why your assessment is important. If these are worrying findings, they must be addressed. Avoid giving anxious relatives false hope of total cure.

Table 24 Paranoid personality disorder: diagnosis and psychodynamic understanding.

ICD-10 criteria	Psychodynamic understanding (Gabbard 1994)
Tenacious sense of personal rights; self-referential attitude with excessive self-importance	Poor sense of self: oversensitive to potential humiliation by others + grandiose ('special') feelings as compensation
Excessive sensitivity to setbacks and rebuffs; preoccupation with 'conspiratorial' explanations of events in immediate environment and the world at large	Assume all relationships will end in disappointment + inability to interpret relationships (e.g. cannot reflect on a relationship setback but decide 'You're just like my cruel mother')
Suspiciousness, pervasive tendency to view neutral actions as hostile	Splitting (extremes of thinking) is common: this is linked to a poorly developed sense of self (Box 8, p. 42)
Tendency to bear grudges; recurrent suspicions of sexual infidelity by spouse or partner – without justification	Thinking and relationship difficulties make them vulnerable to difficult break-ups, in extreme cases erotomania (this is a psychotic condition that is not part of paranoid personality)

This might be a useful time to obtain additional information from Tony's mother: birth and personal history, history of counselling and family history of psychiatric illness (we are told *he* has no *psychiatric* history), home and social factors, recent stressors or changes in behaviour, medical history and current medications. With regard to his psoriasis, how did this present? Did he accept his diagnosis or did he rebel against it? How has it affected him, including impairment of his social life? How does he get on with his dermatologist?

> **KEY POINT**
>
> In the 12 months following DSH, 10–30% of people will repeat DSH and 1% will kill themselves.

| *Tony agrees to be interviewed – without his mother.*

Identify possible reasons why he has been cutting his arms

• These are attempts to cut his radial artery and end his life (for whatever reason):

• To achieve relief from a situation or a problem for which he perceives there is 'no way out' other than DSH. Be alert that this is precisely the mind set of people who complete suicide

• To relieve tension. Some DSH patients who cut themselves see the cutting as the end-point in a series of stressors. It achieves some sort of closure for them in that the wounds/scars, not the stressors, become their focus. For some, the external consequences (e.g. medical interventions, arguments with family) and the guilt experienced are a welcome relief from the original stressors

• Sometimes, cutting, burning and other body mutilations are best seen as a type of self-administered punishment for an internalized sense of badness (e.g. as a result of sexual abuse). The DSH may perpetuate a cycle of guilt and low self-esteem in people with, for example, eating disorders and personality difficulties. Paradoxically, self-punishment is a recognized defence mechanism to reduce feelings of guilt. In depressed patients, guilt is mood congruent and DSH may be provoked by persistent distressing thoughts of suicide – as a defence *against* suicide, rather than a trial of it

• To 'experiment' to see how he feels. Some DSH patients say they harm 'to prove they exist'. He may feel he needs to show 'evidence' of his distress to others to prove how bad things are for him. Many qualitative studies have identified communication difficulties in DSH patients. In Tony's case, remember that the experiment has not finished; his mother brought him to A&E, and he may continue with risky DSH behaviours upon discharge

• Imitation is common in this age group. He may have seen someone with cuts directly, or been exposed to a media item (television, internet, picture or print media) where DSH took place. Up to 10% of DSH attempts and completed suicides have been linked with actual events and media representations of them

• For people who repeatedly DSH, cutting releases endorphins such that the act of cutting becomes partly a pleasurable experience

• It is possible he is trying to remove his psoriatic plaques from his arms rather than cutting as part of DSH? Be alert to the possibility that he may use this as a cover for more serious suicidal or self-harm behaviour

> **KEY POINT**
>
> There is rarely one reason why people cut or harm themselves. Psychosocial assessment records the combination of predisposing and precipitating factors, identifying needs and allowing estimation of the risks of future DSH and suicide.

You find an anxious affect and confirm scars, but there are no other abnormalities on mental state examination (MSE). Tony tells you he first attended the dermatologist with acne 2 years ago and after years of 'useless' creams and tablets, he was finally 'getting rid of it' 2 months ago with stronger tablets. However, then along came new skin problems (psoriatic plaques) which he cannot accept are happening to him.

What are your thoughts?

Self-harm could be an angry/bewildered response to the 'new', second skin illness. He has already experienced acne at a difficult time (early adolescence) and may have had complications (e.g. infections, bleeding, scarring) that caused social difficulties for him. List the consequences of acne for him. Try to identify avoidance patterns as well as more negative experiences such as bullying at school. His actual responses ('Why me? Not again') need to be explored.

There is a clue in the description of his acne (sudden improvement of symptoms on strong tablets) that should alert you to one possible precipitant of low mood.

Isotretinoin (Roaccutane) is a highly effective acne treatment that has been directly linked to low mood (Table 14, p. 47). This acne 'cure' could have been the precipitant of depression and thereby this episode of DSH.

Even if he has plausible explanations for this episode of DSH, clarify previous episodes that may have occurred with precipitants. These, rather than this current episode, may indicate a risk of future suicide attempts.

> **KEY POINT**
>
> The strongest predictor of suicide is a history of self-harm.

Tony does not fully account for this recent episode of DSH. He presents as distressed but denies depression, somewhat unconvincingly. You are worried about him.

What will you do now?

Think about other actions he may have committed prior to presenting, principally overdose. Paracetamol is the most common substance taken in overdose because of its availability. He will need to have visited more than one outlet to buy several packets because of (highly effective) legislation to reduce its lethal use. Many A&E departments take blood for paracetamol levels routinely in all DSH admissions. He may have access to dermatological medications (steroids, methotrexate) and other lethal drugs. Glucometer readings, serum drug levels and urine testing (for legal and illegal drugs) are all easily available in his current setting and these are best considered now, prior to discharge home or possible transfer to a psychiatric setting.

Tony has three of the four individual level predictors of repeated self-harm in the next 6 months: DSH (this episode), being unemployed and being single. The fact that he does not have the fourth risk factor, previous psychiatric treatment, could merely reflect his unwillingness to attend for psychiatric contact. He has already had negative experiences with his dermatologist.

He is distressed and this is his first presentation, with clear risk to himself. His home environment is supportive, but you have seen that he has not been getting on with his mother. Assess for any suicidal intent (Table 27) and any additional risk factors for contemplated suicide (Table 25): your management plan needs to address these.

> **KEY POINT**
>
> While many people who DSH attend voluntarily for treatment, some will conceal their DSH but attend for its consequences: drowsiness, nausea, vomiting, abdominal discomfort, even jaundice (paracetamol overdose), pain or bleeding.

Further disclosures from Tony and normal results from your investigations reassure you that there is no immediate risk of repeated DSH or suicide. Tony is not depressed and you have identified precipitants of his DSH other than his skin condition and poor maternal relationship: he failed to get his 'dream job' despite a second interview with a well-known recording studio.

What are the criteria for the diagnosis of adjustment disorder?

- States of subjective distress arising in the period of adaptation to a significant life change (e.g. migration) or life event (here – the onset of psoriasis and the disappointment of two job interviews)
- The emotional disturbance (anxiety or unhappiness or both) interferes with social functioning, with disability in the performance of daily routine
- Behaviour changes are likely, and in adolescents DSH and violence (to property and people) occur more frequently than other age groups
- Symptoms arise within 1 month of the life event or change, and do not exceed 6 months' duration. About 40% of adjustment disorders fail to resolve and progress to depressive episodes
- There must be presumptive evidence that the disorder would *not* have occurred without the life event or life change
- Individual vulnerability determines the occurrence, nature and severity of adjustment disorders
- Examples and subtypes of adjustment disorders are set out in Table 26

Identify his risk factors for future suicide. How you might remediate them?

While we cannot change what has already happened, we can identify ways to identify future crises earlier, support Tony during these, increase his communication with others, improve existing coping skills and reduce his

Table 25 Risk factors for suicide

Biological factors	
Demographic factors	Men; peaks in adolescence, larger peak in old age
Genetic	Family history of suicide, DSH and psychiatric illness; pathway thought to be serotinergic – also implicated in aggressive and impulsive behaviours
Low birth weight	May act by association with poor obstetric factors, or via its association with later life psychiatric illness
Neurological conditions	All chronic neurological conditions: cerebrovascular accident, epilepsy, multiple sclerosis, head injury, etc.
Medical conditions	Arthritis and other painful conditions, cancer and any terminal illness, HIV infection
Alcohol and substance misuse	Two-thirds of completed suicides have taken these as part of their final act
Medications	Principally, those causing depression (Table 14, p. 47)
Psychological factors	
Childhood losses	Poor bonding/insecure attachments; early losses/bereavement; childhood sexual abuse
Personality traits	Dysfunctional adaptation to adverse events
Problem-solving skills	Higher educational attainment is protective
Life events	Recent losses with a strong subjective component
Help-seeking behaviours	Low in men, higher in women (lower suicide rates)
Inability to change environment	Highest in prisoners, including those awaiting trial
Any psychiatric illness	Primarily depression and schizophrenia
Social factors	
Cultural acceptability	Both unacceptability of suicide and religious beliefs protect people
Social isolation	Divorced, separated and widowed people; motherhood protects, especially if stable partnership
Socioeconomic conditions	Relative poverty, unemployment, homelessness
Imitation (media)	Copycat suicides and suicide pacts common in young
Availability of lethal methods	Highest vocational group suicide rate is among doctors; excess of firearms suicides in USA

access to lethal methods (Table 27). This latter action means direct discussion with his mother about keeping medicines safely in their home.

In the absence of any biological factors save his gender (Table 25), you have identified psoriasis as a major factor here. Close liaison with his dermatologist (copy your correspondence to him/her and offer an interdisciplinary meeting) will help achieve better understanding of his physical illness for Tony. Psoriasis is a common skin condition (1.3% point prevalence) where only 3% of people with the disorder – those with the most disabling

lesions – consult a dermatologist. He may lack a balanced perspective about the illness in general and how it affects him in particular.

A major life event (failure to obtain a job) along with his current unemployment are also risk factors. Having left school prematurely, Tony has reduced employment opportunities. Ideally, a vocational rehabilitation specialist (p. 25) can help him with training, preparation of his resumé, part-time or voluntary work as a bridge from never-worked to the workplace, choice of the best options and interview skills practice. These tasks can be achieved

Table 26 Examples of adjustment disorders (ICD-10).

Example	Criteria	Outcome
1. Grief reaction	Must exceed 6 months' duration; these are best categorized under 3 and 4 below – noting the bereavement as precipitant	Usually good, but can be compounded by additional bereavements during the period of grief. Excess physical morbidity
2. Brief depressive reaction	Mild depressive state that does not exceed 1 month	Self-limiting
3. Prolonged depressive reaction	Mild depressive state of more than 1 month but not exceeding 2 years. Exposure to stressor also prolonged	Good. Social functioning impaired but person can continue to work/study at a reasonable level
4. Mixed anxiety and depressive reaction	Symptoms related to life event or change but do not meet criteria for mixed anxiety and depressive disorder	Good. Social functioning impaired but person can continue to work/study at a reasonable level
In adolescents and children		
5. Adjustment disorders with predominant disturbance of other emotions	Predominant symptoms of anxiety, low mood, worry, tension and anger. In older children, regressive behaviours (e.g. bed wetting and thumb sucking) are common	Good. Collaborative working with patient's family to remove ongoing stressors and minimize their effects achieves results if started early
6. Adjustment disorders with predominant disturbance of conduct	Dissocial and aggressive behaviours – including self-harm	Fair. Apart from DSH, these patients may present to police and probation services first
7. Adjustment disorders with predominant disturbance of emotions and conduct	Combinations of previous two categories	Fair to good
8. Adjustment disorders with other specified predominant symptoms	A diagnosis of exclusion: neither emotional or conduct disturbances feature	Varies

by others, but it is worth noting that his tactics so far (for whatever reason) have failed to deliver for him.

His adjustment disorder has a 60% chance of resolution. You will need to set up periodic monitoring of his mood to identify any new depressive symptoms over the coming weeks. Such symptoms will *increase* his risk of future DSH and suicide. Either mental health services and/or his general practitioner can monitor his mood – preferably with a recognized mood instrument such as the Beck Depression Inventory. Persistent low mood needs to be vigorously treated with a combination of therapy and medication (Table 15, p. 49). You need to

strike a balance between monitoring and giving Tony the confidence to get on with his life.

> **KEY POINT**
>
> At the very least after an assessment, patients who self-harm need to feel 'linked in' to a named professional (a mental health professional, general practitioner, named nurse) who will support them during any future episodes.

Tony agrees to attend a psychologist to talk about his dermatological and other recent disappointments.

Table 27 Circumstances of self-harm suggesting high suicidal intent.

Mental state at time of attempt	Preparation details	Mental state exam currently
Suicidality: Record frequency and severity of **suicidal thoughts** When did **suicidal intent** form? Did this become constant? Define duration from intent to **suicide planning** and execution of plan	Settled affairs: debts paid, projects completed, ensured a written will Said goodbyes to others: often indirectly, but may have left letters for later discovery Suicide note and other statements of why they carried this out: internet sites are increasingly used to communicate finality	Appearance: distress, agitation. Look for evidence of discomfort or pain Speech: usually normal, but he/she might be slow to warm up during the interview Mood: depressed, hopelessness Suicidality: record current intent ('I am going to kill myself')
Record specific MSE findings (see third column) Alcohol and drug use: If intoxicated, was this part of the suicide plan? (lower risk if suicide intent and plan resulted from intoxication)	High risk : rescue ratio: record their perception of chosen method's lethality (violent methods, 'strength' of overdose) and details that made discovery less likely (no-one expected to call by, manufactured a 'cover story' such as going on holiday)	Affect: numb, severely anxious Record thoughts and beliefs about attempt Identify psychotic symptoms: are there delusional beliefs about suicide? If hallucinating are these command ('kill yourself?'), derogatory
Insight: into pre-existing psychiatric illness	High expectation of completed suicide	Lack of insight ('I will never be well again') or full insight (symptoms of psychosis or mood have not responded to treatment)

In the light of what you now know about him, what sort of psychotherapy would you recommend to Tony?

The ideal intervention here is brief, supportive and focused on his existing problems. For some people, DSH reflects relationship difficulties. If there is mutual commitment to the relationship, couples therapy (p. 22) may be a useful way to reduce future DSH.

In young people with adjustment disorders (Table 26), systemic family therapy (p. 22) may be more useful than one-to-one interventions. There is no specific indication for group therapy in cases like Tony's.

Referral to the therapist should detail your assessment of his personality and his motivation for therapy.

There are three broad options for one-to-one therapy:

1 Cognitive–behavioural therapy (CBT) addresses how people think about and react to events using empirical investigation (of maladaptive interpretations) and reality testing. It aims to change the way people respond to disappointments to protect against low mood and anxiety
2 Problem solving therapy (PST) is a variant on CBT that aims to achieve specific goals, chosen by the patient, over eight sessions
3 Psychodynamic therapy has many variations. Its principal focus is on defence mechanisms and previous losses (especially in childhood; Box 8, p. 42)

CASE REVIEW

DSH has a lifetime prevalence of about 5%. It is the most common cause of a general hospital admission in young people although, across most age spans, more women than men carry out self-harm. Over 90% of DSH patients present with overdose, but some people self-harm and overdose in the same presentation. We know DSH patients have difficulties communicating their distress (partly explaining *why* they DSH) and managing their emotions. Judging them to be 'manipulators' is unhelpful. You need to identify underlying mechanisms that lead to self-harm in individuals.

These are difficult interviews, with many outside pressures on them and you; open questions with plenty of time produce the safest assessments. Just because the crisis resolved here does not mean than we can 'play down' impulsive suicidal acts in young people. People will minimize difficulties to get home and we know such patients are poor communicators. Tony's presentation has a beginning, middle and an end, but this is unusual for the majority of cases of self-injury (see Further reading if you are regularly assessing this vulnerable patient group).

Assess DSH patients to define their *needs*, many of which will also be their *risk factors* (Table 25). These are the best potential targets of interventions. Every assessment is different, and so are the management plans and ultimate outcomes.

Reference

Gabbard, G. (1994) *Psychodynamic Psychiatry in Clinical Practice*. American Psychiatric Press, Washington DC.

Further reading

Broadhurst, M. & Gill, P. (2007) Repeated self-injury from a liaison psychiatry perspective. *Advances in Psychiatric Treatment* **13**, 228–235.

Fagin, L. (2006) Repeated self-injury: perspectives from general psychiatry. *Advances in Psychiatric Treatment* **12**, 193–201.

Gunnell, D. & Lewis, G. (2005) Studying suicide from a life course perspective: implications for prevention. *British Journal of Psychiatry* **187**, 206–208.

Johnson, A., Cooper, J., Webb, R. & Kapur, N. (2006) Individual- and area-level predictors of self-harm repetition. *British Journal of Psychiatry* **189**, 416–421.

Ng, C.H. & Schweitzer, I. (2003) The association between depression and isotretinoin use in acne. *Australian and New Zealand Journal of Psychiatry* **37**, 78–84.

Case 9 A 9-year-old disruptive child faces expulsion from school

You are working at a child psychiatry clinic, helping with urgent assessments. A GP phones you about 9-year-old Miguel under her care. He has been suspended from schools on two previous occasions – once for fighting and latterly for stealing. His parents have been keeping him under 'house arrest' for the past 3 months. The current crisis began when he was suspended from school for cruelty to the classroom pets.

What is your differential diagnosis? List likely and unlikely diagnoses
Likely diagnoses

1 *Conduct disorder* (CD) is a pattern of persistent dissocial, aggressive or defiant behaviours. Three discrete episodes and different norm violations have been described in Miguel's behaviour, and you must determine these behaviours are established and not a response to external events, or bad luck (e.g. he was wrongly blamed for stealing). There is frequent comorbidity with other psychiatric conditions (see below). Other examples of dissocial behaviours include destruction of property, fire-setting, lying, truancy and running away from home. CD can be confined to the family context, and it can be **socialized** (good relationships with peers) or **unsocialized** (no or poor peer relationships).

2 *Emotional disorder* seems less likely here: none of the behaviours described above occur commonly in this age group, unless as 'a cry for help' in a highly anxious child. If a child with an emotional disorder refuses to go to school because of fear of events there (e.g. bullying) or separation anxiety, this is *school refusal* rather than truancy. If Miguel has additional symptoms of anxiety with related phobic behaviour, the likely diagnosis here could be *mixed conduct and emotional disorder*. Mixed disorders tend to present and evolve closer to conduct than emotional disorders.

3 *Attention deficit disorder without hyperactivity* (ADD) is best seen as a final common pathway for known and unknown pathologies. There are many neuropsychiatric causes of impaired attention: learning disability, head injury, frontal lobe damage, psychosis, depression and severe anxiety. ADD has a strong genetic component with gene–environment interactions (e.g. excitable, chaotic, inattentive parents raise children with the same behaviours). Deficits in attention must be present in multiple tasks over time, where the child is well rested and not under excessive pressure. The behaviours must occur in many different settings: if they are limited to home *or* school, ADD is unlikely.

4 *Attention deficit disorder with hyperactivity* (ADHD) requires additional signs of restlessness and inability to remain calm in appropriate situations. These children fidget, wriggle, interrupt, make excessive noise, talk excessively and can be reckless to the point of endangering themselves. Be wary of a snap diagnosis; inattentive behaviours could be a response to ongoing stressors. Sustained behaviour of ADHD is difficult to miss, but other causes of development delay must be ruled out before the diagnosis can be made.

Unlikely diagnoses

1 All three behaviours (fighting, stealing and cruelty) could indicate the disinhibition of frontal lobe syndrome. You would expect to observe other signs of this (mood and personality changes, new onset temper tantrums, loss of initiative and socialization) and sequelae of its common causes in this age group (e.g. effects of primary brain tumours, space-occupying lesions, head injury). Careful history and exam with consultation with his GP should rule out this and other *organic pathology*.

2 These 'roller coaster' symptoms could be part of the intoxication and disinhibition caused by *substance misuse*. Depending on his location (urban/rural) and socioeconomic group, available drugs will vary. Consider solvents (glue), stimulants (cough mixtures), cannabis and benzodiazepines.

3 *Oppositional defiant disorder* (ODD) has a peak incidence in 9- and 10-year-olds. Behaviours are defiant, disobedient and/or provocative, but they are not aggressive or violent. Children with ODD tend to be resentful and angry, exhibiting excessive levels of rudeness, provocative behaviours and resistance to authority. They have a low frustration threshold and tend to blame others for their difficulties. Many children with ODD function well with peers and at school, but demonstrate their defiance at home: 'street angels, house devils'. ODD is probably a minor variant of CD. In this case, the highly dissocial and aggressive nature of his presenting symptoms excludes ODD.

4 Common mental disorders, *depression and anxiety*, can be diagnosed in any age group – provided they meet diagnostic criteria. If Miguel had mood and/or anxiety symptoms, mixed conduct and emotional disorder would better describe the nature of his difficulties and help develop an evidence-based management plan.

5 *Psychosis* is most uncommon in this age group and you would have to find good presumptive evidence of links between the aberrant behaviours and psychotic symptoms.

> **KEY POINT**
>
> Avoid stereotyping children with CD as 'bad kids' or 'junior psychopaths'. This is the ideal time to prevent a lifetime of dissocial acts.

How will aspects of Miguel's birth and developmental history help you to differentiate between the two likely diagnoses here, conduct or attention deficit disorder?

Complications in pregnancy/birth and delayed development support a diagnosis of ADD, but neither are essential. CD is best seen as a product of adverse social environments following normal development, although there are probable genetic influences on aggression and temperament.

Although he had normal milestones, Miguel has become a 'difficult middle child' according to his mother. His father wishes he could disown him for the hurt he has caused. He is an army officer, frequently assigned overseas, whose job has resulted in family relocation twice in the past 3 years. Miguel's 16-year-old sister lives alternate weeks with her natural father. Miguel's mother has spent much time recently on hospital visits with her 2-year-old son who has bilateral hip dislocations.

How might this information change your assessment or treatment plan?

If this is CD, it may have had a relatively short course with identifiable *and remediable* precipitants:

- Regular parental separations (father with work, mother with clinic visits)
- Role confusion: does Miguel perceive himself to be the 'man of the house' during his father's absences? Has this role been undermined?
- Anxiety about his father's whereabouts: does he believe explanations about his father's work or is Miguel concerned he is in danger when on active service?
- Separations from his older sibling, who is gaining independence from the family
- Ambivalence about his step-sister's father who may be idealized as 'being there for her' in contrast with his absent father
- Sibling rivalry with younger 'special' brother. One potential explanation for his dissocial behaviour is that he feels ignored and believes he can only achieve 'negative attention' from others
- Multiple moving home and moving school experiences: grief for loss of former friends and/or problems with making new friendships; additional possibilities that the 'new' teachers do not understand his difficulties
- Possibility of adjustment disorder or depression in his mother

His parents describe a chaotic family environment. If anything, they may be understating events. In prioritizing work and their other children, they may have neglected Miguel's emotional needs or increased the risk that he might be exploited by others, unnoticed by them.

We have not yet spoken to Miguel but already there is an impression of a vulnerable isolated child. Always ask a child sensitively about bullying (at school, home or neighbourhood) and abuse (physical, emotional, sexual and/or neglect). In a previously well-adjusted child, torturing animals is associated with childhood sexual abuse.

> **KEY POINT**
>
> Sudden onset dissocial, aggressive or defiant behaviours may have an identifiable cause: abuse of any kind and/or an intolerable family situation.

None of this information excludes a diagnosis of ADD as the sole diagnosis, or that Miguel has a combination of ADD (with or without hyperactivity) and CD. Regardless of which diagnosis he ultimately receives, you can work with Miguel, his parents and his older sister to identify how they can improve their interactions with Miguel, and how his role in their family could be defined better.

The information above hints at a key obstacle to effective interventions – **parental disagreement** about the causes of and solutions to Miguel's behaviour. This is not surprising given the combination of family disruption and the extreme nature of his behaviours. Without knowing it, these behaviours may be reinforced by their actions, despite the best of intentions (Fig. 4). The advantage of identifying a cycle of cause and effect is that you can intervene at any point in the cycle, or make several interventions. It may be useful to show his parents your formulation, making clear that their responses did not cause Miguel's behaviour but might be perpetuating it.

> **KEY POINT**
>
> Identify positive aspects of parenting before making suggestions, change one thing at a time and involve the whole family including the 'patient'.

You find out that Miguel's current school have been concerned about his failure to settle in there, even before the incident with the pets. He has had an assessment by an educational psychologist.

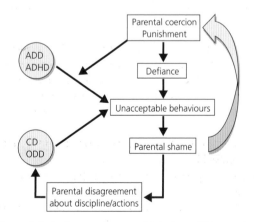

Figure 4 Cycle of repeated unwanted behaviours. ADD, attention deficit disorder; ADHD, attention deficit/hyperactivity disorder; CD, conduct disorder; ODD, oppositional defiant disorder.

What additional information does this offer?

You now have the opportunity to speak to Miguel's teachers, with the permission of his parents. It is likely that several have seen different 'sides' to Miguel. With his previous track record (two suspensions), he will be known to the headmaster and may have been assigned a tutor or mentor. What have they noted in Miguel as different from other children? Are there activities he particularly enjoys or excels at? Is his behaviour always bad? How do they rate his ability to listen and to pay attention?

Neuropsychiatric testing is a valuable and essential addition to your assessment. *Had it not been carried out, you would have requested it.* There is much overlap between what a clinical and educational psychologist measure, but you may need to fill in gaps later. These are key parameters in this case:

- *Intelligence quotient (IQ)* (e.g. the Wechsler Intelligence Scale for Children): this gives an overall IQ, comprising *performance* and *verbal* scores
- *Attention and memory tests* (e.g. the Wisconsin Card Sorting Test, ADHD Rating Scale)
- *Language:* vocabulary and reading tests
- *Perception:* e.g. Thematic Apperception Test
- *Motor functioning:* tests vary and specific comments are useful
- *Descriptions of temperament:* it is far too early to measure Miguel's personality

His parents receive the report from the educational psychologist at the same time you do. His IQ is 71 (Table 28). They are upset that he has scored so poorly.

They ask you whether this the cause of Miguel's problems and if any intervention can make his life better?

Make clear to his parents that this IQ is only a snapshot, taken during a difficult time, and may not reflect his current abilities or his potential. He does *not* have learning disability (LD; Table 28). Explore their fears and the terms they might use for people with LD. They may have a family history of LD with negative experiences of the institutional care of a relative.

While lower IQ did not cause his CD, it contributes to problems with social skills acquisition, school difficulties and understanding the consequences of his actions. Knowledge of his total IQ is useful to some extent in helping Miguel attain his full educational potential, but it will be more productive to identify the individual IQ

Table 28 Clinical features of learning disability.

Category	IQ level	Features	'Mental age' (years)
Borderline learning disability	70–84	Live independently as adults, difficulty sustaining employment. More vulnerable to exploitation	11
Mild learning disability	50–69	Superficially normal social and language skills; appear normal (people with lower IQ tend to be dysmorphic) with minimal deficits in motor skills; may require additional social supports during crises	9–10
Moderate learning disability	35–49	Can learn social and communication skills; self-care with supervision; a minority can lead independent lives	6–8
Severe learning disability	20–34	Very poor social and communication skills; require daily supervision and the provision of structure. Associations with genetic conditions – with reduced life expectancy. Frequent central nervous system pathology: cerebral palsy, epilepsy, hydrocephalus and autism	3–5
Profound learning disability	Below 20	Sometimes no social or language skills; require full-time, often institutional, care	<3

domains at which he scores poorly. Educational and other interventions can then be tailored to address areas of difficulty.

At this point in his assessment, you have some grounds for optimism – and it is good to convey this to his parents, without giving false hopes of 'cure'.

You meet Miguel for the first time, and have two further assessment sessions with him over the next 2 weeks. You have opportunities to ask questions, interact with him and observe him playing.

What behaviours would support the diagnosis of hyperactivity?

To diagnose hyperactivity, ICD-10 requires at least **three** of the following symptoms to be present for at least 6 months. They must be present to a degree that interferes with functioning and be inappropriate to the child's developmental stage:
• Often fidgets with hands or feet, or squirms on seat
• Leaves seat (e.g. in classroom) when remaining seated is expected
• Runs or climbs excessively
• Is often unduly noisy in playing or cannot engage in leisure without much noise

• Exhibits a persistent pattern of excessive motor activity, not reduced by social context or demands

KEY POINT

Adolescents who have ADHD frequently internalize their hyperactivity. They may appear rested, but have a subjective feeling of restlessness.

From repeated assessments, you have identified consistent signs of hyperactivity. His teachers say he frequently fails to complete his homework, having followed instructions poorly. He forgets to keep with him items he needs for this work and becomes upset when his mistakes are identified.

What other features support a diagnosis of ADHD?

• His symptoms have persisted for more than 6 months
• They occur on several contexts: home, school, social life
• They cause distress to him and others
Other symptoms that support ADHD:

- He is easily distracted by external stimuli
- He is impulsive: cannot wait in line, interrupts others
- His relationships with adults are socially disinhibited

What features might exclude a diagnosis of ADHD?

- Late onset: if there were good evidence that Miguel had no signs of hyperactivity or inattention before the age of 7 years
- Predominant features of anxiety, mood or psychotic disorder: if their onset and degree could have a role in producing ADD/ADHD, these should be treated vigorously before any diagnosis of hyperactivity can be made
- Pervasive development disorder (Box 21, p. 152)

> **Miguel is 9 years old and has a clinical diagnosis of ADHD. What clinical features of this disorder are present in the following age groups: 0–4, preschool, school, adolescent and young adult?**

These are set out in Table 29. ADD/ADHD are caused by and cause developmental delay. Their clinical features are also dependent on the person's developmental stage.

You need to find objective evidence of these clinical features (Table 29): collateral from parents, siblings, teachers, school and work reports (typically, patients do not stay in the same job for long) and partners.

One key mediator of their disabilities is communication: when this fails to develop, many other skills (sophisticated emotional responses, stable peer relationships, learning and occupational abilities) fail to be acquired.

Table 29 Clinical features of attention deficit disorder–attention deficit/hyperactivity disorder (ADD/ADHD) by age group.

Age group	Features	Differential diagnoses
Infancy to 4 years	ADD/ADHD cannot be diagnosed in this age group. Non-specific language problems. Mothers may describe common associations (e.g. 'difficult to bond with')	Developmental delay Neonatal/childhood medical conditions Environmental causes
Preschool	Inattentive or very passive; triad of impulsive, inattentive + hyperactive behaviours; may not exhibit this behavioural triad in individual (one-to-one interactions), but will demonstrate this in group settings	Developmental delay: unlike autism, children with ADD/ADHD *want to* interact but lack the social/communication skills to do so
Early school	Poor short-term memory; poor school performance; will not conform to school or household rules; become aware that they are not the same as others → lowered self-esteem → school aversion. Cycles of bad behaviour → punishment → bad behaviours (e.g. Fig. 4)	Developmental delay Conduct and emotional disorders Environmental causes Depression and anxiety disorders
Adolescence	Clumsy, truculent, forgetful: labelled by others as 'lazy'; dislike the more analytical school curriculum; cannot achieve at sports either; hyperactivity is internalized as restlessness	Conduct and emotional disorders Asperger's syndrome Depression, anxiety and psychotic disorders
Young adult – in up to 80%, symptoms persist into adulthood	Struggle to wait, manage anger and organize themselves; hate change; high levels of anxiety; probable low self-esteem; drift into non-academic training and less skilled occupations	All psychiatric conditions are both a differential diagnosis and comorbidity – especially substance misuse

> **KEY POINT**
>
> A new diagnosis of ADD is highly unlikely in an adolescent or young adult who has not shown features of the disorder (Table 29) before the age of 12 years.

Based on what you now know about Miguel's presentation, give a multiaxial diagnosis

This is set out in Table 30.

The team have intervened over 3 months to support Miguel and his family in improving his behaviour. A three-way meeting between the team, his teachers and his parents resolved the issue of harming the school pets. The disruptive behaviours have stopped but he continues to fail at school and this exacerbates his frustration. His mood appears normal and anxiety levels are low, except where homework is involved. There is a team consensus to initiate a trial of methylphenidate.

Outline your preparation plan and the common side-effects of stimulant medication

Preparation

- Speak with his parents. ADHD has a (disputed) 1–3% prevalence, and not everyone is prescribed medication. Of those who are, about 70% respond, provided other supportive interventions are in place. The trial is for 1 month: if there is no response, it will be discontinued. Side-effects are common. Monitoring is shared by health professionals, parents, other family members and teachers
- Confirm physical examination as normal. In particular, note heart rate and blood pressure. No laboratory tests are required for methylphenidate
- Safe practice in all psychoactive prescribing for children is to 'start low and go slow' (Box 5, p. 20)

Side-effects

- CNS effects may be immediate (anorexia, nausea, abdominal pain, weight loss; anxiety, headache, insomnia; dysphoria) or late (motor and vocal tics – these resolve on drug discontinuation)
- Cardiac effects: fixed or labile hypertension
- Stimulants have a high potential for abuse. There may be signs of overactivity (dry mouth, dilated pupils, fast pulse) or of paranoia. There is no syndrome of physical withdrawal but some children experience fatigue, depression and sleep disturbances
- Effects on growth: there appears to be a delay in some children but they achieve expected growth levels following cessation of the drug. Weight loss is common in children who are administered stimulants over long periods of time. Drug holidays and dietary supplements may be required

> **KEY POINT**
>
> There are two extremes of opinion about ADHD: that it does not exist and was invented by drug companies, or that it has a 10% prevalence and everyone benefits from drugs. The truth is somewhere in between.

Table 30 Multiaxial diagnosis.

Axis	Axis description	Description/example	Miguel's diagnoses
I	Psychiatric diagnosis	Depression and other diagnoses of Fig. 1 (p. 7)	ADHD and CD
II	Personality disorders, developmental disorders, intellectual level	Autism, speech delay, moderate LD	No personality difficulties; borderline LD: IQ = 71
III	General medical conditions	Asthma	None known
IV	Psychosocial adversity and environmental problems	Childhood sexual abuse, homelessness	Parental/sibling separations, multiple home/school moves, sibling rivalry
V	Global assessment of functioning	Use of Global Assessment of Functioning scales	Poor: not coping with basic school work despite supports

LD, learning disorder.

Three years later, Miguel attends for review. He has had a good response to medication and this was discontinued without ill effect 2 months ago. He caught up at school, and describes several good friends he has made there. His home life has improved too; his father and his siblings are spending much longer periods at home. He began to enjoy activities with his father, but the last 2 weeks have been characterized by a loss of pleasure in his hobbies and preoccupations about the future. In particular, he cannot imagine what his life will be like when he leaves school at 18.

What are your thoughts?

There appear five broad possibilities here:

1 His loss of pleasure and 'distraction' by what the future holds could indicate the return of the inattention of ADHD symptoms. Other symptoms may have recurred and this would be a useful time to consult with his school

2 Miguel has already experienced anxiety symptoms and these could be the driving issue in this presentation. Clarify what about his future is scaring him. Identify somatic symptoms and subtypes of anxiety (Fig. 2 and Tables 11 and 12, pp. 37–39)

3 Although you have intervened with good intentions, you shared the information of his low IQ. Terms such as 'retarded' and 'slow' could have become common currency at home – or his parents (again with the best intentions) may have conveyed reduced future expectations of him, even that he will never amount to anything. We know little of his relationship with his older sister. From her perspective, Miguel has become the 'special child' – his bad behaviour rewarded. She may be teasing him or indirectly hostile

4 Low self-esteem is a common feature of ADHD (Table 29) and this may be the driving force here. He may have internalized negative expectations of him, despite a high degree of parental, sibling, peer and school support

5 Both anhedonia and loss of hope for the future are reliable symptoms of depression, but other signs, present for longer than 2 weeks, are required to achieve a diagnosis of depression (Table 13, p. 45)

He is depressed. Are you surprised?

It is not surprising that he has developed a second psychiatric disorder. Adult psychiatric morbidity is strongly associated with an early childhood diagnosis of ADHD. Make sure, as you did during his initial presentation, that

recent events and stressors have not preceded the symptoms. If Miguel has either depression or anxiety, these should be treated in the usual way.

> ### KEY POINT
>
> Adult psychiatrists frequently 'inherit' patients who have attended child psychiatrists. While old notes are helpful in describing character and coping skills, the ideal interaction between services is a case conference to achieve safe transition and the passage of all relevant information.

CASE REVIEW

Miguel's presentation and outcome cover many aspects of child psychiatry. Understanding *why* he was behaving badly was central to the diagnostic task. Interactions between the biological (low IQ), psychological (his uncertain role in the family) and the social (chaotic family life) combined to obscure what many believe to be an exclusively biological diagnosis, ADHD. Recent evidence confirms stimulant medication as symptomatic treatment only, and it will only work if adjuvant psychosocial interventions are put in place. These are facilitated by the modest behavioural changes medication can achieve. It is possible to identify different approaches to parenting without assigning blame: *support not censure*. Miguel also illustrates some key differences between child and adult psychiatry:

- Behaviours not symptoms initiated the referral
- Other agencies (teachers, social workers) are frequently involved in the referral process, allowing greater collaboration in future management of undesirable behaviours
- Detailed birth and developmental histories are essential to diagnosis
- Neuropsychological testing is the rule for children, the exception for adults
- Diagnostic uncertainty is better tolerated by child psychiatrists
- In child psychiatry, the pathology is better seen as within the family system, than exclusively in the 'patient' (Fig. 4)
- Medication is used far less frequently than in adults – with other interventions
- In children, treatment *is* prevention

Further reading

Biederman, J., Swanson, J.M., Wigal, S.B., Kratochvil, C.J., Boeller, S.W., Kollins, S., *et al.* (2005) Efficacy and safety of modafinil film-coated tablets in children and adolescents with attention-deficit/hyperactivity disorder: results of a randomized, double-blind, placebo-controlled, flexible-dose study. *Pediatrics* **116**, E777–784.

Coghill, D. (2003) Current issues in child and adolescent psychopharmacology. Part 1: Attention deficit hyperactivity and affective disorders. *Advances in Psychiatric Treatment* **9**, 86–94.

Kramer, T. & Garralda, M.E. (2000) Child and adolescent problems in primary care. *Advances in Psychiatric Treatment* **6**, 287–294.

Lask, B., Taylor, S. & Nunn, K. (2003) *Practical Child Psychiatry: The Clinicians' Guide*. BMJ Books, London.

Case 10 A 48-year-old security guard with new symptoms every day

Stephen returned from a night shift to a distress call from his mother, who lives alone in his former family home in the inner city. Her neighbours had been verbally abusing her, dumping their garbage on her door step. A fight broke out and Stephen was knocked to the ground by two men who kicked him. His brother called an ambulance.

His computer tomography (CT) head scan was normal and he was admitted to the ward later that evening with a diagnosis of concussion. He keeps asking where he is and cannot sleep. His wife is with him and is putting the nurses under pressure to sedate him.

What is your advice?

• It would be dangerous to add a sedative medication to the current setting of uncertainty. Even a sleepless night, with support from his family and the nursing staff, is a better outcome than masking neurological symptoms with drugs. Explain this dilemma to his wife, and try to enlist her help.

• Recommend nursing him in a single room, with adequate lighting and measures to orientate him (Box 10, p. 70). Consider putting up a sign with the hospital's name, the ward, his doctors' names and the day/date for him to read each time he needs reassurance. Agree a simple narrative with his wife and the nurses: some men attacked him, he blacked out and he is in hospital.

• Think about factors that would predispose him to delirium (Table 20, p. 69): previous medical history, current medications, alcohol or substance misuse, intercurrent infection. Has this happened before? Has he had bad experiences of hospital before? Address these in your management plan.

• If he cannot settle, review analgesia and consider special – one-to-one – nursing. This is an excellent option in situations where a period of close observation is required in a secure and calm environment.

The next day, Stephen throws his breakfast at his wife and tries to leave.

What information will you collect?

• Retake his history. Set out his version of the sequence of events. What was his last recollection? He has had a head injury (HI) and you need to clarify either *retrograde amnesia* (loss of memory for a period *before* HI) and/or *anterograde amnesia* (loss of memory for a period *after* HI). In his view, did he black out (lose consciousness)? It is unlikely he has been drinking alcohol during his night work, but enquire about this

• Check all medications

• Get collaborative histories. His brother may have been present for the assault on Stephen. Were there any signs of cerebral irritation (seizures) or focal signs (weakness on one side, loss of speech, visual deficits)? When did Stephen become confused and did this fluctuate? Was there a lucid interval between the HI and his current state? What did the paramedics see? Worrying symptoms are severe headache, focal signs and drowsiness. It is also possible that his mother's neighbours are contactable and can provide useful information about the sequence of events

What signs at this stage would alert you to the possibility of organic pathology?

Of intracranial haemorrhages, subdural haemorrhage (SDH) is the most likely possibility here; about half have a known history of trauma, sometimes weeks before the bleeding. They present insidiously and personality change can be a sign of SDH. Extradural haemorrhage (EDH) is less likely here as it presents early. The most common site where skull fracture causes a bleed is at the temples, just behind the eyes laterally. Usually, consciousness deteriorates and the pupil dilates ('blows') quickly – emergency neurosurgery relieves pressure with burr holes to the skull.

There are other causes of rising intracranial pressure. Trauma can cause an intracranial haemorrhage or cerebral oedema (through changes in capillary permeability). Stephen may have had pre-existing neurological illness, and HI unmasks these.

Table 31 Dependent personality disorder (PD) and psychodynamic understanding.

ICD-10 diagnosis of *any* personality disorder requires that:
• the individual has enduring problematic patterns of *cognition, inner experience, behaviour* and *ways of relating to others*
• traits must have been present in adolescence and persisted unchanged until adulthood
• there must be severe disturbances in character and behaviour, involving several different areas (affect, impulse control, relationships)
• the combination of traits must lead to 'considerable personal and social disruption'
• patterns must be pervasive, and not context-specific
• traits must fall outside cultural norms

ICD-10 criteria for dependent PD
Subordination of one's own needs to others on whom one is dependent; with undue adherence to their wishes
Encouraging others to make one's important life decisions
Unwillingness to make even reasonable demands on the people one depends on
Limited capacity to make decisions without excessive advice and reassurance
Fears of abandonment; exaggerated fears of inability to care for oneself

Psychodynamic understanding (Gabbard 1994)
During childhood, any move towards independence has been overtly or subtly discouraged by parents: low expressiveness, high control parenting style
Excessive need to be taken care of *leads to* clinging and submissive behaviour to achieve this aim (in therapeutic relationships). Therapist experiences excessive demands for approval, advice, interpretation, etc. Dependency develops early in psychotherapy context; towards the end of therapy, extreme emotions including hostility become apparent

Think beyond neurological causes when you consider physical differentials. Has anything been overlooked in history, examination or investigations? (Table 20, p. 69.)

Losing his temper is not a new experience for Stephen. His observations are stable and neurological exam is identical to that on admission. If anything, his level of orientation and his recollection of events are improving. The medical team think it is too early to repeat the CT (head) scan but want to continue to observe him on the general ward. They request that a psychiatrist reviews his diagnosis in the light of his aggression.

What points in his psychiatric history are important?

• Establish what he is angry about. Is it his current environment, the circumstances of the assault upon him or other difficulties? Try to differentiate established traits (his temper) from new symptoms. To achieve this, you will need collaborative history from his family and his GP
• Can he add to the recollections he gave yesterday? Retrograde amnesia should improve with the passage of time. It does not occur without anterograde amnesia, and its degree predicts recovery from head injury
• Does he have psychiatric symptoms? Record all his difficulties. You would expect to find anxiety symptoms at this stage, but not psychotic features
• Define premorbid personality: this presentation may have destabilized someone with dependant PD (Table 31)

Stephen gives a full account of himself. With no previous psychiatric history, he has clear anxiety symptoms suggestive of an acute stress reaction. By the time you review him the following morning, he has been 'twitching' in his face and upper limbs. On several occasions, his legs have 'jolted', one after the other, lasting up to 5 seconds.

What possibilities do you consider, and how will you establish the cause?

• Consider *organic* causes first. Epilepsy seems unlikely from this description. Who has seen these episodes? Repeat your assessment of his orientation level and conduct a detailed examination of his central and peripheral nervous system. If he has not already had one, request a specialist neurology opinion. In this setting, continuous electroencephalography (EEG) would be useful to rule out epilepsy quickly and focus attention elsewhere
• Similar symptoms have been described with post-concussion syndromes. These developments represent deterioration of his previous state, and you must not ignore signs of cerebral irritation, perhaps a *fresh brain bleed*. Be aware that your psychiatric diagnosis of 'acute stress syndrome' may encourage medical and nursing colleagues to ascribe any new symptoms to his 'mental condition'. Continued medical vigilance is needed
• Consider the effects of *drug or alcohol withdrawal*. All his symptoms to date are consistent with the onset of delirium tremens

• Repeat your mental state examination (MSE). A high level of *anxiety and arousal* could explain these new symptoms, but only as a diagnosis of exclusion
• *What has happened* since hospital admission? Are there ward-based factors? Has his family introduced new concerns to Stephen? Is his mother safe? List other consequences of the melée: Stephen may have been interviewed by the police or threatened by his mother's neighbours

Resist pressure to sedate him. You have not separated medical from psychiatric pathology, and have yet to establish a definitive diagnosis.

His twitching continued over the following days, and his EEG is currently being analysed. As the technician removed the leads from his head, he began to cry. He has also been observed laughing loudly at the news bulletins on the radio.

What is your differential diagnosis?

Emotional lability seems likely here. This has a number of established organic causes. It is common after a cerebrovascular accident, head injury or epileptic seizure, and is also common in Parkinson's disease and other dementias, brain tumours (primary and secondary) and multiple sclerosis. It is a prominent feature of frontal lobe syndrome, where it occurs with other signs of disinhibition (bad language, sexually inappropriate behaviour, rage episodes), severe personality change (at the very least, loss of the social graces and consideration for others), loss of initiative and ambition, and reductions in motor activity. Emotional lability also occurs in acute onset anxiety and affective disorders.

These are *new mood symptoms*. Retake mood history (Table 13, p. 45). The possibilities here are depressive episode (very common, but the laughing episodes would be unusual), a hypomanic episode or a mixed affective state. To achieve the diagnosis of bipolar affective disorder – current episode mixed, he must have persistent symptoms for at least 2 weeks. Because he has no history of mood disorder, if he meets these criteria, the likely diagnosis would be an organic mixed affective disorder.

Take the time to understand the nature of his reactions to events around him. Is anything strange going on? Does he know some things (e.g. about items on the news) that

others do not? What did he think was happening when the EEG leads were being removed? Has he seen or heard anything unusual? At this stage, having assessed him on several occasions and gained his trust, you are ideally placed to elicit *psychotic phenomena.*

He slept for brief periods the following night but now complains of aches and pains. The nurses allege he is playing up, looking for stronger medication, but he says the painkillers are useless – in particular, he cannot even do the crossword without pain in his right hand.

They request you transfer him to a psychiatric hospital. What is your response?

Take his symptoms seriously. Chart the areas of pain and observe for any outward marks of trauma. Constant pain, pain on movement and night-time pain suggest *organic causation.*

Aches and pains are common symptoms in *mood and anxiety disorders* but not to this degree. It is likely that his psychological difficulties have lowered his pain threshold but this should not then exclude full medical investigation and treatment of the primary causes of his pain.

Negotiate with the nursing and medical staff. He has had a documented assault and was disorientated on admission, unable to identify his injuries. You (as a psychiatrist) are not the best person to carry out a thorough *locomotor examination.* Tactfully suggest a formal orthopaedic consultation.

The orthopaedic team diagnose a fracture of his right second finger metacarpal bone. It does not require surgery – although there is a possibility of this – but they have fitted a splint and will follow him up with repeated X-rays. He has no other fractures. Stephen's wife wants to sue. She says you are the only doctor to take him seriously.

His EEG is normal as is his repeat CT (head) scan on day 6. A neurologist found no abnormality in his central or peripheral nervous system. Stephen says he cannot walk because he experiences dizziness on standing and falls to his right side. The neurologist thinks Stephen is malingering.

What is your management plan?

Malingering is only one of several possibilities here, and both in general and in the context of this specific case, *the least likely diagnosis*. There are several alternative explanations:

• *Organic pathology* could yet be present. Vertigo has many causes: occipital lobe damage, middle ear disease and infections. Stephen's symptoms raise the possibility of postural hypotension: he is 48 years old and may have diabetic or vascular disease. He has had a recent assault and normal X-rays do not rule out significant soft tissue injury, perhaps to his lower limbs

• Intolerable *anxiety* can have motor manifestations. He may be terrified of a return visit from his assailants or the police. Having a new physical symptom that requires investigation might be a welcome distraction

• People react to trauma and illness in different ways. His behaviours to date could be seen as *unconscious requests* to remain in hospital – ultimately, he may be ashamed that he has let down his mother and his family. We cannot call these conversion symptoms until organic *and* psychiatric pathology are ruled out

Use all available expertise in your management:

• His medical team need to reassure him that there is nothing sinister in his physical or functional neurological investigations. At the same time, they might acknowledge the extent of his injuries and speak of a prolonged period of recovery rather than accusations he is overstating or manufacturing symptoms

• The nursing team can help with practical support, scheduling of treatments and pain relief strategies

• Physiotherapy is an essential part of his treatment. This acknowledges disability (regardless of its cause) and provides a graduated means of recovery without Stephen losing face. As his psychiatrist, you should speak with the physiotherapist to assess his physical symptoms, anxiety, mood and motivation

• Stephen works in an unskilled job where any physical impairment will reduce his earning potential. Consult an occupational therapist (p. 27) for short-term activities (while an inpatient) and medium-term strategies. He may require assistance at home on initial discharge

• The neurologist's involvement has not finished. The remote possibility exists of late bleeding or other neurological disease. Agree a regular interval for review. He may have subtle cognitive deficits: discuss the timing of neuropsychiatric testing

• Implement anxiety-reduction strategies. He can learn tension recognition, relaxation training and sleep hygiene measures (Table 6, p. 16). Most of the suggested changes to improve sleep are far easier to control in community patients. He works nights and readjusting his sleep pattern will be difficult. You have two concerns at this stage in his treatment: (i) that he will generalize his anxiety, and (ii) that he will avoid situations or people to reduce anxiety. Interventions will reduce both outcomes

• Monitor for depression. In patients you are reviewing every day, consider an objective instrument to measure mood – perhaps weekly

• Provided his neurologist agrees, you can prescribe sedation and/or anti-anxiety agents in the short term. If he is not sleeping or is too anxious for interventions, he might gain from low dose prescription of either

• His family are a source of support and if they do not agree with these approaches, they will undermine them. In an ideal situation, where physical and psychological rehabilitation are instituted, a patient's family are ideal co-therapists. Agree a mechanism for discussing progress, setbacks and new findings

You are called to review him after an eventful night. He shouted at the night nurse 'Get away from me!' and reported seeing two tall men at his bedside. The ward is locked by night and no-one else witnessed anything unusual.

Will you need to revise your management plan?

Taking the hierarchical approach to diagnosis (Fig. 1, p. 7), the first three categories seem unlikely. You have not elicited psychotic symptoms (that he is seeing/hearing things or feeling paranoid) previously or in this assessment. He has some mood symptoms but not enough to meet criteria for moderate depression to explain psychotic symptoms.

Speak with Stephen to identify the nature of his experiences. He believed the images were real at the time but does he do so now? These could be nightmares with (normal) hypnopompic visual hallucinations.

They could also be flashbacks: intrusive recollections of his recent trauma. Using open questions, explore the similarities between these experiences and his assault. It would be usual for Stephen to start remembering more details at this stage. Did the images/memories/flashbacks/nightmares provoke anxiety symptoms? Taken together, he is starting to meet the criteria for post-traumatic stress disorder (PTSD; Table 32). It is unusual to have PTSD immediately after a trauma.

PART 2: CASES

A new psychiatric diagnosis of PTSD does not change the management plan. It is especially important to monitor for depression and to prevent the development of dysfunctional strategies (Table 32):

• Cognitive therapy provides essential education and re-education of Stephen about his and the usual response to trauma. Normalizing intrusive phenomena reduces the distress they bring. It will also confer an understanding

Table 32 Clinical features and treatments of post-traumatic stress disorder (PTSD). Based on ICD-10. Note: the incident must be of 'an exceptionally threatening or catastrophic nature'.

Hyperarousal	Intrusive	Numbing
Symptoms		
Sleep disturbances (these occur in almost every case)	Distressing memories of the incident	Feeling flat or numb
	Distressing images of the incident	Loss of interest in usual activities
Concentration difficulties	Flashbacks (usually by day)	Feeling detached from close relationships
Anticipate danger in all situations, not just those similar to original event/situation	Dreams and nightmares of trauma	Loss of hope for the future
	Feelings of guilt as initiator or survivor of the trauma	Gaps in memory, including autobiographical memory
Irritability, easy to startle		
Anger outbursts	Cues to incident (visual, smells, sounds, feelings) invoke intense distress and somatic anxiety symptoms (Fig. 2, p. 37)	
Common dysfunctional strategies		
Misuse of alcohol and substances	Misuse of alcohol and substances	Misuse of alcohol and substances
Angry outbursts at themselves (DSH and suicide) or others	Isolates self from all stimuli (people, media, hobbies and activities)	Avoidance of places, activities, conversations or media items that remind of the trauma
Adopt 'new' cognitive view of the world as unfair and dangerous	Repetitive activities (sometimes addictive behaviours like gambling) to keep oneself from sleeping	Denial or playing down of original trauma
Treatment strategies		
Abstinence	Abstinence	Abstinence
Sleep hygiene (Table 6, p. 16)	Psychoeducation about PTSD	Psychoeducation of family and friends to stabilise supports
Anxiety management	Cognitive restructuring: to address guilt, including survivor guilt	Restoration of routine
Consider anxiolytics, sedatives and SSRI medication	Eye movement desensitization and reprocessing therapy (p. 34)	Reassurance that it is safe to have feelings without the return of distress
Regular reading, tasks	Graded exposure to traumatic memories	Early recognition and treatment of depression
Cognitive reframing	*In vivo* exposure once symptoms are under control	
Anger management		
Relapse prevention		
Plan for future periods of stress	Expectation of future upset with future exposures to new cues	Spread the watch for relapse among family and friends
Practice anti-anxiety strategies	Acceptance of minor setbacks	Close monitoring of mood symptoms

DSH, deliberate self-harm; SSRI, selective serotonin reuptake inhibitor.

of the numbness which is a major obstacle to readjustment and recovery
- Behavioural strategies consolidate his daily routine, reduce dysfunctional strategies (Table 32) and improve symptoms such as poor sleep
- Eye movement desensitization and reprocessing (EMDR) therapy has been proven to reduce the frequency and severity of intrusive images of trauma (p. 33)
- Exposure (including visiting his mother's) forms part of his cognitive–behavioural therapy (CBT) programme
- He will probably require one-to-one psychodynamic or interpersonal psychotherapy beyond these CBT interventions. This will explore previous trauma and losses, his place in the family, past and current relationships and other relevant issues

---

KEY POINT

Anxiety and depression frequently coexist and interact to increase morbidity, and in clinical settings each masks symptoms of the other.

Stephen refuses to see his wife the next day. She is very angry with you. She has read about PTSD and blames you for missing it. She says that if her husband had been 'properly debriefed', none of this would have happened.

What can she tell you?

His *premorbid personality* may indicate difficulties such as dependant personality traits (Table 31). People's vulnerability to PTSD varies depending on their personality and past psychiatric history. Both lower the threshold for developing the disorder and worsen its prognosis.

What will you tell her?

Several possibilities might explain their estrangement:
- His wife may have criticised his behaviour on the night of admission (too tough, not tough enough). He perceives criticism from her about his response to illness
- They were already having difficulties in their relationship, or there may be new practical (e.g. financial) consequences of this admission
- There is disagreement between them about his treatment, his doctors or her wish to sue
- He is trying to shut people out to reduce symptoms of PTSD (Table 32)

Explain these possibilities to his wife, and explore with Stephen whether this is likely to be temporary. Explain that the diagnosis of PTSD is based on symptoms and not everyone who experiences the same trauma goes on to develop it. The idea that debriefing *prevents* PTSD has been *totally debunked*.

KEY POINT

PTSD is a common outcome after severe trauma but its symptoms mimic many other psychiatric conditions. PTSD is beloved of the legal profession as it is the only psychiatric disorder with a definitive single cause – and someone to sue.

Stephen makes a slow recovery and is discharged 2 weeks later. He does not develop more medical complications. Six months later, he has not returned to work.

What are the likely outcomes here? Might he have a new psychiatric diagnosis?

About one-third of patients with PTSD make a substantial recovery (total or virtually symptom free) and a further third make improvements such that they do not meet the criteria to diagnose the disorder (Table 32). It is possible that Stephen is in either group, but for other reasons (charges against him or other litigation prolonging his illness), he has not returned to work.

He may belong to the one-third of PTSD patients who do not respond to treatment. These cases are likely to be complicated by treatment-resistant depression, alcohol or substance misuse.

Some relatives describe a 'different person' or say that he was 'never the same again' after experiences of physical trauma. This is a diagnosis of enduring personality change after catastrophic experience. It is common in former hostages and people who have been tortured, but would be unusual in this setting of a single life-threatening assault.

Most pessimistic of all, he may have gone on to develop a mental disorder as a result of brain damage and dysfunction. He might have retrograde amnesia, indicating the possibility of subtle cognitive impairments. It would be best to repeat neuropsychiatric testing and decide future management on that basis.

PART 2: CASES

CASE REVIEW

Stephen's physical injuries were far more straightforward than his psychological reactions. These interacted with staff's behaviour towards him, sometimes through the prism of his wife's beliefs. With each new symptom, a hierarchical approach (Fig. 1, p. 7) served him well. PTSD, prevalence 1%, developed from an acute stress reaction – you were able to assess him at every turn. The three core PTSD components are:

1 Hyperarousal
2 Intrusive phenomena
3 Pervasive anxiety, with numbing and avoidance (Table 32)

Practical strategies, coordinated by you but delivered by many disciplines, provided better prevention than the (worse than useless) intervention of debriefing. There are no 'quick fix' strategies for PTSD: it requires more treatment interventions (Tables 4 and 5, pp. 13 and 14) than any other psychiatric condition. Legal proceedings, seen frequently in this disorder, will prolong symptoms and may cause a conflict of interest in your treatment plan.

Reference

Gabbard, G. (1994) *Psychodynamic Psychiatry in Clinical Practice*. American Psychiatric Press, Washington DC.

Further reading

Wessely, S. & Deahl, M. (2003) Psychological debriefing is a waste of time. *British Journal of Psychiatry* **183**, 12–14.

Yehuda, R. (2002) Current concepts: post-traumatic stress disorder. *New England Journal of Medicine* **346**, 108–114.

A 28-year-old man has been arrested at the airport

You are called to A&E to see Alex, a 28-year-old single man who is under police escort. It is alleged that he stabbed a security guard in a scuffle which followed his unsuccessful attempt to board a plane without a ticket. He was alone at the airport, shouting 'Revenge to the impostors!' while queuing at check-in.

Before you assess him, what additional information would be useful?

• *Any* collateral history: his relatives, partner, GP, the police or witnesses
• Details of any previous contacts with mental health services
• Some indication from the police about how they intend to proceed
• Results of physical examination and any investigations: he may have been injured in the 'scuffle' or there may be independent signs of an organic cause of his symptoms (Table 16, p. 53)
• Details suggest psychotic symptoms, so a urine drug screen would be useful at this stage

Alex agrees to see you but he is concerned that you are working for the police. He says they are going to 'stitch me up' because of 'the airport thing'. He also tells you that the younger of the two policemen is wearing a false beard 'for obvious reasons'.

Can you guarantee Alex complete confidentiality?

No, you cannot. If Alex tells you any information that puts him or others at risk, you have a duty to act on that. This could be a statement of suicidal intent ('I never thought I'd be caught. I am going to kill myself') or threats to others ('My father must have phoned ahead to the airport to arrange this. If I get out of here, I am going to teach him a lesson'). You should also explain to him that if you identify serious risk you will share your assessment with other health professionals. This is in his inter-

ests. Explain to Alex that you are the doctor asked to assess him, and that you will:
• Keep his information confidential – except if it involves risk to himself or others
• Let the police interview him about alleged offences
• Remind him that he can appoint a lawyer to be present at police interviews
• Provide a report of your findings to his lawyer if requested and with his consent. If someone else (e.g. the Court) requests a report from you at a future time, you will re-interview Alex and obtain his specific consent for this. If Alex's lawyer decides your report prejudices Alex's case in some way, under current guidance his lawyer can choose not to submit your report to the Court.

> ### KEY POINT
>
> If a patient confides in you that they intend to harm a named individual, you have a duty to break confidentiality to inform the police and/or that person of the danger to them. The precedent is set by the *Tarasoff Declaration* from a Californian Court. A psychotherapist was found negligent for failing to disclose a threat from his patient towards the (subsequent) victim.

He cooperates fully with your assessment. Alex has never been seen by a psychiatrist. You identify probable psychotic symptoms of 5–7 months' duration:
• *Auditory hallucinations in the second and third person*
• *Delusions of surveillance*
• *Delusions of thought interference: thought insertion and broadcast*
• *Paranoid delusions that 'actors' and 'impostors' have been placed in key positions to watch on him and harm him*
• *His delusional system appears to involve the police and security guards whom he calls 'uniformed cyborgs'*
• *He is hypervigilant and becomes activated when speaking about the distress 'certain people' have caused him*

> ### KEY POINT
>
> An essential part of assessing risk (to self or others) in clinical practice is **communicating** the degree of **risk** to other professionals. From this point on, **everyone** involved in Alex's care needs to know the links you have made between his psychotic symptoms and violent behaviour.

He does not appear to have any mood symptoms and, by his account, you cannot identify negative symptoms of schizophrenia. His cognition is intact.

What is your differential diagnosis?

- *First episode psychosis*, including drug-induced psychosis. Acute and transient psychotic disorder is unlikely given his 5-month history
- *Schizophrenia:* he meets ICD-10 criteria (Box 9, p. 54) to diagnose this (usually an unwise diagnosis at one meeting), but he is older than the age at which men usually present with first episodes. He may have forgotten previous psychotic episodes (Case 6), or failed to disclose them at this assessment
- *Organic psychosis* appears unlikely given his normal cognitive function. This should be investigated further during his period of assessment
- *Bipolar affective disorder:* his plan at the airport was somewhat grandiose, suggesting a manic presentation
- *Malingering:* Alex has a strong potential gain (e.g. striking out the legal proceedings against him, lesser sentence) in feigning mental illness

Despite the extent of his symptoms, he does not believe any of his difficulties could be caused by stress or psychological problems. Alex tells you that his girlfriend will back up everything he has said. He gives you her mobile phone number and you speak to her. Her English is poor, but even allowing for this, she does not grasp how serious Alex's situation is.

What will you discuss?

Explore if she shares his delusional beliefs (e.g. about the police). Induced delusional disorder ('folie à deux') is rare. One of a close partnership (lovers, parent–child, siblings, friends) persuades the other that their delusional beliefs are real. The characteristic setting is that the couple live an isolated life together, that the 'lead' partner is dominant, perhaps more intelligent and articulate (here, he speaks better English), than the 'led' partner.

Treatment usually involves admission of the lead person to hospital for medication, and supporting the led partner at home without medications – both respond well.

Alex's partner does not share his delusional system. She confirms it began about 6 months ago, but is getting worse. He hangs around the house all day, speaking of a 'big showdown'. He scares her – although he has never threatened or harmed her.

You get the help of an interpreter. What will you discuss with her?

- *Risk:* has Alex spoken to her about specific plans to challenge 'the impostors'? What else has he done so far? Are there named people he believes are leading events? What has he told her about people in uniform? Has he armed himself? In view of the solo nature of Alex's airport visit, has he discussed suicide with her? Has he harmed himself?

> ### KEY POINT
>
> Acts of suicide occur in people who perceive there is **no** other **way out** of their stressful situation. Suicide is higher in prisoners than any other group – this is not about 'guilt' and includes those on remand who have not been convicted of any offence.

- *Forensic history:* all previous offences and charges, especially history of violence to others
- *Evidence for a prodrome:* a prodrome is a definable period prior to the emergence of psychotic symptoms where social functioning becomes impaired (Box 14). In this age group, ask about the sequence of jobs to identify a decline in performance or gaps in employment. By definition, prodromal symptoms are hard to pin down. They come and go over several weeks, but a close confidant (parent, partner) can usually recall the time when changes occurred
- *Illegal drug use:* cannabis, amphetamines, cocaine, ecstasy (and alcohol)
- Confirm this is his first episode
- List other indicators of poor prognosis (Table 17, p. 58)

> ### KEY POINT
>
> The best single predictor of violence is a history of previous violence.

Box 14 Identification of a prodrome of psychotic illness

Prodromal symptoms are vague and frequently suggestive of other disorders. The common unifying result is a clear deterioration in social functioning at home, school or work. The following non-specific features of prodrome have been described:

- Loss of concentration and attention in late childhood (ADD begins in early childhood) or early adult life
- Reduced motivation and ambition
- Loss of interest in usually enjoyed activities
- Loss of energy
- Sleep disturbances: insomnia or sleeping excessively
- New onset low mood and/or anxiety symptoms
- Irritability
- Increased suspiciousness
- Social withdrawal: change in previous routine as a 'passive' choice by the person
  Factors indicating likely transition to psychosis: '**at-risk mental state**'
- Positive family history of psychosis
- Definite loss of social functioning
- Attenuated (subthreshold) psychotic symptoms: bewildered thinking (but not with full psychotic force), perhaps with repetitive 'silly' questions to the spouse/relative: 'What's all that about?'
- Actual psychotic symptoms that are shorter than 2 weeks: if these persist beyond 2 weeks, this should be defined as a first psychotic episode

The police tell you that the airport security guard required emergency surgery for multiple cuts to his face, arms and stab wounds to his chest, but is medically stable. The assault by Alex had 12 witnesses and was filmed on closed-circuit television. They will charge Alex with attempted murder. You have diagnosed a first episode psychotic illness with a preceding prodrome of 5 months and, in other circumstances, would be arranging for transfer to a psychiatric hospital.

What will you advise?

The police should charge Alex, based on the evidence they have. This can take place either in a police station or a detention centre. Make clear that Alex needs psychiatric treatment, but do not obstruct the process of justice.

Give the police your contact details so that the police surgeon (the duty doctor at the detention centre) can speak directly to you about Alex's management and the degree of risk he currently poses to others and himself.

Once he has been charged, Alex needs to be moved to a psychiatric facility as soon as possible. Given his symptoms, the risks identified, the seriousness of the index offence and his total lack of insight, Alex needs to be in a secure forensic setting – under mental health legislation.

Alex was charged with attempted murder and bail was refused. He has been assessed in prison by a forensic psychiatrist who recommended to the Home Office that he be transferred to a high security forensic unit. The Home Office agreed to this. He will appear again in Court to face this charge. The Court asks you about his fitness to plead.

How will you determine he is fit to plead?

You need to explain to Alex that the circumstances of your assessment are different to his first assessment. All information must be shared with the Court.

The test for fitness to plead is set out in England and Wales in the Criminal Procedure (Insanity and Unfitness to Plead) Act of 1991. The accused person must be able to:

1 Plead to the charge(s): guilty or not guilty
2 Understand the course of Court proceedings such that they can make a proper defence
3 Know that s/he can challenge the appointment of a juror (i.e. object)
4 Comprehend the details of evidence presented to the Court

Being fit to plead is essentially about establishing that the defendant's mental state meets a minimum standard such that he/she will receive a fair trial. Patients with delirium or mania are not fit to plead. It is not enough to have paranoia or that the defendant is likely to conduct his defence poorly.

Your report is your professional opinion, based on key facts (Table 33).

You decide that Alex is fit to plead. He accepts antipsychotic medication in hospital and has several meetings with his solicitor over the following weeks. Alex says he did not wish to kill the security guard and feels remorse for his actions.

Table 33 Key features of court reports.

Item	Essential	Desirable
Introduction	Who requested the report?	A summary of diagnosis and recommendations
	What specific questions have you been asked to address?	Circulation list for this report
	Confirm details of confidentiality have been explained to the defendant	
Collateral history	Informants	School reports
		Employers' reports and references
	Previous psychiatric reports: check with the authors that they are willing for you to quote their findings.	Discuss and clarify reports with colleagues
	GP records	
Details relating to the charges	The exact nature of the charges made against the patient/client	Witness statements, police taped interviews
	Reports from probation services, forensic assessments: ask solicitor about all other available information	Discuss with these colleagues
Symptoms	At time of alleged offence	Contemporaneous reports
	Current symptoms	—
Other points of history	Birth, personal, sexual, family, medical and psychiatric history	Psychometric testing: IQ
	Previous treatments	Dates and doses of all medications
	Social history: lifestyle, alcohol and substance use	Urine drug screens as evidence
	Forensic history	Previous forensic assessments
Signs	MSE at time of alleged offence	Contemporaneous reports
	Current MSE	—
Opinions (as requested by the commissioner of the report)	Diagnoses of mental disorder(s) if any	For a lay reader of the report, the conclusions are clearly linked to the evidence
	Your conclusions of links (if any) between this and the offence(s) in question	
	Available treatments for their mental disorder(s)	
Recommendations (as requested by the commissioner of the report)	About fitness to plead	—
	About your opinion of the best treatment options	If you are to be the treating psychiatrist, state the specific settings, bed availability, etc.
	About the basis of detention: voluntary treatment, under section (state which one), probation order, etc.	—

MSE, mental state examination.

Had Alex killed the guard, his solicitor might advise him to plead not guilty to manslaughter 'by reason of insanity'. What are the criteria?

This plea is based on English legal precedent (McNaughten Rules, 1843) that some people with severe mental illness are not responsible for their actions, and need to be detained in hospital, not in prison (Box 15).

Alex's defence may fall outside the McNaughten Rules if at the time of the assault, he knew what he was doing was wrong. He had specific ideas (delusions) that the people at the airport were against him, and there is some evidence that Alex assaulted the guard as a direct result of his delusional system. According to this system, this was an act of self-defence – consistent with the third point of the McNaughten Rules.

Alex would have the option of this plea providing psychiatric reports to the Court identify psychiatric hospital, not prison, as the best *disposal* (the Court's term) of his

---

Box 15 The McNaughten Rules

Background: these apply only to homicide cases. McNaughten, during an episode of paranoid psychosis, attempted to kill the British Prime Minister, but killed his secretary and was convicted on a plea of insanity. To be found guilty but insane, the accused person's defence team must prove in a higher court that at the time of the offence:

1 By reason of such defect from disease of the mind, he did not know the nature or quality of his act; or

2 By reason of such defect from disease of the mind, he did not know what he was doing was wrong; and

3 Where 'an insane delusion' prevents him from appreciating the true nature of his act, he is under the same degree of responsibility as if the facts were as he imagined them to be

Outcome: in the original case, McNaughten believed his life was in grave danger (from the then Prime Minister's political party) and was treated as acting in self-defence. If his motives had been revenge against or hatred of the Prime Minister, he would have been punished according to the criminal law.

The McNaughten Rules result in a 'special verdict' and automatic transfer to a psychiatric facility. For more 'minor' offences (short of murder and homicide), defendants are found guilty 'under disability' and can be sent to hospital under appropriate section of the Mental Health Act.

---

case. Remember that Alex has previously shown no insight and he may decline to accept legal advice.

l *The charge will be attempted murder.*

Do you think the charge should be dropped because he has mental illness?

No. He should be charged. From the perspective of future public safety, it is better that Alex has a conviction for his stabbing of the airport guard. This will identify his history clearly to health and probation services in the event of future deteriorations, following treatment and subsequent release. Were he not charged, future assessments could play down the 'airport incident' rather than consider it as a near-lethal knife attack on an unarmed man.

Alex will be charged. Can he plead guilty with diminished responsibility?

Yes. For example, under the English Homicide Act (1957), a person with mental illness can enter this plea if:

• He has an 'abnormality of mind' such that a reasonable man would deem him abnormal (this is for a jury to decide based on medical reports and the evidence before them), and

• The *abnormality* arises from either 'arrested development of mind' or has been induced by disease or injury (case law has seen these interpreted as severe learning disability, psychosis, depression, female victims of domestic violence, alcoholism and severe personality disorder); and

• The *abnormality* substantially impaired his responsibility for his acts

Under current law, if the person is found guilty with diminished responsibility but there is no proven treatment for the 'abnormality' (e.g. a defendant with dissocial personality disorder), the sentencing judge can decide to send the convicted person to prison rather than hospital.

KEY POINT

Where homicide has been committed under the intoxication of alcohol or drugs, this is no defence in law. If sustained alcohol or substance misuse has caused gross brain disease (e.g. Korsakoff's syndrome) this could be argued as an 'abnormality of mind'.

You prepare a report that links his offence to his psychiatric diagnosis of schizophrenia. Your recommendation is for involuntary admission to a secure psychiatric facility. He pleads not guilty, but is convicted of attempted murder. The judge makes an order that he be sent to a secure unit under Section 37/41 of the Mental Health Act (1983) of England and Wales.

What is different about his management in this setting from treatment in a general psychiatric hospital?

Similar to a general hospital setting, he will be managed by an interdisciplinary team of psychiatrists, psychiatric nurses, psychologists and occupational therapists. These professionals have additional training in forensic psychiatry/nursing/psychology, etc. The ratio of staff to patients is higher than on general adult wards.

Patients receive the same medications, but the degree of supervision of their concordance is even higher than in a general facility. Routine monitoring is likely to include serum drug levels to provide empirical proof the patient is taking psychiatric medication as ordered. Equally, documentation of treatments and progress is more rigorous as future legal review is inevitable.

Security is an additional priority. In addition to locking and checking routines, there will be additional outside restraints to prevent escape. Part of this will include thorough searching of all visitors for drugs, weapons, etc.

The usual processes of granting leave of the ward are restricted. They will depend on thorough risk assessment (Table 34) and communication with the Home Office who must agree to every leave application. Discharge planning will take months and years, not weeks.

Partly as a result of these differences and in the context of the (necessary) isolation of special forensic units, recent inquiries have identified institutional problems there of overcrowding, cultures of *control not care* of patients and, on occasion, abuse of patients. The current trend is to 'step down' suitable patients into smaller regional secure units. These medium secure facilities can be seen as intermediate between general wards and special hospitals, and aim to balance security (control) with treatment (care) priorities.

Alex remained in a medium secure hospital for the next 5 years. He seemed to settle in well initially but was found inducing vomiting of his risperidone syrup. This was changed to an injected depot preparation, at maximum dose. Three months later, he attacked an army officer who was visiting

the ward. He subsequently revealed deep-rooted delusions similar to those of his presentation. He was changed to clozapine medication and had regular blood tests to check his white cells (Table 8, p. 18) and to monitor serum clozapine levels. A period of sustained low mood followed for 3 months: he did not receive medication for this, and his mood restored itself by the anniversary of his first year's admission. CBT helped him control his voices – these had continued but he had always denied they were present. He participated well in occupational therapy and completed a foundation course that led to studying history at the Open University. Five years later, he was transferred to a general psychiatric ward. Recently, he has had regular overnight leave to his elderly parents' second, country house (60 miles away) – some of this has been unsupervised – and these seemed to go well. On one occasion, he returned to the ward drunk, and later expressed remorse for this lapse. A team meeting is considering his transfer to a supervised group home in the city, where he will be free to come and go during the day.

What do you think are risk factors for a third violent attack?

This is a complex assessment of two groups of parameters, the *risk factors* that predict violence (Table 34) and the nature and degree of potential violence, *harm*, combining to a third variable, the *risk*.

The potential **harm** Alex could inflict is *considerable*, given his index offence. He has *seven* prominent **risk factors**:

1 Young
2 Male
3 Single
4 He has been hospitalized for schizophrenia following a violent offence
5 His circumstances on discharge will likely place him into a *lower socioeconomic category*
6 He is likely to misuse *alcohol* in the context of an unstructured day on his release (Table 34)
7 The use of alcohol to reduce stress raises his risk, as does the *lack of any vocational activity*: in effect, these latter two are the only remediable risk factors here.

We are assuming that his personality is not psychopathic, with no adverse traits, and that he will not misuse substances.

Evidence supports the lack of other adverse factors (Table 34) and he appears to be from a well-off family.

Table 34 Predicting violence by actuarial methods (risk factors).

Variables	Factors	Proven predictors of violence
Dispositional	Age	Peak age is mid-adolescence to middle age
	Gender	Men
	Race	–
	Marital status	Single, separated and divorced people
	Social class	People from poorer socioeconomic backgrounds
	Personality	Traits of impulsivity, problems with anger control
	Neurological factors	Head injury
Historical	Family history	Separation from parents under the age of 16; childhood abuse; family history of criminality
	Psychiatric history	Numbers of hospitalizations
	Criminal history	History of violent offence
		Juvenile delinquency; history of offences against property
Contextual (i.e. current variables)	Social supports	No supports increases risk and close (e.g. family) ties may act as a cue
	Stress	Environment has a key role as a trigger for violence: prison or ward confinement
	Access to weapons	Restricted access reduces risk
Clinical	Mental disorder	Personality disorder diagnosis: psychopathy checklist strong predictor
		Any substance and alcohol misuse: intoxication and dependence
		To a much lesser extent than the other factors in this table, schizophrenia has been linked to violence, depression with homicide
	Level of functioning	Employment, meaningful daytime activity protective

The **risk** is therefore moderate that he will re-offend, and it is unlikely he will be released now, but risk will change over time. His discharge should be phased and under the supervision of familiar staff who are aware of his ability to conceal symptoms and his potential for harm. Regular assessments, perhaps as an inpatient, will monitor his progress.

CASE REVIEW

Alex provides an example of the rare but proven association between psychosis and violence. In the public's mind, care in the community has failed and psychiatrists have released violent offenders on to the streets without adequate supervision. In reality, the number of homicides carried out by people with psychosis in England and Wales each year has remained stable (50 per year) over the past four decades. A far more potent predictor of violence is alcohol and substance misuse. We know too that people with schizophrenia are far more likely to be victims of violence, including homicide, than others with the same demographic profile who do not have mental illness. This said, we need

Continued

to identify risk in all patients with psychosis, and set out clear risk prevention strategies, communicated to all.

There are clear links in Alex's case between his symptoms and his violent actions. Throughout your assessment of him, issues of consent, confidentiality and risk were prominent, and his management took place in the context of the laws of the land. Wherever you work, you need to be aware of these, and of recent changes or legal precedents: stop and ask if you are in doubt.

Alex had concealed his delusions prior to his attack at the airport and later, when committed to hospital. Although not illustrated in this case, you would have consulted with colleagues who have experience of homicide, forensic colleagues and lawyers where you work. Your roles were to identify and treat his mental condition, advise his counsel and the Courts, and to manage the risk he presents to others. Just as we saw 'step downs' in Alex's incarceration, he will ultimately be discharged from specialist forensic outreach programmes to a generic adult community team and a general practitioner. This could be you.

Further reading

Frampton, A. (2005) Reporting of gunshot wounds by doctors in emergency departments: a duty or a right? Some legal and ethical issues surrounding breaking patient confidentiality. *Emergency Medicine Journal* **22**, 84–86.

Monaghan, J. (1996) Violence prediction: the past twenty years and the next twenty years. *Criminal Justice and Behavior* **13**, 107–120.

Stone, J.H., Roberts, M., O'Grady, J., Taylor, A.V. & O'Shea, K. (2000) *Faulk's Basic Forensic Psychiatry.* Blackwell Science, London.

A 24-year-old new mother in distress

Margaret has been 'inconsolable' since the birth of her first child, an as yet unnamed boy, 3 days ago. He was born with a cleft lip and palate (incidence is 1 in 700 live births) which had been undetected prior to delivery by Caesarean section. Margaret has been crying almost continuously since his birth. Although disfigured, he is feeding well with a special teat, but Margaret has not yet taken an active role in this.

What are the factors in her history (other than her presenting complaints) relevant to possible diagnoses here? State why they are relevant
Medical and personal history
• *History of depression or other psychiatric illness*: depression predicts further episodes of depression; over half of women with a history of psychosis will develop psychiatric symptoms in the year after childbirth
• *Antenatal depression* is a frequent antecedent of postnatal depression
• *Medical history*: some medical illnesses (e.g. diabetes, hypertension, cardiac illness) complicate both pregnancy and labour
• *Family history of psychiatric illness and suicide*: always useful in supporting a particular psychiatric diagnosis
• *Family history of congenital abnormality*: these factors are associated with increased risks of congenital anomalies, but explore carefully *her perceptions* that she may have *caused* her son's birth defects. Enquire about her experience of congenital abnormalities in family or other contacts; congenital anomalies tend to cluster in some families, and she may have known babies who died prematurely
• *Supports*: partner, family and friends, housing, financial status – these are key determinants both of her developing mental illness and ultimate outcome

Pregnancy and childbirth
• *Planned or unplanned pregnancy*: the latter is associated with poorer mental health outcomes, although there are several confounders for this
• *Difficulties conceiving, infertility treatments* (more relevant to older women): pressured/precious pregnancies by their nature have higher anxieties in both parents, sometimes even the wider family
• *Previous pregnancies*: this is her first child, but she may have been pregnant before. Ask about miscarriages and terminations
• *Medical complications* during pregnancy
• *Use of medications at conception, pregnancy and current medications*: know the list of teratogenic medications – in psychiatry, the common ones are lithium, carbamazepine, sodium valproate, monoamine oxidase inhibitors and benzodiazepines. Caution is urged with all 'new' psychotrophic agents because of the lack of prescribing experience. In general, tricyclic antidepressants are safer in pregnancy than selective serotonin reuptake inhibitors (SSRIs) but both can cause a withdrawal syndrome in neonates. The most harmful drugs in late pregnancy are benzodiazepines
• *Alcohol and substance misuse at conception/during pregnancy*: as above, although fetal alcohol syndrome is a rare event (incidence is 1 in 2000 live births) that results in severe disability with fatalities. For all drugs (prescribed, legal and illegal), the associated guilt in the mother may be overwhelming
• *Details of labour*: duration, interventions, indications for her Caesarean section – this goes to the state of mind of the mother. She could be traumatized by these events, or guilt-ridden that during labour she did not 'try hard enough'
• *Details/complications of Caesarean section*: up to one-third of postpartum psychoses have organic causes; infection, retained products of conception, emboli, metabolic disturbances

You are the liaison psychiatrist asked to assess her on day 3. Before you are able to ask her questions, she wants to know everything you know about cleft lip and palate.

How will you proceed?

There are two extremes of approach to these challenges for liaison psychiatrists. First, it would be wrong to evade all of her questions. The second extreme is to respond *as if* you have far more knowledge than you do and give guestimates of what *might* happen. In effect, any information you give is based on imperfect knowledge. In general, this means conveying pessimistic outcomes as psychiatrists have completed their general medical training some years previously, and are unaware of newer treatments. Similarly, guestimate psychiatrists, with the best of intentions, can paint an overly optimistic picture that encourages false hope, and will reactivate anger when disappointment comes later.

The correct approach lies in the middle of the two extremes. Passing on *accurate information* is the humane approach, and it would help establish rapport here.

> ### KEY POINT
>
> Get briefed by your medical/surgical colleagues when faced with rare/unusual diagnoses. 'I don't know the answer to that, but I will try to find out' is the best answer to some questions. In difficult settings (breaking bad news, terminal illness, angry patients), record in the notes exactly what you told them – so others will know.

For parents, the occurrence of a congenital abnormality, prematurity or neonatal medical illness can precipitate a grief reaction: Margaret has lost her hopes of 'the perfect child'.

List the stages of grief and relate these to Margaret's experience

Exaggerations of normal grief (Box 16), or where a person gets 'stuck' in a particular phase of grief, represent pathological grief, usefully described as an adjustment disorder (Table 26, p. 93). ICD-10 defines *any* grief

---

Box 16 Normal reactions to loss, as applied to Case 12

Shock and **denial** precede the expression of grief. She may be unable to 'take in' what has happened: subjectively, *people* (not patients) describe feeling '**numb**' or even their inability to feel anything. This could explain her reluctance to help with her baby's feeding. Margaret may claim, without delusional intensity, that there has been a mistake and she has been given the wrong baby.

Anger that the loss happened is frequently directed at medical staff: in the person's view, they should have saved life or prevented an unwanted outcome. It can also be directed at others, frequently those closest to the bereaved person. Because she took her doctors' advice about everything during pregnancy and had regular ultrasound scans, she may feel let down by the system. As anger resolves (it can persist in a prolonged grief reaction), it may give way to **anxiety**.

Disengagement from usual activities (self-care, eating, work, hobbies) and from social contacts except a few intimate friends – typically those who have experienced the same grief. This period is culturally determined, although work requirements may intervene, but is usually days rather than weeks. Margaret may be retreating from medical staff and feeding duties as part of this.

Searching for the lost object. This is more relevant to bereavement for a close family member or intimate relationship. Pangs of grief are briefly relieved by imagining we hear or see the deceased person, and hallucinations (abnormal perception *but* good insight) are common and are a normal psychopathological experience.

Bargaining can accompany the severe restlessness, both motor and psychological (going over the sequence of events repeatedly), and yearning. This can involve prayers and petitions, based on religious belief. In Margaret's case, she might request second opinions or emergency surgery for her baby. In people who are grieving their own terminal illness, they may seek new explanations and interventions (doctor shopping, alternative therapies) in order to reduce their distress and restore their previous equilibrium. This might be seen as a **denial** of the outcome, not the loss.

Acceptance implies resolution of the grief and re-engagement with usual activities. While the person still thinks about the lost object, the resultant anxiety and mood symptoms are less intense, and he/she can function at their former level. Margaret would be able to speak about her child's cleft palate without becoming distressed, but she would nonetheless continue to reflect on it as a sad event.

Future episodes of grief are common, especially at anniversaries: in Margaret's case, this could be her son's birthday, the birth of another's child or her next child. Here, anxiety and sadness are less intense and self-limiting.

lasting longer than 6 months as a 'prolonged depressive reaction'.

KEY POINT

Emotional reactions to loss are not sequential (Box 16). Different cultures experience grief differently – in what is culturally acceptable and the religious rituals practiced. Factors such as blaming of others and self-blame make it more likely to be a prolonged, so-called pathological, bereavement.

Margaret seems reassured by the information you have given her about cleft palate, and on the basis of your first assessment has anxiety appropriate to her current situation, is not depressed and has no psychotic symptoms. Her mother arrives on the ward the following day and, with Margaret's permission, asks to speak with you. She is very concerned about her daughter and describes her as 'a different person' – right now, she insists, Margaret could not cope with anything, much less a 'demanding, handicapped child'. Added to this, despite your intervention yesterday, Margaret has not yet fed her son. She watches as others feed him and the nurses describe her as 'miles away'.

What are your thoughts about likely diagnoses?

Clarify what 'different person' means: is this about symptoms (1–5 below), odd behaviour (addiction or psychosis), abnormal affect/seeking reassurance (anxiety), lack of social reactivity (depression), irritability (mania) or loss of usual personality features (schizophrenia)? Take the time to reassess Margaret, including observation of her interactions with her baby, with the following differentials in mind:

1 Non-psychiatric diagnoses are unlikely here. Where mood symptoms are prominent and/or others have raised concerns, *baby blues* should *not* be diagnosed, as the label will play down her difficulties and fail to alert others to the potential seriousness of her condition. Baby blues (labile mood of crying with euphoria, impaired *subjective* concentration) are related to sudden changes in hormones, but are benign and will resolve with support.

KEY POINT

Baby blues are present in between half and two-thirds of postpartum women – their peak is day 4.

---

2 *Adjustment disorder* or other anxiety disorder (Tables 11, p. 38 and 26, p. 93). For example, up to one-quarter of pregnant women develop a severe fear of childbirth, more likely in older women having their first child.
  These fears are thought to contribute to rising rates of Caesarean section in Western settings, and once women have experienced this surgery, the fear is even more intense in subsequent pregnancies.

3 *Post-traumatic stress disorder* (PTSD) remains a possibility: at this point in its evolution, anxiety symptoms will be prominent and these could lead to PTSD (Case 10). Some PTSD cases in women have had a traumatic event related to pregnancy or childbirth. Of pregnant women with PTSD, each of suicidal thoughts and substance misuse occurred in up to one-third. Screen for traumatic events, including partner violence. Maternal PTSD has been associated with poor fetal growth and other complications that compound anxiety symptoms further.

4 *Postnatal depression* (PND) occurs in 10% of live births. PND diagnosis is based on symptoms and signs, supported by collateral history and predisposing factors (Table 35). It is worth noting her mother's description of the child as 'handicapped' and her strong prediction that Margaret will not cope. Both, of themselves, reinforce Margaret's negative feelings about her future, and will contribute to symptoms and likely outcomes.

5 *Postpartum psychosis* occurs in 1 in 1000 live births. This may be rare but this diagnosis has the highest risk potential of all.

KEY POINT

In the first year postpartum, the most common cause of maternal death in Western settings is suicide.

It is now day 8 since Levin was born. You had advised your obstetric colleagues to keep Margaret in hospital but once she 'got the hang of' feeding and her mother agreed she could stay with her, they discharged her. On meeting Margaret at home, she appears exhausted and speaks hesitantly. You screen her for mood and psychotic symptoms, backed up by collateral history from her mother and any health professionals (public health nurse, GP, paediatrician) who have seen her in the past week.

Table 35 Risk factors for postnatal depression (PND). Odds ratios (OR) are from study by Dennis et al. (2004).

	Factor	Risk factor
Mother		
Sociodemographics	Age	Very young and over 30 years
	Social class	Lower income: more depression in general in this setting
	Supports	Absent or abusive partner; lack of a confiding relationship; poor access to transport
	Migration	Immigration in the past 5 years: OR = 4.9 (i.e. strong association)
Medical and psychiatric history	Obstetric history	History of complicated labour, previous miscarriage, abortion, child death. Infertility problems: birth of long-awaited precious child; weak evidence of a difficult switch between wanting a baby and being pregnant; premenstrual tension
	Psychiatric illness	History of depression independent of pregnancy; antenatal depression
Personality	Non-specific factors	Anxious, avoidant and dependent traits; problems in relationship with own mother
		Vulnerable personality: OR = 1.2 (i.e. weak association)
Life events/stressors	Job satisfaction	Absent or low job satisfaction
	Domestic stress	Partner abuse/domestic violence
	Hospital discharge	Lack of readiness for discharge from hospital: OR = 3.8 (as here)
Pregnancy	Parity	Primiparous women; young women having a third or subsequent child
	This pregnancy	Obstetric events; pregnancy-induced hypertension: OR = 3.6
Infant		
Medical illness	Prematurity	More common with assisted reproduction and complicated pregnancies
	Congenital illness	Any anomalies, Down's syndrome and other learning disabilities
	Acquired conditions	Jaundice (even if short-lived, physiological jaundice), neonatal medical illness
Temperament	(?as a cause or an effect of PND)	Baby described as 'fractious, fussy, unadaptable'

Identify risk factors for postnatal depression. How do these differ from the risk factors for postpartum psychosis?

Table 35 sets out common risk factors for postnatal depression. In many cases, these are associations not causes, but taken together contribute to the onset and maintenance of persistent low mood for up to a year. As with other risk factor settings (self-harm, delirium, addictions) many are potential points of intervention as prevention or treatment.

Being single of itself does not directly lead to PND, but

is usually accompanied by other risk factors (poverty, poor supports, younger age; Table 35).

Odds ratios (OR) give an estimate of the increased chances of a particular event – where the chances of this event (here, PND) without the risk factor are 1.0. Personality raises the risk slightly, but being a migrant carries nearly a five times risk of PND (Table 35).

> **KEY POINT**
>
> Avoid an 'either/or' approach to diagnosis: it is PND *or* psychosis. She may have mood congruent psychotic symptoms (delusions of worthlessness, derogatory second person auditory hallucinations) and treatment must *include* vigorous treatment of depression (Table 15, p. 49), but with additional attention to the interests of the child.

Postpartum (puerperal) psychosis has far fewer risk factors.
- It is not a disorder in its own right, and is associated with bipolar affective disorder, where the trigger for relapse is labour. Women present with either mania or depression with delusions, confusion, even stupor
- A family history of postpartum psychosis is common, and/or patients may have a family history of bipolar disorder
- Women with schizophrenia may relapse around labour but with a postpartum presentation that is atypical for them
- Organic causes of postpartum psychosis are common and highly treatable

If Margaret has postnatal depression, with no psychotic features, set out strategies that would prevent and/or treat PND

Table 36 lists these in detail. Many interventions are directed at wider society, but they are useful to know when you meet with Margaret's mother and her wider support network. Educating them about PND will reduce any stigmatizing attitudes to Margaret, not least her mother's declaration of no confidence in her, as well as suggesting practical measures to reduce the burden on her.

You identify psychotic features in Margaret's mental state examination: she thinks there have been items on the television about her private life (delusions of reference) and she believes people she has never met are making her think 'horrible things' about Levin (delusions of thought interference). When she thinks she is alone, several people have seen Margaret responding to voices: mostly she gets angry and shouts for them to stop, but she was heard saying: 'I'll do it, and that will show the lot of you'. She told a student nurse that the Devil 'did this to Levin', but she has 'a secret plan to fix it'.

Given what you now know about Margaret, set out the issues concerning Levin's well-being and safety – clarify in each case what you would do to reduce that risk

Try to group these into separate categories. Many things need to happen to sustain Levin, physically and emotionally. If they do not happen, even for a few hours, the risk is neglect – with serious consequences. The key issue here is a psychotic mother but there are other risks. Here is a potential risk matrix, based on current information:

1 *Physical needs of the baby*: the priority here is feeding – that adequate nutrition and hydration are achieved every day. Will Levin be warm enough and nursed in a secure setting? If he wakes frequently, will his mother or another person be able to attend to his needs? Can they feed him correctly and how will they recognize choking or aspiration? Mindful that some weight loss is normal for neonates, set out how often and which professional will weigh the baby. How will this be reported and acted on?

2 *Emotional needs*: these centre on bonding between mother and baby. There will be wide variation in the behavioural consequences of psychiatric disorders. Women with PND may be emotionally unavailable for the infant – unable to experience pleasure in their interactions. By contrast, women with psychotic symptoms could be highly engaged with the child, having separated out their bizarre symptoms – where the baby might be seen as a welcome relief from these. This does *not* appear the case with Margaret: she has linked Levin's cleft lip to the Devil, and spoke of a secret plan.

> **KEY POINT**
>
> Mothers with hypomania can be intrusive and stressful to babies with their attention; mothers with psychosis may be emotionally incongruent, and this bewilders the infant.

Table 36 Levels of prevention of postnatal depression (PND).

Level	Target group	Examples
Primary 'To reduce the incidence'	Universal strategies 'for all women of reproductive age'	Education to increase public awareness of PND, health promotion (sensible drinking, no smoking or substances during conception and pregnancy), family planning, high quality antenatal care, awareness of differences between baby blues and PND
	Selective strategies 'for at-risk women'	Promote antenatal care and make it accessible to women without good income, transport or supports (Table 35). Regular antenatal and postnatal depression screening for all women thought to be at increased risk of PND. Consider therapy and/or prescription of safe antidepressant for antenatal depression
Secondary 'Early detection of morbidity'	Universal strategies 'all postpartum women'	Increased awareness for all health professionals, reduced stigma, use of screening instruments in hospital and community: Edinburgh Postnatal Depression Scale
	Selective strategies 'for women with PND'	Assertive treatment programmes: shared care between hospital, social services, GP and health visitors – with community mental health team if necessary. Proactive measures: reduce stressors, encourage resilience, treat medical conditions likely to promote PND. Reactive measures: increase supports (e.g. child care), coordinate care, and optimize income and housing
Tertiary 'To reduce disability caused by the disorder'	Selective strategies	Agree with patient a comprehensive multidisciplinary programme of treatment of her PND. Rule out comorbid medical illness (e.g. thyroid disorder) and psychotic symptoms (antipsychotic required), combine antidepressant with psychological therapy, treat comorbid anxiety with CBT or relaxation therapy, assess bonding and the needs of the child regularly, maximize supports, and consider best setting: mother and baby unit if indicated. In severe cases, consider ECT early on in the course of treatment. Once responds, devise clear relapse prevention strategy

ECT, electroconvulsive therapy.

3 *Potential emotional abuse*: this is harder to monitor. Other family members and people in contact with Levin need to understand the nature of his cleft lip. His intelligence and needs, if not his appearance, are just the same as every newborn baby. He needs social interaction (eye contact, smiles, conversation, games) to develop: ignoring him could be just as damaging as shouting at or mocking him in arresting his development. Absence of this or direct negative comments both inflict emotional abuse on Levin.

4 *Potential physical abuse*: this is often so unthinkable that it is missed by health and other professionals. Parents under pressure can assault children, but you have been made aware of psychotic symptoms that could directly impact on this child. Even if these are fleeting and the reassurances are convincing, she cannot be left unsupervised with him until they resolve.

> **KEY POINT**
>
> A parent with psychiatric problems should not be denied access to children based on a psychiatric diagnosis (label), but rather, it is their actual behaviour and potential risks to the child that should be taken into account.

Table 37 Levels of prevention of childhood distress and mental disorder, applied to Case 12.

Level	Measure	Examples
Primary 'To reduce the incidence'	Direct	Management of cleft lip and palate in a coordinated, timely way; speech and language therapy if required; nutritional advice; regular milestones checks for developmental delay
	Indirect	Assertive management of his mother's mental health (see text and Table 36) to prevent abuse, or (strongly associated with later mental health problems) Levin going into Care.
		Financial/housing support and parenting skills' training for Margaret
Secondary 'Early detection of morbidity'	Direct	Interventions to improve mother–infant and social interactions: each are more predictive of poorer outcomes than low birth weight; support for and liaison with staff at preschool and school; anticipate bullying by other children; psychotherapy for Levin is indicated for early symptoms
	Indirect	Encourage maternal resilience; family therapy for Margaret and her own mother; anticipate future challenges: new episode of psychiatric illness, new relationship, new baby
Tertiary 'To reduce disability caused by the disorder'	Direct	Comprehensive treatment of childhood mental health problems (Cases 9 and 15)
		One-to-one (psychodynamic, CBT) and/or group-based therapy (family therapy, CBT)
	Indirect	Independent meetings with mother to reduce her guilt and promote his recovery; regular liaison with child minders, teachers and other professionals involved in their care; devise a consensus-based relapse prevention protocol for Margaret's psychiatric disorder and coping strategies

CBT, cognitive–behavioural therapy.

Margaret accepts voluntary admission and antipsychotic medication. Her family are a traditional Christian family: they have a strong belief in God and the Devil, but Margaret believes what a priest has told her–that the Devil has not acted to harm her or her son. She knows it would be wrong to harm a defenceless person and 'killing is always 100% wrong' – even if a voice tells her to do it. She became pregnant outside of marriage and her mother has told her she will never recognize the child as belonging to their family. Her mother, but not Margaret, considers Levin's 'deformity' a punishment from God.

What are your management options, specifying which treatment setting in each case?

Postpartum psychosis is the diagnosis, but you have not yet ruled out *organic illness*. What is her thyroid status?

Could she have an infection? Have you carried out a urine drug screen? She needs to stay in a *general hospital/obstetric* setting until these disorders are ruled out.

Margaret has a new onset *psychotic illness* that requires treatment. She should be offered an *admission to psychiatric hospital* to reduce her symptoms, ensure all symptoms and the functional consequences of her illness are addressed, and maximize her psychosocial treatment (Cases 3 and 6). This may require admission under mental health legislation should Margaret refuse admission. She retains the right to appeal, but she should be allowed supervised access to her baby every day.

Bipolar affective disorder could be the underlying process but you have not established either a high or low mood component (Table 13, p. 45) in this presentation. If this is suspected, she will require *admission to a psychiatric facility* to establish her diagnosis and stabilize her mood. The least restrictive option here would be home treatment, but she does not have enough reliable supports and there are identifiable risks to her baby. Extensive multiagency cooperation must be established before home treatment could safely happen.

At this time, there is no obvious carer for Levin (other than his grandmother) and he may be facing a prolonged 'social' admission to a *paediatric unit*. The ideal setting here is a specialist psychiatric mother and baby unit. Margaret can have treatment for her illness and Levin's needs be met in full – with regular supervised interactions between them.

> ### KEY POINT
>
> Medication for postpartum psychosis must take into account unwanted sedative and hormonal effects in addition to the issue of breastfeeding (e.g. lithium reaches a higher concentration in breast milk than its serum levels). Check the most up-to-date advice about medications.

Maternal psychiatric illness increases risks of emotional disorders in children. 'Cure is costly, prevention is priceless.'

Taking Levin's perspective, how would you prevent distress and/or psychiatric disorders in the first 7 years of his life?

General strategies to prevent PND (Table 36) will support his mother and continue to have benefits for him. Levin is already at risk of emotional disorder: the normal attachment between mother and infant is disrupted with PND, which can leave the infant with an insecure sense of self and less capacity to manage their own emotional experiences. Table 37 identifies these and other interventions that would prevent adverse outcomes in Levin. The evidence base for these is poorer than for PND interventions.

You are general practitioner to 7-year-old Levin and his 31-year-old mother, now married with a 2-year-old daughter. She stopped her antipsychotic 3 years ago on the advice of her psychiatrist – she has been declared well at her review last month. Her husband gets on very well with Levin. Levin achieved normal milestones, is fully well and thrives at school. Four years' ago, he was discharged by the child and family team: no intervention was thought to be required. Given his mother's history, a colleague wonders about getting him 'checked out' from a psychiatric point of view.

Should you re-refer Levin to child psychiatry?

No: you have no reason to refer him. He can be followed up by you as their family GP. If difficulties arise, his parents are likely to report these. However, you must make clear to all people involved in his mother's care that should her illness return, this might put Levin and his sister at risk.

CASE REVIEW

Margaret had many risk factors for PND (Table 35), and the birth of a child with cleft palate seemed the 'last straw' that precipitated low mood. Multiple risk factors are usually prominent in women presenting early (before day 10) with PND: they 'bring forward' their depression, but the peak incidences of PND are at 3 and 9 months' postpartum. Most cases are successfully treated by GPs in collaboration with health nurses/visitors, consulting mental health services only for complicated cases (e.g. Margaret's). That said, her final diagnosis was psychosis: its treatment is identical to other psychoses, except for interventions to protect the interests of the child.

This case unites the reactive approach of adult psychiatry with the proactive/preventative ethos of child psychiatry. In preventing distress in children, many interventions are indirect – for the parents' benefit and thereby helping the child (Table 37). Do not be surprised by the happy ending here. At almost every turn in this case, the worst possible event intervened (unsupported pregnancy, congenital abnormality, rare psychosis, obstacles to bonding, lack of support from Margaret's mother, and hospital admission). These are highly unusual: there is nothing pathological about pregnancy, and even among those women who experience postnatal depression and/or psychosis, outcomes are good or excellent.

Reference

Dennis, C.E., Janssen, P.A. & Singer, J. (2004) Identifying women at-risk for postpartum depression in the immediate postpartum period. *Acta Psychiatrica Scandinavia* **110**, 338–346.

Further reading

Chandra, P.S. & Ranjan, S. (2007) Psychosomatics and gynaecology – a neglected field? *Current Opinions in Psychiatry* **20**, 168–173.

Eberhard-Gran, M., Eskild, A., Samuelsen, S.O. & Tambs, K. (2007) A short matrix-version of the Edinburgh Depression Scale. *Acta Psychiatrica Scandinavica* **116**, 195–200.

Paykel, E.S. & Jenkins, R. (eds) (1994) *Prevention in Psychiatry*. Gaskell, London.

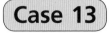 **Case 13** **A 15-year-old head prefect with pneumonia is behaving secretly**

Sharon is a 15-year-old schoolgirl, the second eldest of four girls. Her asthma specialist Dr Conor started her on antibiotics 2 weeks ago when she complained of breathlessness, cough and purulent sputum. She did not respond to the antibiotic and her chest X-ray 3 days ago showed right middle lobe pneumonia. Dr Conor admitted her immediately for a second course of oral antibiotics, but has asked for a psychiatric review. Sharon cooperates with all requests but does not share information with staff. She 'disappears' from her room frequently, especially after meals – any questioning of her behaviour makes her tearful and even less forthcoming with information.

You are the on-call psychiatrist and Dr Conor says he needs to know now what is going on. What areas will you explore with Sharon?

Sharon has pneumonia not responding to treatment for whatever reason, and she may be experiencing some psychological difficulties. Before you can assess her you need to gain the <u>consent</u> of her parents to a psychiatric examination. You cannot assume that they will both automatically welcome your assessment or that the medical team have explained the referral to them. Speak to both parents. In exceptional circumstances (parents unavailable or emergency circumstances), you could take consent verbally by phone but you are well advised to get a senior colleague to witness the phone call and verify consent for him/herself with the person on the phone.

KEY POINT

Any treatment of a minor (a child under 16 years), including physical and mental state examinations, that takes place without the consent of parents or guardians could be legally construed as an assault – unless it is justified by a recognized emergency. Where parents are separated, or there is known disharmony between them, it is best to obtain the written consent of both parents.

Approach Sharon with sensitivity. Consider seeing her with the member of the ward staff with whom she gets on least badly. Remember that Sharon may not have been told who you are, just that 'someone is going to speak to her about things'. Many liaison psychiatrists in similar situations may tentatively introduce themselves as doctors working in the hospital who specialize in psychological matters. Even in some young people, the word 'psychiatry' has negative connotations. Several diagnostic possibilities arise here:

• *No psychiatric diagnosis:* she is on her second antibiotic, and this is likely to be less well tolerated than the first line agents. It may be erythromycin for example – known to cause nausea and therefore administered at meal times. Sharon is a young girl perhaps experiencing her first hospital admission. She may be too embarrassed to tell staff that the tablets are making her sick

• *Adjustment disorder:* to her current infection, this admission, or to being separated from her family and friends

• *Acute stress reaction:* events around family/school/friends/admission, etc.

• *Prodrome of a psychotic illness* (Box 14, p. 113). Sharon is a little younger than the peak incidence of first episode psychosis in women but always consider prodrome in vague presentations or where others complain of symptoms, not the person themself. Her strange behaviour and lack of trust in staff might be psychotic symptoms or part of a 'transition' to psychosis

• Given the information of odd behaviour at mealtimes consider the diagnosis of an *eating disorder*

• *Other diagnoses* are possible here, although less likely: a *mood disorder* (look for symptoms of mania and depression; Table 13, p. 45), other *anxiety disorders* (Table 12, p. 39), delirium (rare, but possible in this age group; Table 19, p. 68), and substance misuse. Just because Sharon is a head prefect does not mean she is not subject to the same peer pressures, influences and temptations as others. Always consider *alcohol and substances* in people with erratic and/or secretive behaviour. Common *disorders of adolescence* have been set out in Case 9.

> *Sharon confides in you that for the past 3 years she has been inducing vomiting on a regular basis, mostly after she has eaten a 'feast'.*

How might you explore possible features of bulimia here?

First clarify her *behaviours* in a neutral non-judgemental way:
• What does she mean by a 'feast' (quality and quantity of food) and how often does she have a feast?
• Does she control her weight in other ways?
• Identify outside triggers (stress, past/current abuse of any kind)
• Facilitating factors (alcohol, shared bulimic activity with friends)
• Associated activities (self-harm, risky behaviours)
   At this point, the interview should be going well, and you can use open questions to explore her *beliefs* and establish she has the mental state examination features of bulimia (Table 38)
• *Morbid fear of fatness* has been described as a 'weight phobia', short of a delusional belief: patients believe that the worst thing that could happen to them is for their 'ideal' weight to be exceeded, even by a tiny amount.

These patients usually impress upon others their need for absolute control over their weight
• Many beliefs are *shared by peers*, perhaps by a wider internet community of specialized websites and chat rooms that encourage food restriction

> *Sharon has been examined by physicians. The only positive findings have been abnormalities on her chest examination and hyperpyrexia on admission.*

What essential part of the physical examination must you establish right now?
Her weight
• This is best done in privacy by an experienced female nurse
• She should be weighed in her nightclothes and without footwear
• Choose a time of day (ideally pre-breakfast) where this can be repeated over the course of her admission
• If weight is low, she should be weighed at least three times each week
• When patients' weights are low, or have fallen over a short period of time, consult with physicians and dietitians
• If there is confrontation around weighing, deal with this early

Table 38 Diagnostic criteria for bulimia nervosa (all 1–3 required). From ICD-10.

Domain	Mental state examination	Behaviour
[typical bulimia] 1. Food	Preoccupation with eating Craving for food, typically carbohydrates	Episodes (binges) where large amounts of food are consumed in short periods of time
2. Solution	Overvalued ideas/concerns that food consumed is 'fattening' and needs to be removed from their body	Action to reduce food effects: self-induced vomiting; periods of restriction of food; abuse of purgatives/appetite suppressants/diuretics/thyroxine, etc.
3. Belief	Morbid fear of fatness: a belief, held to the intensity of an overvalued idea but not delusional, that they will become fat with regular eating	Sets a carefully defined weight as target: this is usually below healthy BMI (18.5–25). There may have been a short history of anorexia nervosa and/or transient amenorrhoea
Atypical bulimia nervosa Food solution belief	Lack one or more MSE findings	Patient is overweight (BMI 25–30) or obese (BMI above 30)

BMI, body mass index; MSE, mental state examination.

• Some patients attempt to 'beat the scales': jumping on quickly, supporting her body other than on the scales, secreting heavy objects on her person or overloading with fluids prior to being weighed. In this context, unpredictable 'spot' checks on weight are useful

> **KEY POINT**
>
> Body mass index (BMI) is calculated as weight (in kilograms) divided by height^2 (in metres). A healthy BMI is 18.5–25. In children under 16 years' old, it is better to use a weight–height centile chart.

She has been vomiting excessively. What electrolyte abnormalities concern you?

Potassium levels: hypokalaemia is a medical emergency.

Mary is the asthma nurse who has known Sharon since she was 10. She is very angry at the time she 'wasted' teaching her how to use her inhalers to manage her asthma. She confiscates Sharon's magazines from her bedside convinced they have made her sick with this 'new condition', wanting to be like 'all the other size zero, silly, young girls'.

What are your thoughts?

There is nothing 'new' about eating disorders: they were described by Lasègue and Gull (independently) over 130 years ago. They are strongly culturally bound, and highly unusual outside Western medicine. Public confusion may arise in that *bulimia* (Table 38) was under-recognized until about 30 years' ago.

It is one thing to acknowledge the high prevalence of bulimia in young women from higher socioeconomic groups, but stereotypes are not helpful. There are associations between bulimia and exposure to certain women's 'fashion/lifestyle' magazines but this relationship does not prove reading the magazines *caused* problems with eating – it is plausible that people who are developing concerns about eating search out and selectively attend to images of thin women in the media.

Negative attitudes to people with mental illnesses among health care personnel (including psychiatrists) are well described. Although there is a limited literature here, people with eating disorders are judged even more negatively by medical staff than they judge people who overdose and misuse substances. Drivers of this appear to be blaming the patient, and believing they could make themselves better if only they tried.

Mary's reaction is extreme. Two possibilities arise: either she knows someone with bulimia (relative or friend) and/or she has allowed her personal feelings towards Sharon to drive her actions. In this case, Mary has known Sharon for 5 years and may have powerful feelings of hurt and anger that Sharon has let her down. Mary's maternal feelings for Sharon may have facilitated asthma education and medication adherence, but in this situation, they have worked against Sharon's best interests.

> *Dr Conor is unhappy. He tells you his job is to look after patients 'who are really sick – not the ones who make themselves sick'. He wants her moved to a psychiatric facility.*

Convince him that Sharon still needs medical care

Sharon was admitted to a medical ward for good reason: pneumonia. Your findings may explain why oral medication has not worked (e.g. she has vomited her antibiotic tablets). Even this will not guarantee that the vomiting will stop, that she will now comply with prescribed medication or that this second antibiotic will work. It would be unsafe for her to leave hospital until she has responded to treatment for her pneumonia.

There could be a direct link between her psychological disorder and the presenting physical complaint. Aspiration pneumonia is a common complication of purging, and the site of Sharon's pneumonia is the most common site for aspiration, the right middle lobe. While medical admission for psychiatric problems is not desirable, she was admitted for a medical complication of a psychiatric disorder. In this difficult setting, it is in Sharon's best interests to be managed medically, but with psychiatric care alongside.

Taking all psychiatric disorders over a lifetime, people with eating disorders have the highest physical morbidity and mortality from all causes. Impress upon him that these are not theoretical risks. Sharon is currently at risk of dehydration, hypokalaemia, cardiac arrhythmias and epileptic seizures.

As a psychiatrist, you need his team's help in excluding a physical illness as a cause of her presentation. Upper gastrointestinal disorders (hiatus hernia, oesophageal or gastric ulcers, gastric obstruction) can mimic the behaviours of bulimia. In these cases, the characteristic psychopathology (Table 38) will be absent, but they are also absent in bulimic patients who deny their disorder.

There are additional medical conditions that mimic bulimia: side-effects of medication, metabolic disturbances and infection. Another cause of regular vomiting in women is pregnancy – this should be considered in all female patients between the menarche and the menopause.

> Sharon has a normal BMI, recovers from her chest infection and is discharged home to psychiatric follow-up.

What treatment do you advise for bulimia without low mood or features of anorexia?

Cognitive–behavioural therapy (CBT) should be the main treatment offered to people with binge eating. NICE guidance recommends 16–20 sessions over 4–5 months. The beliefs (second column of Table 38) lead to the behaviours (third column), but behaviours have adverse consequences and reinforce the beliefs. It is not just that the C and B of CBT act on these two initiators of bulimia, but parallel interventions can help break the cycle. Establishing regular eating should of itself reduce the craving for a binge that will cause a relapse in behaviours. Early response to CBT in bulimia is predictive of better long-term outcomes.

There is good evidence that self-help programmes empower patients to long-term recovery from this disorder. The major component of this is psychoeducation, identifying the patterns of dysfunctional ideas about eating that lead to the behaviours that in turn cause adverse emotions (guilt, low self-esteem, anxiety and depression).

Assessment by a dietitian will establish how best the patient can switch to healthy eating choices with a diet they actually like. Despite extremes of control of their diet, these patients frequently do not understand the fundamentals of a balanced diet – even if they can count calories to the nearest decimal point.

Family therapy, adapted to eating disorder issues, should be offered to everyone under 18 years presenting with any eating disorder. There are several types of family intervention and these are best delivered by specialist centres.

Recent studies have shown promising results with other individual therapies, principally cognitive–analytic therapy (CAT), focal psychodynamic therapy and interpersonal therapy.

Medication should only be a supplement to the interventions above. The use of selective serotonin reuptake inhibitor (SSRI) medication in bulimia has the best evidence for medication use in eating disorders. No other drugs are recommended here: they do not work, and many (e.g. tricyclic antidepressants, antipsychotics) could potentiate the medical complications of cycles of starvation–binges–vomiting.

Even if patients are not prescribed SSRI medication, their overall management should be coordinated by a psychiatrist. Attendance at therapies, other life events, relationships, physical health and comorbidities (anxiety and/or depression are the rule rather than the exception in people with long-term eating disorders) need to be monitored – with changes to maximize the benefits of interventions. While the first four interventions listed above have social components to them, an additional challenge is to support Sharon through her adolescent milestones.

> Sharon has been taking 20 mg/day fluoxetine for 3 months along with a combined programme of CBT sessions, guided self-help and regular family meetings. You have been asked to review this medication by her GP. Her parents are concerned that it is not doing her any good and that she will become addicted to it.

What will you say?

You will need to assess Sharon again to see what progress she has made in her behaviour and her beliefs on food/body weight (Table 38). With her permission, confirm with her parents that she is giving a true reflection of what has been happening. In these situations, most parents are overvigilant and unlikely to miss out on continuing purging, other counter weight gain measures or new index symptoms. If she has improved, it is unlikely that 20 mg/day fluoxetine can take much credit for this (see below). If she has *not* improved significantly, or has become worse, consider:

• The parents' views here. Are there concerns other than the medication?

• The patient's views. Has she placed excessive hopes on the medication or does she share her parents' concerns that she will become addicted to it?

• Fluoxetine is an antidepressant: it is not addictive (Table 7, p. 17), but it is standard practice when stopping it to reduce the dose over a period of weeks

• Fluoxetine 20 mg is an effective antidepressant dose, but 60 mg is required for effective treatment of bulimia, as indeed this higher dose is required for people with obsessive-compulsive disorder. Try to persuade Sharon and her parents that the medication is safe, non-addictive and effective at higher doses.

The consultation uncovers previously unknown details of Sharon's illness. She has had two previous prolonged episodes of amenorrhoea, known only to her mother who promised she would keep quiet about it if Sharon ate properly again. She did not. Sharon's BMI is 14, having lost 5 kg in the past 4 weeks.

What are the diagnostic criteria for anorexia nervosa?

These are listed in Table 39, and it seems likely that she meets these criteria. Low weight drives amenorrhoea and endocrine changes as her body shuts down. Major sleep and low mood disturbances frequently accompany low weight. These latter two symptoms provoke help-seeking behaviour in people with anorexia.

She has anorexia nervosa. She looks terrible and has a resting pulse rate of 60 beats/min.

What are you going to do right now?

Admit her to hospital at once. This is justified by:
• *Bradycardia* – a sinister finding here. She is not an athlete and her body is shutting down. In conjunction with likely electrolyte abnormalities (she reduces her weight primarily by vomiting), she is at immediate risk of cardiac arrhythmias
• *A rapid fall in weight:* 5 kg, or 4 points in her BMI, over 4 weeks
• *Electrolyte and other abnormalities* are likely here: hypokalaemia, dehydration, anaemia and multiple endocrine abnormalities (Table 39). Together with her poor physical health, these are life-threatening
• This is a *new disclosure of anorexia nervosa* that must be acted upon
• The past 2 months of coordinated treatments have not improved her clinical condition and can therefore be described as a *failure of community treatment*

> ### KEY POINT
>
> **External motivations** for eating disorders involve factors such as the influence of significant others (e.g. friends, family) and the wider social context (e.g. a culture that celebrates thinness as an achievement). From a psychodynamic perspective, **internal motivations** may include a strong need to remain in control, with the focus for that becoming physical. Weight preoccupation may also protect against (i.e., help avoid) uncomfortable emotional experience.

Table 39 Diagnostic criteria for anorexia nervosa (all 1–4 required). From ICD-10.

Core symptoms and signs	Criteria	Unusual patient groups
1. Actual weight	BMI of 17.5 or less	Children fail to achieve expected weight on centile charts
	Weight at least 15% below expected weight	
2. Self-induced weight loss	Food restriction and *one of:* excessive exercise; self-induced vomiting; purging (laxative use); appetite suppressants/diuretics	Diabetic patients may use insulin to excess in an effort to reduce body weight
3. Disorders of thinking (overvalued ideas)	Body image distortion (perceives self as heavier than objective evidence shows)	
	Morbid fear of fatness (Table 38)	
4. Endocrine disorder	Amenorrhoea; in prepubertal patients, puberty is delayed or arrested	In men, loss of sexual interest and potency
	Laboratory findings: low levels of gonadal hormones; elevated levels of growth, cortisol, and thyroid hormones	
Atypical anorexia nervosa	Lack one or more of 1–4 criteria	

Sharon refuses to come in to hospital and her parents say they do not want to force treatment on her. They say they will bring her in every day – even for breakfast – but want to take her home with them to rest. Her father says he will give her £100 if she eats a family dinner this evening.

What are your options?

You have a duty of care to Sharon. Her father's suggestion of rest and rapid feeding at home, with a cash bribe, indicates a complete lack of understanding of the seriousness of her situation. His good intentions could kill his daughter. In this context, given her lack of insight, actual and potential medical complications, she may need a Mental Health Act assessment. A stand-alone psychiatric facility would not be a safe option here. Either she can be admitted to an age-specific psychiatric hospital close to a general hospital with facilities to give intravenous feeding, or admitted to a general hospital where care can be jointly delivered. Weight gain must be planned carefully (p. 32).

> **KEY POINT**
>
> Under mental health law, feeding is deemed a medical (psychiatric) treatment of starvation that has caused psychiatric symptoms. Feeding can therefore be administered to a patient with anorexia against her/his will as part of treatment of a mental disorder.

Sharon is placed under Section 2 of the Mental Health Act. She complies with a feeding programme and forced feeding (nasogastric tube feeding, intravenous fluids), although legal, is not necessary. By 2 weeks, her BMI is 16 and she seems to be getting back to her usual self. Her parents want to know the likely long-term outcome.

> **KEY POINT**
>
> Admission of people with anorexia is frequently a necessity to save life. Involuntary admission to psychiatric hospital is associated with worse outcomes and higher mortality in eating disorders.

Table 40 Long-term complications of anorexia nervosa.

	Mechanism	Complications
Metabolic	Hypoproteinaemia	Oedema, renal damage
	Vitamin deficiencies	Depend on deficient vitamin
	Hypercholesterolaemia	Cardiovascular and hepatic damage
Endocrine	Decreased sex hormones	Infertility
	Decreased growth hormone	Retarded growth, especially if prepubertal
Cardiovascular	Hypotension, heart/valve damage	Congestive heart failure, heart valve damage
Gastrointestinal	Gastric dilatation	Dumping syndrome
	Induced vomiting	Peptic ulceration, gastritis
	Malabsorption	Constipation, folate/B_{12} deficiencies
Renal	Renal calculi (stones)	Acute and chronic renal failure
Neurological	Malnutrition, electrolyte abnormalities	Epilepsy, autonomic and peripheral neuropathies
Musculoskeletal	Hypocalcaemia, hormone changes	Osteoporosis: broken bones, spinal injury; myopathies
Haematological	Malnutrition, iron and vitamin deficiencies	Anaemia (especially iron deficiency)
Other	Malnutrition	Chronic susceptibility to infection, poor skin and hair (lanugo: infant-like hair)

What will you advise them?

In broad terms, one-third of people with anorexia will recover fully, one-third will have an intermediate outcome and one-third will not recover to a significant degree. The latter two groups contribute to the 18% mortality (all causes) reported for all people with anorexia. Now that Sharon has admitted the extent of her eating disorder, there are some grounds for optimism, but the average time to recovery is 5 years, and late complications (Table 40) are described even in those who recover fully.

KEY POINT

Many people with anorexia nervosa can be treated as outpatients, but treatment is not a short-term option (minimum of 6 months) and must include physical and psychological health monitoring.

Further reading

Harrison, E.C. & Barraclough, B. (1988) Excess mortality of mental disorders. *British Journal of Psychiatry* **173**, 11–53.

National Institute for Clinical Excellence (NICE). (2004) Eating disorders – core interventions in the treatment and management of anorexia nervosa, bulimia and related eating disorders. National Institute for Clinical Excellence Clinical Guideline 9 (www.nice.org.uk).

Palmer, B. (2006) Come the revolution: revisiting the management of anorexia nervosa. *Advances in Psychiatric Treatment* **12**, 5–12.

Wilson, G.T. & Shafran, R. (2005) Eating disorders guidelines from NICE. *Lancet* **365**, 79–81.

CASE REVIEW

Between 3% and 5% of young Western women have an eating disorder. Self-rated surveys of US women attending college have reported that up to 20% have binged and vomited at least once over the previous 12 months. Despite this prevalence and the highest mortality of any psychiatric disorder, few come to medical attention and those who do present with physical complications. As in this case, you are likely to encounter resistance from patients, families and health professionals.

Anorexia is less prevalent (0.3%) than bulimia. It is characterized by comorbidities and poorer engagement with health services: some studies concluded that outcome is independent of whether treatment is accepted or not. Treating these patients safely and effectively will test your medical knowledge, relationships with medical colleagues and your ability to integrate multiple psychological therapies. At this time, best evidence supports CBT interventions, psychoeducation and family therapy.

Case 14 Insomnia in a 26-year-old successful City man

Nick is a 26-year-old business studies graduate, working at the Stock Exchange. He works 10-hour days during the week and frequently goes into the office on a Saturday and works from home on Sundays. For the past 3 months, he cannot get to sleep and sleeps no more than 3 hours each night, lately even less. He says he has been to two different GPs and 'tried all the usual stuff' but still cannot sleep.

It is Sunday morning of a Bank Holiday weekend in A&E. You are asked to see him. The department is busy and a colleague suggests you sort him out with a quick word and a week's supply of something.

What areas will you explore with Nick?

> **KEY POINT**
>
> There is no such thing a quick first assessment of people with mental health problems. Approaching patients with an open prescription pad means misdiagnoses and missing serious disorders.

Begin with clarification of his difficulties sleeping:
- Is this a new problem?
- Has the pattern changed lately?
- Insomnia can be one or a combination of *initial* insomnia (difficulty getting to sleep), *middle* insomnia (poor or no sleep between getting to sleep and waking) and *late* insomnia (early morning wakening, EMW).
- Has insomnia been progressive, and if so, what has made it worse?

> **KEY POINT**
>
> Chronic insomnia is poor quality sleep or relative lack of sleep that lasts longer than 1 month. People require less sleep as they grow older: some older people can function on 4 hours nightly.

In relation to GP treatments, spell out what he means by 'all the usual stuff'. Begin with a check that his lifestyle, already defined by overwork with the probability of deadlines and late nights in front of a computer screen, might be the major contributant to his sleeplessness (Table 6, p. 16). His help-seeking suggests a strong desire for a 'quick fix'. Clarify self-help measures he has initiated, from home and lifestyle changes to over-the-counter, legal (prescribed, borrowed and alcohol) and illegal drugs.

What are the likely diagnoses?

Medical causes are sleep disorders: enquire about sleep-disordered breathing (snoring, obesity, nocturnal wheezing or coughing), nightmares (as a side-effect of medications, notably β-blockers), symptoms of thyroid disorder, myoclonus and/or restless legs at night. If these causes seem likely, speak with the patient's partner to identify abnormal behaviour indicative of these or other medical causes of insomnia. They may also identify possible psychological symptoms.

Anxiety disorders: carefully explore for other anxiety symptoms (Table 12, p. 39) some precipitants may suggest a particular anxiety disorder (Table 11, p. 38).

Ask about symptoms of *low mood and mania* (Table 13, p. 45). EMW is not unique to depressive illness, but in the context of other indicators of low mood, supports a diagnosis of depression. EMW is both a symptom and risk factor for the development of depression: its treatment prevents depression. Use open questions to establish EMW. It comprises waking up consistently ahead of that person's usual getting up time *and* the inability to get back to sleep. People's usual rising time needs to be established. It will vary over time and at different stages of their lives. You are unwise to diagnose EMW in people on shift work patterns or those who have taken long-distance flights.

Many *other psychiatric disorders* are associated with insomnia. Take a full psychiatric history, while considering the hierarchy of possible conditions (Fig. 1, p. 7) across the lifespan: insomnia in children may mirror stress at home or even abuse. Think of prodrome and emerging psychosis in adolescents and younger adults. In young women, insomnia may be the only intolerable symptom of anorexia nervosa, where other symptoms are inconvenient but fit with the person's wish for control.

> When you ask Nick for the name of someone to speak to for collateral history, he says everyone (his partner, family and friends) are enjoying the holiday weekend – except him. He does not want them disturbed. Nick denies 'excessive' worrying and is unhappy about his lack of sleep, but not depressed. He assures you he has cut out everything – alcohol, nicotine and caffeine – that acts against restful sleep, and already tried many common remedies (Table 6, p. 16). He accepts that stress goes with the job he holds, but he cannot give it up and nobody in his office is a part-timer. His first GP prescribed a week of zopiclone medication that he says was 'worse than useless'; the second opinion GP refused to help him with a prescription. He tries to convince you that you are both busy people and a month's supply of a strong sedative, 'temazepam, for example', will help restore his sleep habit.

What are your thoughts?

So far, you have not found any reason for his sleeplessness, and the purpose of prescribing would be to give symptomatic relief only with the *possibility* (in his mind at least) that he could reverse the pattern.

Nick's 'doctor shopping' should alert you to a number of possibilities: he is impatient, desperate or worse. He might be using a brief period of insomnia to score some tranquillizers that would help him reduce work pressures. People tell untruths for lots of reasons: often it is in their interests to do so.

In short, you are in a clinical setting where history has not elucidated an underlying cause of insomnia, and collateral history is unavailable. As with every patient, but especially in this setting, start with a thorough mental state examination (MSE).

KEY POINT

Step back when you have strong feelings of being pressurized to prescribe. Pressure can come from patients, relatives or fellow professionals. You may pressurize yourself to prescribe something, anything – even if it is unhelpful.

> General appearance and behaviour: sweating (handshake cold and sweaty); did not present as tired but yawned throughout the interview, rubbing his eyes frequently; agitated towards the end of the interview; seems highly alert to outside (A&E) noises
>
> Speech: fast with no mistakes; no evidence of thought disorder
>
> Mood: subjectively 'fed up', objectively he has an anxious affect, but does not look for reassurance; no suicidality
>
> Concentration: poor subjectively and objectively
>
> Thoughts: denies these as 'racing' by night; no delusions or overvalued ideas with minor preoccupations about his health; became guarded on close questioning about some aspects of his personal life
>
> Perception: no hallucinations; illusions or misinterpretations
>
> Cognition: normal
>
> Insight: into causes and treatments for insomnia: aware he has a problem (insomnia) and familiar with its treatment

What essential investigation must you carry out immediately?

Urine drug screen.

Something does not add up when he denies anxiety but presents with multiple MSE features of it. Other pointers to substance abuse are the inconsistency of his symptoms (overdoes the tiredness but denies anxiety), implausible claims (no one who knows him can be disturbed) and his direct pleas to prescribe (even naming a particular drug).

KEY POINT

The first presentation of a substance misuse problem, even with physical addiction, represents the best opportunity for successful interventions.

> The A&E nurse tested a supervised urine sample. Nick's urine tests positive for opiates, cocaine and alcohol. It also shows traces of benzodiazepines. When she confronted him with the results he said it must be a mistake as he has never been prescribed benzodiazepines. She chides him for wasting everyone's time and wants you to discharge him with the telephone number of a drugs advice line. She reminds you how busy the department is, and suggests if you keep him waiting, he will probably abscond.

What aspects of his drug use need to be ascertained?

Approach Nick with sensitivity. He has been 'economical with the truth' on this occasion – specifically he has lied about using alcohol and benzodiazepines – but direct confrontation will result in a loss of face for him. If he is humiliated, he will leave A&E to suffer the consequences of substance misuse (see below) or to attend other professionals. Establish a rapport for best results.

Starting with **alcohol** (Box 1, p. 4), and for **each substance** subsequently:

• Record the age of first use
• Why did he consume it?
• Was it for only hedonistic reasons (to get drunk or high), or to suppress/compensate for an event/loss or a feeling? With whom did he consume?
• Try to measure amounts consumed: with alcohol, this is units per week (one unit is a glass of wine, small measure of spirits, or half pint of regular strength beer or cider)
• Record the doses of prescription drugs, joints per week of cannabis and the total spent on each drug on a weekly basis

With each substance, screen for features of **physical dependence** (Table 41). These differ between substances, and may take regular use before they are established (Table 42). Using more than one illegal drug regularly, polysubstance misuse, is the rule not the exception – most users know the after effects of the cocktails they have taken.

Could there be any other psychiatric diagnoses here?

When did he begin to consume progressively more? Try to note any stressors or psychiatric symptoms that triggered this. Just as we misdiagnose depression in someone misusing alcohol, there is frequently hidden depression behind the high or blank façade of an addict. With persistent cannabis use, psychotic symptoms mask other psychopathology. In Nick's case, and all patients where substance misuse is part of their difficulties, the combination of erratic mental states and hidden psychiatric illness increases the risks of self-harm and suicide.

He has already presented with insomnia and objective anxiety features. In seeking tranquillizers, he may merely have been acting to reduce withdrawal effects. However, if he walked out without your careful clarification of potential physical addiction and hidden illnesses, you would have missed an opportunity to help him.

KEY POINT

Identification of physical dependence is an essential part of assessment of all patients who misuse substances and/or alcohol. Alongside broader public health aspects of substance misuse, physical addiction could potentially result in fatalities.

Table 41 Seven features (**bold**) of physical addiction: 'the dependence syndrome'.

Before	During	After	
Strong desire to consume: →	**Neglect** of other activities in favour of taking substance, or recovering from its effects →		*Vocational*
			Medical
compulsion, craving	**Narrowing** of repertoire of substances misused: e.g. swaps beer for spirits	**Persistent use** despite harmful effects →	*Personal*
			Financial
			Legal
Difficulties controlling use			
When to consume?	How much to consume?	Difficulties stopping once started	
	Tolerance (tachyphylaxis): as time passes, the same amount does not achieve the same effects – more substance is required	**Withdrawal** state (physiological symptoms vary by substance): relieved by taking substance or similar agent (e.g. diazepam to prevent alcohol withdrawals)	

Table 42 Acute effects and withdrawal symptoms of commonly misused substances.

Drug	Intoxication	Adverse effects acutely	Withdrawal symptoms
Amphetamines	Euphoria, confidence Fast talk, agitation Poor judgement Hallucinations: all modalities Anorexia (used as slimming pills)	Hypertension (rare) Cardiac arrhythmias Anxiety, insomnia Acute dysphoria Paranoid psychosis – especially among IV amphetamine users	**Lasts up to 5 days** No physiological withdrawal: can be stopped abruptly, safely. Benzodiazepines may lessen psychological effects. Phentolamine if ↑ BP
Benzodiazepines	Sedation mostly. Disinhibition: can paradoxically provoke aggression or induce a 'high' at lower doses	Respiratory depression: give *flumazenil antagonist* Cognitive impairment Confusion/delirium	**Lasts weeks not days** Anxiety, insomnia Irritability, depression Nausea and vomiting Tremor, tachycardia Seizures can be fatal
Cocaine	Euphoria, high energy ↑ Sexual activity 'speeding' = rapid speech 'snowlights' = flashes of light in peripheral visual fields 'formication' = tactile hallucinations	Damage to nasal mucosa Cardiac arrhythmias ↑ BP and stroke Bronchitis (esp if free basing = inhalation) Anxiety, insomnia Severe depression Psychosis	**Lasts up to 7 days** No physiological withdrawal but support and sedation needed to help with 'crash' of severe low mood and extremes of anxiety
Narcotics/opiates	Euphoria State of blissful calm Associated sedation varies with real dose taken	Complications of IV use at sites and distant (emboli, infection) Aspiration Respiratory arrest: *naloxone antagonist* Dysphoria	**Lasts 5–10 days** Sweating, excess lacrimation, rhinitis. Dilated pupils, yawning Tremor, fast breathing Mostly anxiety and mood symptoms

Nick has no significant medical history and has no family history of mental illness, alcoholism or substance misuse.

From an ethical standpoint, what aspects of his social and other history need to be established?

His *occupation* has additional ethical implications. If Nick was a health professional or had responsibilities for the care of others, you would be required to report this presentation to his professional body. You are expected to report fellow doctors in this position to the General Medical Council; from your colleagues' perspective, it is far better for them to voluntarily report themselves and indicate they are seeking help for their addiction. There are profound implications for public safety if you 'turn a blind eye' to substance misuse in key professional groups.

For people with a *driving licence*, you have additional responsibilities to report medication misuse (e.g. benzodiazepines) to the licensing authority. You are bound by law to report him if, for example, he worked as a long distance lorry driver or drove a school bus.

You may need to inform his GP if he has been using *needles*. Anyone who has shared a needle is likely to be antibody positive for hepatitis C, less so HIV. His *sexual partner* must be informed if he does not disclose an infectious disease.

You must also take a full *forensic history* here (Table 1, pp. 2–3):
• Has he been arrested, cautioned or convicted for intoxicated behaviour or possession of illegal substances? Clarify if there are any charges pending
• Does he have convictions for supplying others? These and drink driving convictions indicate both the seriousness of an alcohol/drug problem, and could imply impulsivity or psychopathic traits
• Does he owe money to his dealer or others? Do not assume that just because he is in a highly paid job that he has not been forced to steal to buy drugs. Most people taking cocaine or heroin will eventually resort to crime to feed their habit
• Screen for episodes of violence, although you will need collateral history to be more certain
• Drug dealing subcultures are frequently underpinned by threats of violence, but users present an increased risk of violence to others when intoxicated or in withdrawals (Table 41). To put this in context, the attributable risk of violence to others by someone with psychosis is 1.2%, but this rises to 21.7% and 29.8% in alcohol and drug dependence, respectively.

At this point in the interview, Nick is cooperating fully with you and you need this information. Your documentation must include accurate risk assessment.

> **KEY POINT**
>
> The two most common deficiencies in risk assessment of psychiatric patients (as determined by homicide inquiries) are that the assessment was not carried out properly early in the treatment course, and that risk findings were not communicated to everyone involved in the patient's care.

Nick has been taking cocaine for 4 years. It began as a 'Saturday night' experience, but within months he was spending at least £100 a week on it. The benzodiazepines had been prescribed by his regular GP but Nick left the practice when his GP said he would no longer prescribe them. Nick has stolen benzodiazepines from his mother and bought 'D5s' (diazepam 5 mg tablets) on the street for the past 18 months. They help him calm down after cocaine, especially now that he takes it during the week. He does not misuse alcohol, but when he goes out with workmates, all it takes is three drinks and he loses his willpower: he 'has to' score that night. Because he works late, he finds it hard to get cocaine and travels to the wrong part of town late at night to get some. He is not surprised his urine showed opiates – he knows the cocaine he buys is laced with heroin when the supply is low. He has never injected himself and would 'run a mile from methadone' as he has seen it ruin lives. For the past 2 months he has spent over £250 every week on cocaine, D5s and codeine tablets.

How will you manage him?

1 Clarify physical dependence (Table 41) on any of alcohol, benzodiazepines, cocaine or narcotics (Table 42). Dependence is defined as a cluster of physiological, behavioural and cognitive phenomena in which a substance takes on a higher priority than other behaviours. All seven features are usually present (Table 41), but tolerance and withdrawal symptoms indicate the need for medical intervention.

> **KEY POINT**
>
> Prescribing for withdrawals should only happen in a planned treatment programme: ad hoc prescribing is likely to perpetuate cycles of substance misuse.

2 Central nervous system (CNS) depressants sedate during intoxication but cause agitation when withdrawn. CNS stimulants hyperexcite during intoxication but withdrawals are characterized by sedation. Check he is not taking other drugs (e.g. designer drugs, barbiturates) that routine urine screens do not detect.
3 Insomnia is probably explained by the cycle of intoxication–withdrawal but be careful to consider psychiatric disorders. A careful screen for these (mood, and anxiety conditions, less commonly psychosis) will alert you to possible suicide risk as Nick 'comes down' from various substances.

4 Physical examination is mandatory here to detect the harmful effects of drug use (Fig. 5). This is the ideal opportunity to check his physical health and carry out blood investigations. Positive findings should help persuade him towards cutting down: his lifestyle has caught up with him. You have a wider public health role here of harm minimization for Nick and his sexual partner.

5 Assess what stage of recovery Nick is at (Table 43). He may not even see his drug use as a problem in itself or for its effects upon him. Were he still 'partying' with cocaine but inconveniently separated from his usual suppliers and having a bad Bank Holiday weekend, he would be precontemplative. All you could do then is 'patch him up', ensure against withdrawals, communicate with his GP, give him some phone numbers and send him off.

KEY POINT

Alcohol and cannabis are 'gateway drugs': even moderate amounts disinhibit/impair judgement and facilitate the person to try stronger, even more harmful substances. A relapse prevention plan that does not address gateway drugs will probably fail.

Nick has psychological dependence on cocaine but is not physically addicted to it. His benzodiazepine use has led to dependence – and he has being buying these and dihydrocodeine from the internet. Despite signs of weight loss and ulcers on his nasal musosa, he is otherwise physically fit. Your history and examination confirm features of opiate dependence. He is not looking for methadone maintenance, but is requesting a brief prescription to stop him going 'cold turkey'. The most he can take off work is 2 days.

PART 2: CASES

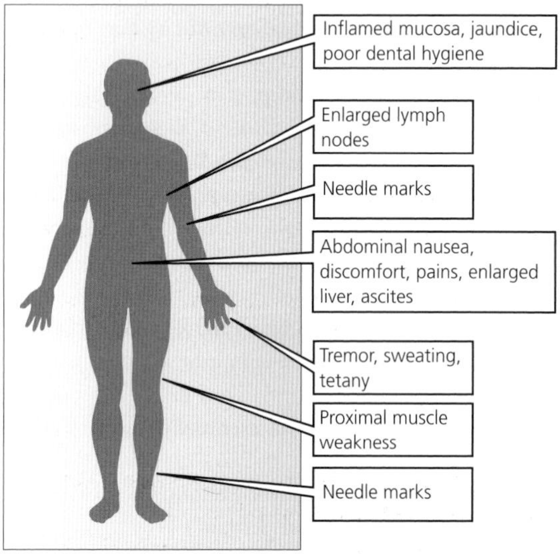
Inflamed mucosa, jaundice, poor dental hygiene
Enlarged lymph nodes
Needle marks
Abdominal nausea, discomfort, pains, enlarged liver, ascites
Tremor, sweating, tetany
Proximal muscle weakness
Needle marks

Figure 5 Physical examination of a patient known to misuse substances including alcohol.

Table 43 Stages of change in the path to recovery from addiction. Based on Prochaska & DiClementi (1984).

Stage	Description of mindset	Potential healthcare interventions
1. Precontemplation	Not thinking of cutting down, or that he/she has a drug/alcohol problem	Educate about risks: police contacts, damage to health, loss of job, broken relationships, etc.
2. Contemplation	Thinking about stopping but no current resolve or plan to achieve this	Inform about options Identify benefits of change for each individual; contrast with effects of use
3. Determination: ready for action	Clear statements of intent to stop using	Help to formulate a concrete plan: gradual reduction, withdrawal effects
4. Action user	Has stopped using for a significant period of time	Identify what is necessary to maintain this positive change
5. Maintenance	Continues to abstain	Relapse prevention strategies
6. Relapse	Starts to use again	Support to restore addict to the second, contemplative phase: 'don't quit quitting'

How might you begin to approach the first steps of breaking his addictions?

It is better that the substance misuse team, or their on-call cover, prescribe a short course of methadone for him. Many services will ask him to return for urine testing (to verify his drug use) prior to any methadone prescription. The prescription is usually written on a day-by-day basis for collection. Once the upper dose is established, this is reduced gradually to zero – with clear follow-up. If, and this can only be decided if he fails a withdrawal programme, he requires methadone maintenance, he must attend a specialist centre. Many GPs have developed an interest in this area and can prescribe methadone in safe supervised settings.

> Nick is frustrated with your decision not to help him there and then. Despite your best efforts, he self-discharges from A&E and refuses any follow-up. One week later, Nick has returned and requests to see you to apologize for his behaviour. He is far more forthcoming about the degree of his difficulties and you both agree on referral to an addictions counsellor.

Detail a brief intervention, based on motivational interviewing

There is a mnemonic, FRAMES, to describe these:
- **F**eedback about the consequences of substance misuse: damage and risks of damage
- **R**esponsibility: remind him it is his personal responsibility to make changes
- **A**dvice to cut down or quit harmful substances
- **M**enu of alternate options for changing his behaviour (relationship, exercise, hobbies)
- **E**mpathic interviewing
- **S**elf-efficacy: each meeting should aim to enhance this in Nick. This concept refers to Nick's ability to achieve change in himself through his own efforts.

Box 17 Potential therapies for substance misuse

- One-to-one drugs counselling
- Motivational interviewing, FRAMES (see text)
- Self-help group interventions: *Alcoholics Anonymous* and *Narcotics Anonymous*. Regular attendance predicts better outcomes
- Formal group therapy (open and closed groups): these may be linked to treatment settings
- Meetings and possible interventions with friends and family: they have a key role in maintenance of sobriety. In this case, he excluded them initially, but this does not mean they will not be essential players in his future recovery
- Treatment (as usual) of psychiatric comorbidities
- Couples'/relationship therapy
- Monitoring of misuse (e.g. self-report diaries, urine screens), physical and mental health: these are best combined in a specialist psychiatry of substance misuse setting
- Some intravenous drug users require specialist medical treatment of the medical complications of drug use: hepatitis C and HIV infections. Both illnesses have common psychiatric complications, and these may require specific therapies
- Other supports: many women are forced into prostitution by their drug habit. They may require physical protection from pimps and drug dealers; with child care issues, it is better to involve social services early – on a voluntary and transparent basis. These and similar interventions help break the cycle of intimidation–poverty–despair–using

CASE REVIEW

Treating people with substance misuse is a constant challenge. They seldom present in a straightforward manner. If you assume all they want or need is more drugs, by this definition you can never give them what they want. In Nick's defence, it is hard to ask for help for substance misuse directly, and when he agreed to a urine test he must have known it would test positive. It is difficult for people who have never had an addiction to understand the intensity of craving, and how this overwhelms them at the expense of honesty and their usual behaviours (see Further reading, p. viii). You should not suspend judgement on addicts, but it is never your role to punish them for their actions.

Continued

At every stage of addiction, it is difficult to separate drug symptoms from psychiatric symptoms, but it is important that you try. You need to combine your skills as a physician to manage adverse consequences of addiction safely (for your patient and the wider community) and to apply your best judgements as a psychiatrist about how and when to treat root causes/maintainers of addiction. Part of this is to establish 'where they are at' – the stage of change (Table 43) – and link patients in to the best talking treatments for them (Box 17). Use the 'FRAMES' method in each contact with people who are misusing alcohol or drugs. We have not given Nick's story beyond 1 week, and it is likely he will require multiple interventions over time to keep him sober.

References

Prochaska, J. & DiClementi, C. (1984) Stages in the modification of problem behaviors. In Hersen, M., Eisler, R. & Miller, P. (eds.) *Progress in Behavior Modification*, Vol. 28. Sycamore Publishing, Sycamore, IL.

Further reading

Bien, T.H. (1993) Motivational interviewing with alcoholic outpatients. *Behavioural and Cognitive Psychotherapy* **21**, 347–356.

Coid, J., Yang, M., Roberts, A., Ullrich, S., Moran, P., Bebbington, P., *et al.* (2006) Violence and psychiatric morbidity in the national household population of Britain: public health implications. *British Journal of Psychiatry* **189**, 12–19.

Crome, I.B., Bloor, R. & Thom, B. (2006) Screening for substance misuse: whose job is it? *Advances in Psychiatric Treatment* **12**, 375–383.

Kupfer, D.J. & Reynolds, C.F. (1997) Management of insomnia. *New England Journal of Medicine* **336**, 341–346.

Swadi, H. (2000) Substance misuse in adolescents. *Advances in Psychiatric Treatment* **6**, 201–210.

Case 15 A 15-year-old child assaults his foster mother

Five days ago, 15-year-old Joe had a tantrum during which he hit his main carer, Jodi, who had been looking after him for almost a year. Jodi's husband brought her to A&E with a black eye and scratches to her face. She was discharged without follow-up: no X-rays or other investigations were ordered. Joe was not seen in A&E; he was looked after at home by his social worker who noted that he remained silent all afternoon.

You have been asked to see him. They say the assault on his foster mother was minor but want to know if this behaviour is likely to recur.

What areas will you explore with Joe?

Clarify who is the responsible guardian for Joe. This could be either his foster mother or his social worker – or a third unnamed person. You *must* get his guardian's consent, preferably in writing, before you interview Joe.

His guardian, a social worker, gives you verbal consent by telephone, and arranges to fax you written confirmation of this. She says Joe has been in care for most of the time since his mother died 11 years ago. She had thought this placement was working well. You will wait until you receive her fax.

What are your objectives here?

Your priority here is to gain Joe's trust. For whatever reason, things got out of hand at home and he needs to explain what happened.
• You need to hear the full sequence of his dispute with Jodi
• How did he feel afterwards?
• Explore his home situation from his perspective
• Was this the first blow up?
• Who else lives there other than his foster parents and him?
• Does anything point towards a mental health disorder of childhood (Case 9)?
• Are there other factors that will help you establish a multiaxial diagnosis (Table 30, p. 101)?

Joe is brought to see you by Paddy, his foster father. He wishes he had been at home when it happened. He tells you he is not angry at what Joe did but wants some guidance as to what to do to prevent it happening again. Joe has been prone to tantrums for longer than he has known him. He says Joe is well able to 'tell a good version of his side of the story'. He asks to sit in on your interview so he knows what you hear.

What will you do?

To achieve full disclosure from Joe, and to understand his perspective – even if this includes Joe telling untruths to you – the better option here is to interview Joe without Paddy. You can supplement this with collateral histories from Paddy and Jodi later. Parents and foster parents should understand their voices will always be heard. You will also need to speak to his social worker. It is likely she has access to Joe's longer history, perhaps previous assessments and interventions. Joe must have been the subject of a multidisciplinary case conference and notes from these will give you a picture of what Joe is like and may even document previous similar problems. At some point, you should convene a meeting with everyone to establish the full version of events and test your working hypotheses of how events turned out so badly.

Joe tells you that 5 days ago he knew he was not allowed play his video game but he turned it on anyway. When Jodi and Paddy asked him to stop, he ignored them. When she unplugged his game, he scratched her. Nothing like that has happened 'before or since'. He has been very happy with Paddy and Jodi, and would hate to leave. His lip is cut and he has bruises on his arms. He says this happened playing football.

What are your thoughts?

You have uncovered a contradiction in the sequence of events. Paddy says he was not in the house at the time of the argument but Joe says he was. In the circumstances of a row, most teenagers would express at least ambiva-

143

lence to their carers. In addition, a child is unlikely to use so succinct a phrase as 'before or since'. It is quite a defensive statement, and it could have been picked up from his foster parents' lexicon, or it could have been rehearsed with them to project a certain version of events.

You are still gathering evidence. With any child of this age, frequent confrontations at home are the rule not the exception. You would expect these to be more common in someone who has been fostered for a relatively short period of time. Even if Paddy and Jodi are experienced foster parents, they may have had disagreements about limit setting for Joe.

The most negative part of Joe's story so far is the number of years he spent in care as even the best settings fall considerably short of nurturing parental relationships. Set aside your prejudices:

• Joe could be the sole aggressor here, he could be a victim of physical abuse (from either parent or someone else at home, neighbourhood, school, etc.), or this could be a mixture of both his aggression and others'

• If you have not already done so, interview Joe in the presence of another colleague from your team. There may be further subtle phrases and signs that help point to the truth here. Your colleague and you can document properly and improve objectivity

> **KEY POINT**
>
> Do not to turn a 'blind eye' to non-accidental injury (NAI) in children. Balance your instincts with due process to the people who are the subject of allegations.

How will you document possible non-accidental injury?

If NAI is suspected, arrange for photographs of the direct physical evidence and carefully document investigation findings (Table 44).

Even if the child has disclosed physical abuse, he/she frequently thinks that it was deserved punishment and may play down injuries.

Any head injury where NAI is suspected is both a medical and social care emergency. The child is admitted to a paediatric ward, without judgement or accusations, and managed medically – while gathering evidence about the causes of the trauma. Children fight frequently, but

Table 44 Factors that raise suspicion of non-accidental injury (NAI) in children.

	Factors
Previous history	Repeated visits to GPs or A&E with injuries; documented failure to seek medical care for significant injuries
Past physical evidence	Multiple established injuries: exam and X-ray evidence (e.g. rib fractures, many fractures at different stages of healing)
This presentation	Inconsistent details; reluctance to give any details; well 'rehearsed' story of events; direct accusations common in older children
This examination	Nature of injuries: defensive or offensive; child upset, nervous: 'frozen watchfulness'; burns or scalds; any head injury: check for retinal haemorrhages
Parents/carers	Hostility to questions; lack of guilt about injuries; requests to take child home before investigations
Other collateral accounts	Concern from teachers (recent deterioration in grades), other relatives, neighbours, doctors (growth charts), etc.
X-ray investigations	CT or MRI of brain to rule out life-threatening injury; full skeletal survey
Blood tests	To confirm NAI, you must rule out bleeding or other medical disorders

CT, computed tomography; MRI, magnetic resonance imaging.

a child is unlikely to inflict significant head trauma on another child.

> **KEY POINT**
>
> NAI is a common cause of death in children, especially infants. The most common finding in inquiries into deaths of children is the identification of several points in past medical presentations where doctors should have intervened but did not do so.

Joe does not appear to be in any distress. The cut to his lip is fresh and could have been either a sports injury or

PART 2: CASES

self-biting. He has no other injuries, investigations (Table 44) are normal and computer records confirm he did not have multiple presentations to GPs or A&E departments locally. Paddy and Jodi are interviewed separately. They are a middle-aged couple (each in their fifties) who have been fostering children for 20 years. They have never been the subject of allegations of mistreatment, despite taking on challenging children. Last Thursday, Joe had said he had 'tummy pains' and stayed home from school. He recovered quickly and started playing video games and swearing loudly. Jodi rang Paddy at work, but he could not leave until 4 PM. Jodi says she did not provoke Joe by unplugging his game but that when he broke it himself, he 'went for' her. She was relieved when the social worker arrived as she was 'shaken' and it was a relief to go to A&E where she was joined by Paddy.

What are your thoughts now?

At this point, NAI seems less likely but you must document the areas where suspicion arose and have a direct conversation with Joe's social worker.

The *paramount principle* is that the child's interests come first (Table 5, p. 14). Separate objective information (foster parents' age, school attendance record, Paddy was at work – *verify this directly*, Jodi's injuries) from subjective judgements (they are a nice couple, they have a blame-free record, Joe appears vulnerable).

You should consider childhood sexual abuse (CSA) in children displaying new psychological or behavioural symptoms, especially if these are sexualized or brutal in nature (e.g. torturing animals in Case 9). Other presentations include unexplained deteriorations in school performance, self-harm, adolescent encopresis/enuresis, school refusal or running away from home.

KEY POINT

Victims of CSA tend to be anxious vulnerable children who are less likely to speak up for themselves. Perpetrators target 'quiet' children, especially those in care, knowing they are less likely to disclose the abuse and also less likely to be believed.

The case is not made for either NAI or CSA. You receive objective evidence that Joe exhibited violent behaviour in his previous two placements. Paddy and Jodi had raised concerns about Joe, but because he has had multiple placements, a consensus decision was that Joe would attend anger management sessions through the school's counselling service and everyone would document his behaviour. Two weeks later, Joe was discovered destroying their wedding album with a sharp knife. He said they needed a 'makeover' and he was doing them a favour. Paddy said Joe 'did not even pretend' that he was sorry for doing something so nasty. His bad behaviour has been escalating.

What is your differential diagnosis here?

You are working with a small amount of information and during one assessment Joe failed to volunteer symptoms suggestive of any particular disorder. In such cases, give a broad differential highlighting common conditions for the patient's age and gender:

• *Conduct disorder* (CD) is a strong possibility (Case 9)

• *Emotional disorder* seems unlikely given the lack of anxiety or emotional symptoms. He may have had these in the past

• *Attention deficit disorder* without hyperactivity (ADD) and attention deficit disorder with hyperactivity (ADHD) should have become apparent at an earlier age (Case 9). You should be reassured by Joe's ability to sit still when he is doing what he wants to do, and his calm presentation to you. His foster parents are under considerable pressure (damage to their property, assault, placement breaking down, suspicion of NAI) and may not provide the reflective history necessary to identify ADD. Talk to Joe's teachers

• You should rule out *organic pathology* (nothing in his history suggests this)

• His behaviour could be part of cycles of intoxication and disinhibition caused by *alcohol and/or substance misuse*: carry out a urine screen. Cannabis is a major cause of both depression and psychosis in adolescents. When these occur in early life, both are more likely to become lifelong conditions

• *Depression* is the most common psychiatric diagnosis at all ages, beginning in early teens. Even if Joe has normal mood on this occasion, intermittent mood symptoms could have contributed to the behaviours highlighted above. Try to see mood disorder on a spectrum of severity with distinctive temporal patterns (Fig. 6). In your enquiry about mood symptoms (Table 13, p. 45), steer towards impairments in his enjoyment of hobbies and

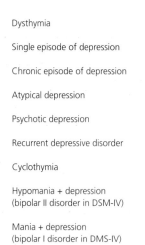

Dysthymia

Single episode of depression

Chronic episode of depression

Atypical depression

Psychotic depression

Recurrent depressive disorder

Cyclothymia

Hypomania + depression
(bipolar II disorder in DSM-IV)

Mania + depression
(bipolar I disorder in DMS-IV)

Figure 6 The affective spectrum. From Smith & Blackwood (2004).

deficits in social function rather than the more 'adult' discussion of lowered mood
• *Anxiety symptoms* should have declared themselves by now
• *Psychosis* is less common in this age group, but it can present as a non-specific prodrome (Box 14, p. 113)

KEY POINT

Diagnosis is always helpful but not essential in devising management strategies in children and adolescents.

Joe does not have psychotic symptoms, nor does he misuse alcohol or substances. He had a difficult time following the death of his mother from cancer when he was 4. He was an only child who never knew his father, and spent his early years in care. Everyone hoped that this placement 1 year ago would be an ideal setting where he could thrive. His behaviour continues to challenge the limits set for him by his foster parents. The pattern is that he 'strikes out' at them or household objects, usually at bedtime or at weekends. The consensus diagnosis is that Joe has a conduct disorder.

Do you have any concerns about the diagnosis of CD in this case?

Yes. Adolescent onset CD is unusual and may indicate comorbidity (ADD, substance misuse, depression, learning disability) or has been brought on by adverse events: disappointments (perceived as important by the child),

parental disharmony and intolerable home situations through to abuse of all kinds. Prodrome and/or early symptoms of psychosis remains a possibility and you should continue to observe for any signs of this (Box 14, p. 113) or transition to psychosis. Joe may be exhibiting psychopathic traits for the first time.

The diagnosis is CD. His foster parents enrol on a parenting course, his social worker agrees to weekly visits to monitor his behaviour, and staying with a maternal aunt is arranged for Joe on alternative weekends. Joe is sent for individual therapy.

What different forms of psychological treatment can be taken?

Broadly, there are three therapeutic alternatives:

1 Supportive therapy is the least 'invasive' option while psychodynamic therapy addresses more deep-rooted issues
2 Cognitive–behavioural therapy (CBT) is usually seen as an intermediate option (Table 45)
3 Psychodynamic therapy helps make links between current difficulties and past losses

Most therapists are familiar with all three modalities and may have an eclectic approach to using several elements in combination with others. Table 45 is a useful conceptualization of therapies' commonalities and points of departure – a similar approach is useful for adults.

Joe's difficulties are too complex for a support-only intervention, although these techniques (brief meetings, immediate gains, simple explanations, confidence building) are an excellent way of beginning the process of engaging him.

A CBT approach could chart his thoughts and feelings as antecedents of his (unwanted) behaviours. Remember that he may gain in the short term from these behaviours: negative attention is better than no attention, he may be controlling others' actions towards him by invoking their fear of another episode, or he could be modelling his aggressive behaviour on his idea of how 'real men' behave. Previous cases (Cases 1, 4 and 10) have demonstrated how patients can confuse the distress of anxiety symptoms (Fig. 2, p. 37) with anger feelings, and this may be relevant here. Joe has already been exposed to anger management therapy, and he may have his own views on this CBT-based approach. However, CBT on its own will

Table 45 Three broad approaches to psychotherapy. After Lask *et al.* (2003).

	Supportive psychotherapy	Cognitive–behavioural therapy	Psychodynamic psychotherapy
Who?	Vulnerable children with poorly developed psychological strategies	Children who prefer educational/thinking approaches	More resilient children who want to understand their emotions and relationships
What?	Emphasis on coping skills: strength to solve the problems the client has right now	Focus on unrealistic thinking: problems as a model for future ones. How feelings and thoughts affect us now	Discussion of patterns of past struggles: how losses and past relationships influence current feelings
Why?	To get through this To keep going To gain confidence	To show that the way they think influences how they feel Change thinking style to protect against future stresses	To understand why they feel the way they do To understand patterns of difficult times To change style of feeling and coping via their relationships
How?	Build trust through listening Brief interviews Limited sessions	Feeling finding, thought spotting, symptom searches, schemata Fixed number of sessions	Greater emphasis on therapeutic relationship, transference, process More sessions, length of therapy may not be fixed

not help Joe with several past losses and relationships, for example:
• His lack of a father figure
• Maternal bonding: what was the impact of his mother's illness on her capacity to bond with Joe prior to her death?
• How has he coped with her loss?
• What effect did multiple care settings have on his ability to develop and sustain relationships?
• Does his relationship with Paddy or Jodi remind him of previous relationships?
• Does he have any regrets about his behaviour with his foster parents?

Eighteen months later, Joe is living in his own room in a supported hostel. His placement broke down with Paddy and Jodi, although Paddy calls by every week to see how he is. Paddy spent 2 months in hospital for a heart condition but Joe did not visit him. Joe had over a year of psychodynamic psychotherapy which he found annoying and upsetting. He says on his good days he likes to think his past is behind him. He stopped psychotherapy on his 17th birthday. He wishes he was 18 so he could say goodbye to 'everyone in the mental health services'. New hostel residents and staff find him charming, but those who get to

know him become wary of his requests for money – he never pays them back. The local police know him well. They have cautioned him for threatening behaviour and he will be charged with stealing a car and driving it recklessly without a licence, smashing a glass into a woman's face in a public house and for an alleged aggravated assault on the arresting officer. Joe says he will plead 'not guilty' even though they caught him on camera. He wants to make it worth their while taking him to court.

You have been asked to compile a report on Joe for his upcoming court appearance.

What approach will you take?
You are well placed to give a detailed historical account of Joe's childhood and what has led him to where he is now, and Joe has reached an age (17 years) where he can directly consent to this.

To achieve a comprehensive report (Table 33, p. 114), it would be useful to talk to other professionals involved in his care, especially the psychotherapist who saw him. If interventions were not completed, state this.

Joe is not claiming mental disorder as a defence, but his difficulties in the context of childhood adversity may go towards mitigation.

Record what the working diagnoses were throughout his contact with services: there was no evidence of either a mood or sustained psychotic disorder, and he did not have ADD. He was not therefore prescribed psychoactive medication. This is an important negative in that the Court may link medications with severity of disorder. It will look negatively upon an individual who was prescribed medications but did not take them.

If you have objective evidence that he did not misuse substances or alcohol, this is useful information to report. It is also useful to indicate appointments kept and incidences where Joe complied with advice given or treatments recommended.

What's the diagnosis?

Joe does not have a definitive diagnosis. Conduct disorder does not fully explain how he feels and acts, and he cannot be said to have a conventional treatable psychiatric disorder. Nor is he fully 'well', and psychopathy is a possibility but you cannot recommend specific treatments for this. Your report may evoke the Court's sympathy with a view towards mitigation, but it will not give the Court any opportunity for disposal of the case other than through a Referral order (for a first offence) or a Detention and Training order (prison equivalent for young people).

What should you do?

Seek the advice of a consultant forensic psychiatrist. While you may suspect psychopathy (Box 18), this is a complex specialized diagnosis best made by a forensic specialist. This 'second opinion' could also recommend specialist interventions with which you are unfamiliar. It is not in Joe's interests to receive a label of psychopathy from a non-specialist (you) who views the 'disorder' as untreatable, and has no positive suggestions to treat it. The worst outcome here *from Joe's point of view* is a Detention and Training order. A forensic consultant is best placed to ensure transfer to the best setting for Joe, and that he receives treatment likely to benefit him and reduce any risks to society.

Box 18 Item content of the Hare Psychopathy Checklist: Youth Version (after Forth *et al.* 2004)

1 *Impression management*: conforms with notions of social desirability, presents him/herself in a good light, is superficially charming

2 *Grandiose sense of self-worth*: is dominating, opinionated, has an inflated view of own ability

3 *Stimulation-seeking*: needs novelty, excitement, is prone to boredom and risk-taking behaviours

4 *Pathological lying*: exhibits pervasive lying, lies readily, easily and obviously

5 *Manipulation for personal gain*: is deceitful, manipulates, engages in dishonest or fraudulent schemes that can result in criminal activity

6 *Lack of remorse*: has no guilt, lacks concern about the impact of his/her actions on others; justifies and rationalises their abuse of others

7 *Shallow affect*: has only superficial bonds with others, feigns emotion

8 *Callous or lacking empathy*: has a profound lack of empathy, views others as objects, has no appreciation of the needs or feelings of others

9 *Parasitic orientation*: exploits others, lives at the expense of friends and family, gets others to do his or her schoolwork using threats

10 *Poor anger control*: is hotheaded, easily offended and reacts aggressively, is easily provoked to violence

11 *Impersonal sexual behaviour*: has multiple casual sexual encounters, indiscriminate sexual relationships, uses coercion and threats

12 *Early behavioural problems*: lying, thieving, fire-setting before 10 years of age

13 *Lacks goals*: has no interest or understanding of the need for education, lives day-to-day, has unrealistic aspirations for the future

14 *Impulsivity*: acts out frequently, quits school, leaves home on a whim, acts on the spur of the moment, never considers the consequences of impulsive acts

15 *Irresponsibility*: habitually fails to honour obligations or debts, shows reckless behaviour in a variety of settings, including school and home

16 *Failure to accept responsibility*: blames others for his/her problems, claims that he/she was 'set up', is unable and unwilling to accept personal responsibility for own actions

17 *Unstable interpersonal relationships*: has turbulent extrafamilial relationships, lacks commitment and loyalty

18 *Serious criminal behaviour*: has multiple charges of convictions for criminal activity

19 *Serious violations of conditional release*: has two or more escapes from security or breaches of probation

20 *Criminal versatility*: engages in at least six different categories of offending behaviour

KEY POINT

In patients you know well, it may be wrong to act as sole medical expert. Your patient would benefit from a report by a professional who has not been involved and can act as an independent expert.

Joe is convicted of all the offences, but not sent to prison on the condition he attends the community forensic service. A month later, he has stopped attending. He is filmed on closed-circuit television carrying out an unprovoked attack on a father and daughter. The man has multiple cuts to his face and was being kicked in the head by Joe when the police arrived. His 6-year-old daughter is in a coma. At his trial, you are praised for your efforts to help Joe. He gave no reason for the attack and he is given a Detention and Training order to reflect the seriousness of his escalating violent behaviour.

Box 19 Criteria for dissocial personality disorder (ICD-10)

Refer first to the definitions of Box 13 (p. 89) before diagnosing *any* personality disorder. Dissocial personality disorder is characterized by the following persistent feelings and behaviours:

- Callous unconcern for the feelings of others
- Persistent attitude of irresponsibility and disregard for social norms, rules and obligations
- Incapacity to maintain enduring relationships although no difficulty in establishing them
- Very low tolerance of frustration and low threshold for discharging aggression, including violence
- Incapacity to experience guilt or to profit from experience, particularly punishment (e.g. prison)
- Marked proneness to blame others, or to offer plausible rationalizations, for behaviours that have brought him/her into conflict with society

CASE REVIEW

You cannot help everyone. From what we now know, dissocial personality disorder seems likely (Box 19). Inevitably, you looked for treatable disorders at each point in his history: *if all you have is a hammer, every problem you see is a nail* (Mark Twain). Not only did interventions fail to reduce his behaviours, they did not prevent escalation of them. Psychopathy is the pursuit of one's goals without regard to the feelings of others. Joe gets little pleasure from human contact and his lack of empathy may reflect his lack of normal childhood attachments. Efforts to help him understand his feelings, and how his behaviours impact on others, may have worked only partially, or he could have chosen to ignore them. Some prevention strategies (Table 37) might have helped Joe following his mother's death, but this is less likely in the absence of one secure relationship. The ideal intervention should have been to support his mother as a lone parent *before* cancer intervened, throughout her illness, with a managed transition between her care of Joe and his planned carers after her death. Resources needed at this early stage would be considerable, but only a fraction of the material resources required to address and latterly contain Joe's behaviour since that time, even without counting the cost of the distress he caused to others.

References

Forth, A.E., Kosson, D.S. & Hare, R.D. (2004) *The Hare Psychopathy Checklist: Youth Version (PCL–YV) – Rating Guide.* Multi Health Systems, Toronto, Ontario.

Lask, B., Taylor, S. & Nann, K. (2003) *Practical Child Psychiatry: The Clinicians' Guide.* BMJ Books, London.

Smith, D.H. & Blackwood, D.H.R. (2004) Depression in young adults. *Advances in Psychiatric Treatment* **10**, 4–12.

Further reading

Dolan, M. (2004) Psychopathic personality in young people. *Advances in Psychiatric Treatment* **10**, 466–473.

Gerthardt, S. (2004) Original sin: how babies who are treated harshly may not develop empathy for others. In *Why Love Matters: How Affection Shapes a Baby's Brain.* Routledge, East Sussex.

Case 16   A 42-year-old woman insists she is pregnant

Louise is a 42-year-old woman admitted to your psychiatric ward. She self-presented this morning at a GP practice where she was not registered, demanding to see a doctor and saying she was pregnant. Reception staff told her she would have to wait, and in response Louise started to shout at them. When a member of staff approached her she started screaming and began to scratch her own arms, drawing blood. The police were called. Louise was taken to A&E where she was given sedative medication (diazepam), which calmed her down a little. A psychiatric liaison nurse saw her but did not get an account of recent events. Louise had several outbursts of shouting in A&E, insisting she was pregnant despite a test being negative. She also answered 'yes' when asked whether she was hearing voices. She was given a provisional diagnosis of schizophrenia with delusions of pregnancy and auditory hallucinations.

Louise agreed to being admitted to the psychiatric ward where you will see her.

What are your first thoughts?

Louise has had difficulties negotiating with the people she has met so far today and containing her reactions to them – few people would turn up unregistered at a GP surgery demanding to be seen and then have such a catastrophic reaction to being told this was not immediately possible. Since being in A&E she has been unable to give any account of herself and has continued to appear unable to manage her emotions.

It is unlikely that this is Louise's first presentation with such difficulties. If Louise remains unable to give a comprehensive history, prioritize finding out who can give you a collateral history and how to contact them.

A diagnosis of schizophrenia at this point is hasty. Louise says she is pregnant. Can we be certain this is a delusion? Does she have any other physical problem that she is misinterpreting as pregnancy?

Louise has been scratching her arms and making them bleed. Is this deliberate self-harm (Case 8)? Is there a risk of suicide?

Louise has already had a long day. She is likely to have already been interviewed several times already, which is tiring for anyone at their best. Given how difficult she has clearly found being questioned, you need to consider what you need to establish today, and what can wait until tomorrow. If possible, allow her to settle on the ward first, eat and drink something, before you approach her with your key questions.

Louise lashes out at a ward nurse who tried to take her arm. The nurse is not hurt but Louise is distressed. You go to see her and find her pacing the interview room, repeating loudly that she is pregnant while continuing to scratch her arms.

What are your priorities at this point?

• To reassure Louise she is safe and calm her down
• To clarify whether she is physically unwell
• To establish her risk of further self-harm, suicide or harming others
• To discover whom you can contact for more information

How will you proceed?

• Conduct the interview with a nursing colleague
• Familiarize yourself with the room's alarm system
• Tell other staff you are about to interview a patient who may become aggressive towards you
• You may wish to leave the door of the interview room open, with other nurses nearby in case assistance is needed
• Introduce yourselves by name and your positions and explain why you have come
• Some patients are reassured by seeing a photo ID badge. It is better to wear this than flash it before them
• Speak in a calm measured way
• Reassure her she is safe, she is in a hospital and that you are here to help her

- Suggest you all sit down
- Choose your territory: nearer the door, adjacent to alarm, with space between you
- Avoid sustaining eye contact for long periods

KEY POINT

Be aware of your use of eye contact and body posture when patients are aroused and aggressive. Try to turn your body slightly away from the patient and look downwards in between glancing at the patient. When aroused, patients can find a direct stance towards them and sustained eye contact provocative. It can trigger violence.

Louise stops shouting but continues to pace the room. She is clutching her handbag. She does not look at you at all, and is not physically threatening towards you.

What will you do next?
- You may wish to sit down to try and put her at her ease. Let her continue pacing if she wants to – this may be a stereotyped behaviour of hers that helps her manage tension. Physical confrontation at this point is likely to aggravate her and increase her anxiety
- Repeat your explanation of who you are and why you have come to see her
- Ask how she is feeling: is she in pain?
- Ask if there is anyone she would like you to contact

Louise sits down and tells you again she is pregnant. You ask her if she is hurting anywhere. She points at her lower abdomen and starts to cry loudly again. She also tells you that she would like to see her 'worker' Sarah. She cannot recall Sarah's details.

Will you examine her straight away?
- You need to examine Louise physically but this can wait. It might be helpful to get some collateral history from Sarah before you do so
- Louise is carrying a handbag – suggest she might look in it to see if she has Sarah's contact details, you can offer to help her if she likes
- See if you can get Louise to tell you her own address and phone number – she may live with someone who could help

Louise tells you she lives alone. She manages to find a card in her handbag that lists her name, address, telephone number, her prescribed medication and Sarah's contact details. It identifies Sarah as a community psychiatric nurse (CPN) with a local Learning Disability (LD) mental health team.

Box 20 Terminology, epidemiology and aetiology of learning disability (LD)

Approximately 2% of the population have a LD.

LD terminology
Within psychiatric diagnostic systems (ICD-10, DSM-IV) learning disability is referred to as mental retardation. In everyday clinical use in the UK, the term 'learning disability' is preferred. The term 'mental handicap' is no longer used.

What is the difference between learning disability and learning difficulties?
In UK psychiatry, LD specifically refers to pervasive developmental disorders with global intellectual impairment with an IQ of less than 70, whereas learning *difficulties* refers to specific cognitive deficits (e.g. dyslexia). In US psychiatry and the UK educational system, learning difficulties are referred to as LD, which can result in confusion between doctors and teachers as to what is meant by the terms. In the USA, what is called LD is referred to as developmental disability. Throughout this book, LD means only learning disability.

The following factors cause, or contribute to a LD either singularly or in combination:

Genetic: Down's syndrome (IQ often around 50) is the most common LD of specific genetic aetiology. Others include fragile X (mild–moderate LD, associated with autism), Duchenne muscular dystrophy (most borderline IQ but 10% severe LD) and phenylketonuria (LD across range).
Prenatal toxic insults to brain development: maternal excess use of alcohol (fetal alcohol syndrome) and illicit drug use, congenital hypothyroidism ('cretinism'), intrauterine infection.
Obstetric complications: perinatal hypoxic brain injury, premature birth, infections.
Infancy (all examples here are preventable): malnutrition, phenylketonuria, lack of intellectual stimulation from care-givers, experience of abuse – any type.

Note for any individual, especially at the higher LD range of IQ, it may be that no causative factors are identified. Molecular genetics may identify more specific LD syndromes.

On learning this, what questions about her LD occur to you?

• What degree of LD (Table 28, p. 99) does Louise have?

• How does this normally impact on her functioning?

• Is her LD part of a specific syndrome and/or associated with any psychiatric disorders? For example, she might have a genetic cause of LD associated with a particular constellation of physical or psychological problems (Box 20).

Does Louise's LD explain her presentation?

Not as such. It might help explain why she has presented in the *way* she has, but not why she has presented now.

KEY POINT

The term 'diagnostic overshadowing' describes the phenomenon of a diagnosis of a LD obscuring diagnosis of other disorders – physical and mental.

Her LD alerts you to several potential interactions (Box 21):

• She has an increased vulnerability to physical and mental illness coupled with a decreased capacity to cope with it

• She may have communication difficulties

• She may behave or communicate in idiosyncratic ways that appear unusual and mimic psychiatric illness, but are normal for her

• She will be more sensitive (perhaps exquisitely so) to social difficulties and change in her circumstances. Her presentation may be brought about by changes or stress in her social system, rather than 'illness'

• She is likely to be more suggestible at interview. Here the received history of her hearing voices must be questioned

You contact the team and are told Sarah left her job as Louise's support worker without warning 3 weeks ago because of illness. Louise's care is under a locum CPN called Roger who has not managed to meet her yet. Roger accesses Louise's records on computer and tells you over the phone that Louise has a moderate LD and lives in warden-supported sheltered accommodation. Sarah has put a crisis plan on the system that states that Louise is sensitive to changes in her routine and when she gets upset she tends to complain of physical problems. Roger asks you if there is

any other specific information you need him to look for at this point.

Box 21 Associations with learning disability (LD): the impact on physical, mental and social domains

Physical
Specific
Genetic disorders such as Down's syndrome will be associated with particular physical problems such as cardiac deficits, increased rates of sensory deficits (deafness), etc.

Epilepsy in particular is more common; as the association increases the lower the IQ score. Seizures and post-ictal confusion may complicate the diagnostic picture in the acute situation.

General
Overall physical health problems are underdetected and more poorly managed. Individuals are less able to identify and/or proactively seek help for physical problems and the phenomena of 'diagnostic overshadowing' may occur (as described above). Adhering to investigations and treatment regimes may also pose more of a challenge.

Mental
Psychiatric disorders are more common but may be more difficult to diagnose given less information about a patient's subjective experience. Objective observation of changes in behaviour and level of functioning can therefore be crucial to diagnosis.

Behavioural disorders are more common, including challenging behaviours (e.g. aggression); self-injurious behaviour (e.g. scratching, head-banging, biting) and motor stereotypies (e.g. rocking; hand-wringing). The frequency of behavioural difficulties increases with both lower IQ and autistic spectrum disorders.

Social
Social disadvantages can be manifold due to actual impairments and/or the reaction of others to them. Educational needs may not be met and the normal developmental milestones (e.g. forming friendships and becoming independent from caregivers) may be delayed or simply not achieved.

Note there will be a complex interplay between difficulties in the above domains, which can negatively impact on each other, thus compounding the disabilities experienced. In turn, interventions at the level of one domain may well positively impact on the other two.

What might you ask Roger at this point over the telephone?

• Is she known to have any mental or physical illness (Box 21)?
• Does she have any established behavioural/communication difficulties?
• Doses of medication? Recent changes?
• Does she have a history of self-harm?
• Contact information available – GP, family?

Louise has a support package that includes Sarah visiting her once a week to monitor her mental state, deliver her medication and offer her support. She also has a community support worker (Rachel) who visits twice a week to help her with cleaning and shopping. The warden in the hostel makes contact with her daily. Roger cannot find the details of psychiatric or physical diagnoses on their system. He does find her risk assessment, which records she has no history of deliberate self-harm, but she is known to scratch herself when distressed. Louise's regular medication is as follows:

Risperidone 4 mg nightly – increased 3 weeks' ago from 2 mg
Sodium valproate 1 g/day in divided doses

What does this information about her community support tell you?

• Louise already has a considerable degree of support in place
• Sarah's departure may have been a trigger for this episode

What does the information about her medication suggest?

Her medication has been reviewed relatively recently and she is under active psychiatric follow-up:
• Risperidone (an atypical antipsychotic) is prescribed primarily for *schizophrenia*, but it might have been prescribed as a *mood stabilizer*. It also has non-specific *sedative* effects. In people with LD, it is sometimes prescribed for challenging behaviours, backed up by a weak evidence base that it is effective for hyperactivity, aggression and repetitive behaviours
• The medical response to her 'illness' three weeks ago (her CPN left) was to increase her risperidone
• Her sodium valproate might be prescribed for *epilepsy* or as a *mood stabilizer*. It might be given on an empirical basis for aggression

> **KEY POINT**
>
> Psychiatric medication is sometimes prescribed 'off-licence' in patients with severe behavioural disturbances. The use of medication in this way is not based on research, and is therefore best left to specialists with more clinical experience in this field.

The fact that Sarah usually delivers Louise's medication suggests Louise might have run out of tablets recently, or stopped taking them. This could have contributed to her presentation. Either of her medications, alone or in combination, could have side-effects that she cannot articulate.

Do you still want to carry out a physical examination of Louise at this point?

Yes. The above history does not rule out a physical problem either precipitating or complicating her current presentation.

Alongside your examination, perform routine blood tests (at least full blood count [FBC], urea and electrolytes [U&Es], glucose, liver function tests [LFTs]) and if possible obtain a urine sample to check for infection.

The nurses have given her tea and biscuits. Louise is considerably calmer and has some rapport with them. Louise agrees to a physical examination, including palpation of her abdomen, which is unremarkable.

How might you progress your assessment at this point?

Keep her talking. This is an opportunity to take a more detailed history:
• How does she know she is pregnant?
• Can she tell you more about the pain in her abdomen?
• Does she have any associated gynaecological or urinary symptoms?
• Has anything else happened recently to upset her?

Louise tells you she knows she is pregnant because her period has stopped.

What else in her history might explain her period stopping, other than pregnancy?

She is on risperidone, which was recently increased. Risperidone is a potent prolactin-elevator via dopamine antagonism: dopamine inhibits prolactin production and release. Other pathology such as polycystic ovary disease cannot be ruled out. It would be helpful to take a prolactin level at this time.

What else would be helpful to explore around this topic?

• Is Louise sexually active? She may need advice (no doubt previously given) about protecting herself from unwanted pregnancy and sexually transmitted diseases (STDs), and having routine check-ups for the latter
• Does she understand how pregnancy can result from sexual activity?
• Has she been 'warned' about sex in such a way that her anxieties are provoked even following innocent activities? This may underlie her pregnancy worry

KEY POINT

Patients with LD tend to be more vulnerable to exploitation from others, including sexual exploitation. This issue needs to be explored sensitively, alongside their awareness of sexual health and contraceptive issues.

You attempt to examine Louise's mental state as things are going well, but notice that she begins to answer 'yes' to all your questions.

How do you approach this situation at interview?

You need to make a conscious effort to think – even more carefully than usual – exactly how you are phrasing your questions and whether or not she is actually able to understand the language you are using (Box 22).

KEY POINT

People with LD can be suggestible at interview and may automatically agree with what is put to them as a result of anxiety and/or a wish to please. They may have limited understanding of what is being asked and, as with all patients, the more stressed they feel, the less likely they are to understand: it is your role to make sure they do.

Box 22 Good communication in people with learning disability (LD)

Core principles, which can be usefully applied to all patient groups:
• Use the person's preferred name as a prompt before asking a question
• Use simple language
• Be consistent with your use of terms
• Repeat questions
• Avoid using closed questions too early (e.g. 'Are you hearing voices?)
• Do not frame questions as negatives (e.g. 'You don't hear voices do you?') or, even worse, double negatives (e.g. 'You don't not want that do you?')
• If you are unsure whether someone has understood your question, ask the question in a different way to see if you get the same answer
• Visual information may be more easily comprehended than verbal information. Rather than ask someone to tell you where their pain is, ask them to show you, demonstrating how they might do this by pointing towards parts of the body

You are satisfied that Louise is not experiencing auditory hallucinations. There are no other psychotic symptoms. She is oblivious to the scratches on her arms and denies thoughts of self-harm. She continues to appear anxious, still clutching her handbag and gently rocking in her seat back and forth. Her eye contact in conversation remains poor.

How would you describe the scratches on her arms?

They are best described as 'self-injurious behaviour', rather than deliberate self-harm (DSH) because there appears to be no self-harm intent as such. *Self-injurious behaviour* includes stereotyped behaviours: biting, scratching or head banging.

The intent is not self-harm, although there may be underlying mechanisms that overlap with that of DSH (as discussed in Case 8):
• Depending on the context, it could be a form of self-stimulation or self-management to cope with stress
• Physical sensations can help the individual 'block out' external stress and internal anxieties. People with lower IQ have more limited cognitive resources to understand and manage stress psychologically
• Self-injurious behaviour releases endorphins that may reinforce the behaviour

Louise tells you that she ran out of tablets a week ago. She says she has been having a lot of fits since then, and had three when she arrived on the ward.

How do you respond to this information?

• You need to clarify exactly what she means by 'fits'
• Check with staff if they observed any episodes suggestive of seizures
• Her aggressive behaviour may have been caused by a partial seizure. Post-ictal patients may have automatisms and can become violent if others try to interrupt their unconscious execution of these actions

From Louise's history it sounds like she has had generalized seizures in the past but these did not happen on the ward. It transpires that she uses the term 'fit' to describe episodes of strong emotion that she finds difficult to manage. As we know by this point, these 'fits' involve her screaming and sometimes lashing out at people. Staff observed her earlier sitting herself down on the floor and waving her arms and crying.

Have you excluded current mental illness by this point?

No. While you are now satisfied that she does not have a psychotic illness, you are not yet clear whether she has a mood or any other psychiatric disorder requiring intervention.

It may be difficult to obtain a clear history of mood symptoms from Louise. You get more from collateral history from people who know her.

KEY POINT

Collateral history helps identify features that might suggest the onset of mental disorder. For example, in LD patients depression might present with behavioural change, decline in functioning or changes in appetite or sleep (Table 13, p. 45).

Louise's warden, Rachel, contacts you. She confirms that Louise had been very unsettled by Sarah's leaving, but she only became agitated this morning when she ran out of medication (not a week ago). Rachel says she is happy to come to the ward tomorrow and talk to her about coming home, now she has her medication again. Overnight the nurses have difficulties encouraging Louise to go to bed –

she is restless on the ward and starts screaming and scratching her arms again when another patient tries to strike up conversation with her.

What is your differential diagnosis now?

It is reasonable at this point to diagnose an *adjustment disorder* (Table 13, p. 45). She has had particular difficulties adjusting to recent events, mainly the departure of her CPN, with the change in her medication routine as the immediate precipitant to this presentation. Changes in her social system appear to be the main problem to be addressed at present. Note that her adjustment disorder has occurred in the context of underlying *moderate learning disability*.

Thus far, there is no clear evidence of a *mood disorder* as such, but she is vulnerable to developing one, especially if her current social difficulties continue.

Although a remote possibility, *substance misuse* might be relevant here if Louise tried to replace her lost medication with street drugs. Illegal drugs continue to be available on many psychiatric wards, and she may have been given these by other patients.

Her behaviour might suggest she has traits of an *autistic spectrum disorder* in addition to LD. This would explain her degree of difficulty:
• Managing changes in her social system
• Being in the novel situation of the ward – adding to her distress
• Mixing with other patients
• Eye contact that has been persistently poor
• Communicating her distress in any psychologically reflective way
• Placing events in time with accuracy (e.g. saying she ran out of medication a week ago)

KEY POINT

Autistic spectrum disorders are pervasive developmental disorders broadly characterized by deficits in the domains of: (i) language and communication; (ii) reciprocal social interaction, with (iii) associated restricted repertoire of interests.

Rachel and Roger come to the ward to take Louise back home. Louise is relatively calm now Rachel is with her and is keen to leave. Roger is happy to offer Louise increased support over the next couple of days. You are not satisfied that you fully understand the nature of her difficulties, or whether Louise needs any changes to her medication – unchanged since admission.

Should you keep Louise on the ward?

No. The immediate crisis leading to admission has been resolved. Louise has a support package in place and will be closely monitored. Staying on the ward is likely to increase her distress. She attends a psychiatrist who is a specialist in learning disability. They can review her mental state and make any decisions with regards to longer term medication. The results of her prolactin levels will take several days and only then can her risperidone dose be reviewed in relation to her late menstruation. On discharge, you should provide them with a comprehensive account of her presentation, your examinations and findings, including investigations.

CASE REVIEW

Over half of those with learning disability will have enduring psychiatric illnesses throughout their lives. With hindsight, the key omission in treating Louise was finding evidence of her LD late on in a sequence of events. Staff reacted to, rather than managed, events. Additional challenges were:

- The absence of her family (potential partners in management)
- No GP input (to clarify past treatments: we knew her medications but not their indications)
- The departure of the CPN who knew her best
- Her aggressive behaviours and how to manage these
- Self-harm that did not conform to its usual presentation (Case 8)

Several principles of management of LD patients are demonstrated:

- It would have been wrong to characterize her as aggressive and deluded, needing medication – just as her arm scratching could have been misunderstood as DSH
- Although not spelt out in this case, a multiaxial diagnosis (Table 30, p. 101) is frequently helpful in these patients
- Familiarity with LD patients reduces misunderstandings (e.g. that she has a delusion of pregnancy)
- The core issue here is to understand her diffuse communication difficulties and improve communication to match the patient's intellectual level

Further reading

Bradley, E. & Lofchy, J. (2005) Learning disability in the accident and emergency department. *Advances in Psychiatric Treatment* **11**, 45–57.

Cooray, S.E. & Bakala, A. (2005) Anxiety disorders in people with learning disability. *Advances in Psychiatric Treatment* **11**, 355–361.

Fraser, W. & Kerr, M. (eds.) (2003) *Seminars in the Psychiatry of Learning Disabilities* (2nd edn.) Royal College of Psychiatrists.

World Health Organization. (1980) *International Classification of Impairments, Disabilities and Handicaps.* WHO, Geneva.

Case 17 The wife of a 66-year-old GP with Parkinson's disease is worried about him

Daniel, a 66-year-old recently retired GP, is referred by his GP Dr Harvey to the outpatient clinic of Mental Health of Older Adults. Diagnosed with Parkinson's disease 3 months ago by a neurologist, his only complaint is stress. Dr Harvey has been contacted by Daniel's wife, Jill, who says Daniel is 'not himself'. His GP knows Daniel through past professional contact and is unsure whether psychiatric assessment is actually required, but asks you to see Daniel briefly as 'a favour to a colleague'.

What are your first thoughts?

It will not be brief. You need to be wary of being unduly influenced by Daniel's position as a former GP. Doctors can make bad patients. In turn, their doctors' assessment and management of them can be compromised. Problems occur as a result of omitting to ask the obvious, embarrassment about enquiring about professionally sensitive topics for a doctor (e.g. substance misuse) or failing to explain what they assume the other doctor will be aware of (e.g. recent treatment advances).

> **KEY POINT**
>
> If your patient is a 'celebrity' (e.g. powerful well-known doctor), make sure you do not change your standard approach to history, examination and treatment.

There is a lack of any clear history here, probably reflecting Daniel's celebrity status.

If Daniel is having mental health problems, there are four possibilities (Box 2, p. 7):

1 His Parkinson's may be causing brain-related change leading to an organic psychiatric disorder
2 Its treatment may be causing adverse psychological side-effects
3 He may be having psychological difficulties adjusting to his declining physical health and recent diagnosis of Parkinson's (principally, *adjustment* or *depressive disorders*)
4 Independent of Parkinson's, he may have a history of mental health problems preceding this diagnosis or this could be an unrelated problem

> *Daniel attends but is a reluctant historian. He appears hostile to your questions about recent events, and how he is feeling. He tells you that yes, unsurprisingly, he has felt stressed about his diagnosis but there is nothing wrong with him mentally. He never dreamt in all his years he would have to see a 'head-shrinker', and he's not happy about seeing one now. He confesses the only reason he came was because his wife (who is sitting outside) insisted.*

> **KEY POINT**
>
> Doctors as patients may strongly identify with an idea of themselves as invulnerable and always in control. Following the ancient dictum *physician heal thyself*, doctors present late and do not accept help. All health professionals are motivated by helping others in need and can feel uncomfortable when this situation is reversed.

How might you approach this situation?

As he appears to be finding seeing a psychiatrist humiliating it is important to acknowledge, rather than directly challenge, his reluctance. Making him confront why he might need to see you will only shame him more and thus alienate him further from engaging with you. State you appreciate he has only come out of respect for his wife's wishes.

> **KEY POINT**
>
> Do not expect doctors to be any less uncomfortable around mental health problems than the lay public.

Focus initially on the less emotive topic of what physical problems he is having with his Parkinson's. Ask routine questions about the nature of his physical symptoms of Parkinson's (*tremor*, *rigidity* and *bradykinesia*). These lead naturally to more general questions about the impact of the illness on his functioning and the more sensitive question of how he is managing (or otherwise) to cope.

Remember, as a retired GP he is likely to have had considerable direct clinical experience of patients with psychiatric disorders related to their Parkinson's. His hostility may reflect underlying and realistic anxiety about what the future holds. You might try and address this indirectly at first by asking about his experience of this area, and then gradually move towards questioning whether this has led him to wonder about his own prognosis.

Do not forget his hostility may itself be a manifestation of underlying psychiatric illness, in addition to the above possibilities.

> *Daniel reports the first symptom of Parkinson's he noticed 18 months ago was a resting tremor. He then had difficulty getting out of a chair and turning in bed. Gradually, he developed a marked tremor in both arms, his walking became affected and he was annoyed when he had to give up playing the piano. His symptoms have improved since he started medication (a dopamine agonist) 2 months ago. He insists he is generally feeling more positive about things now, and not worried about 'mental symptoms'.*

How might you approach his resistance?

You might switch tack to asking what he thinks his wife may be concerned about.

> *He tells you he has been married to Jill for 40 years and she has always been a worrier. Recently, she has been nagging him about 'some financial matters'. He is very vague as to what they are. He goes on to mention his considerable past experience in neurology, he name-drops several prominent psychiatrists, and tells you he has 'every confidence' in his 'excellent' neurologist, a world expert in Parkinson's. You have the strong sense you are being implicitly contrasted with his neurologist, and found to be lacking. Daniel looks at his watch several times when you are speaking and makes a comment about how young you look. He dispatches your attempts to explore any other concerns.*

How should you respond to Daniel?

Rather than respond defensively with natural irritation to his dismissive attitude, take an objective view. His manner of relating and the response he invokes in you (countertransference, p. 24) are potentially useful tools for informing you about his mental state and personality, and therefore how best to approach this situation. He is coming across as narcissistic. This may be his habitual manner of relating, it may reflect how he acts defensively when he is anxious or it may represent a grandiosity secondary to psychiatric illness.

This is not the time to challenge any narcissistic defences (this is a psychiatric assessment, not psychotherapy), but you can adapt your interview style accordingly. Whatever is underlying his grandiose manner, your best chance of engagement is to appeal to his clinical professionalism.

Refer back to clinical protocol: preface your questions with a simple statement that your questions are – 'as I'm sure you know' – routine elements of every assessment you conduct in your clinic.

At this point you need to complete your mental state examination (MSE), including a cognitive assessment (Table 19, p. 68) – essential here given his diagnosis of Parkinson's. He is unlikely to agree to answer these and personal questions in front of his wife.

Following these, speak to his wife to get a clearer idea of what is happening.

> *Daniel cooperates with your questions, saying he enjoys a 'good quiz'. MSE notes his Parkinsonian gait and a course tremor in both hands. He does not have Parkinsonian facies. There are no other findings of note and he scores 29/29 on mini MSE (MMSE): his tremor prevented him from copying the drawing. There are no other findings.*

Does a score of 29/29 on the MMSE mean neuropsychiatric deficits are excluded?

No. People with above average intelligence can score well on tests despite cognitive and functional decline having occurred as their cognitive reserve is greater. People with high levels of education will always score relatively better on MMSE (Folstein *et al.* 1975), and this can distract clinicians. You need to combine a MMSE with examination of frontal/temporal/parietal functioning, including specific neuropsychiatric tests and collateral history.

> *Daniel is reluctant to bring his wife into the discussion.*

Should you insist?

Yes. She wants him to see a psychiatrist *now*, after 40 years of marriage. Why? Gently suggest he will understand your curiosity as to why that is. Tell him you would appreciate the opportunity to hear from her directly why she is concerned.

> *Daniel's wife Jill comes in and tells you Daniel has lost their savings gambling. She is concerned that he has lost thousands of pounds over the last month on internet gambling sites, which he is now visiting every day. She says this has only happened relatively recently and she thinks 'he must be depressed' about his illness and 'this is his mad way of coping with it'. Daniel tells Jill to 'shut up, you stupid woman' and she bursts into tears, saying he never used to speak to her like that.*

What are the possibilities here?

• Daniel's gambling habit is a new, significant problem, associated with personality change and causing tension in their relationship
• Daniel's Parkinson's may be causing brain-related personality and behavioural change
• There may be adverse psychological side-effects from his medications
• He may be having psychological difficulties adjusting to his diagnosis
• His behaviour, and her opposition, might be complicated by wider long-standing problems in their relationship, unmasked by his recent retirement and/or the burden of his illness

> *Daniel does not apologize to Jill and he adamantly denies debt is a problem. His gambling started soon after his medication was titrated up. There is no evidence of depression or other psychological difficulties.*

What are the likely explanations here?

Pathological gambling was precipitated by a combination of his Parkinson's and medication. Pathological gambling is a recognized, although unusual and poorly understood, complication of Parkinson's.

Daniel's uncharacteristic abrasiveness with his wife and his apparent lack of awareness about the gambling being a problem is also of note here. Pathological gambling is one example of an *organic impulse control disorder* that can occur in Parkinson's; impulsiveness and disinhibition in other domains such as shopping, sex and eating can also occur. There may therefore be organic

reasons for his apparent personality change: lack of *insight* (awareness of change) and/or *judgement* (appraising his behaviour and its consequences).

His irritation may simply be a normal psychological reaction to the situation, involving anxiety and guilt, reflecting his *premorbid personality*.

What might you do at this point?

Explain that gambling is a recognized complication of Parkinson's and dopamine agonists. Daniel is likely to respond more positively to this 'medicalized' (rather than psychological) view of his difficulties, which hopefully will come as some relief to them both as a way of understanding the situation.

You need to speak to his neurologist to discuss this presentation and how his medication might be adjusted as a result. It is to be hoped that reduction of his medication or alternative combinations will bring some relief. Prescribing for Parkinson's routinely involves difficult decisions about balancing drug benefit with side-effects (physical and psychological) and needs to be carefully monitored, with good communication between the professionals involved.

Daniel and Jill need advice as to what practical steps can be taken to reduce Daniel's debt and future contact with internet gambling sites. Cognitive–behavioural therapy (CBT) may have a role here, but you would need to convince Daniel. You might consider couples therapy (p. 22).

Depending on the success of other strategies, selective serotonin reuptake inhibitors (SSRIs) have been reported to ameliorate compulsive or disinhibited behaviour in *some* similar cases, but there is a lack of research evidence.

It is worth taking this opportunity with both Daniel and Jill together to try and reduce the stigma of possible future psychiatric reviews. Alternatively, he might prefer to carry out more private research himself first about the intersections between Parkinson's and psychiatry.

> *Daniel's neurologist reviews his medication and he does well on an alternative regime. You do not have further contact with Daniel until he is referred to you again by Dr Harvey 5 years later with the complaint of increasingly disturbed behaviour since his wife's death. Jill died 6 months ago and Dr Harvey has become increasingly concerned about Daniel's safety in the home. He has been hoarding rubbish, refusing to throw out rotten food and going out to the shops leaving the front door open.*

What is your differential diagnosis?

• *Dementia* sounds likely (Box 23). Prior to her death Jill may have been caring for him and able to contain his behaviours

• *Depression* or a pathological grief reaction to Jill's death must be excluded

• *Alcohol or substance misuse*; perhaps benzodiazepines in a health professional

You visit Daniel at home and are struck by the degree of his physical decline. He is stooped, his posture is very stiff and his face is mask-like with no emotional range. The house is in a terrible state, his self-care is poor and there is a strong smell of urine. He makes no spontaneous speech, there is a marked delay in answering your questions and he scores 18/29 on MMSE. Points lost are as follows: five points on orientation, three on attention and calculation, two on recall and one for writing. You then attempt frontal lobe testing – tests of word generation, proverb interpretation (abstract thought) and estimates – but he stops answering your questions when Nancy (his housekeeper) enters the room.

Other than dementia, what might explain his poor performance on neuropsychiatric testing?

• Non-demented patients with *Parkinson's disease* often experience slowed thinking and execution of actions. You may have rushed him through questions that he needed more time to process

• This could be *delirium*, possibly superimposed on a dementing illness. Potentially reversible causes of his decline need to be excluded (Table 20, p. 69)

• He may be *depressed*. Severe depression mimics dementia: 'pseudodementia'. Depression is common in Parkinson's and is understood to be caused primarily by brain changes brought about by the illness (rather than as a psychological response to it). Depression can be difficult to diagnose in these patients given the constriction of affective reactivity that can occur, combined with the other features of subcortical brain change associated with psychomotor retardation

• He may be *physically* tired, in pain or discomfort

• *Psychotic experiences* might be interfering with his answers (e.g. possible visual hallucinations). These can develop in clear consciousness in Parkinson's and unlike in schizophrenia, insight into their morbid nature may be maintained, at least earlier on in the illness course. He may be deluded about Nancy

---

Box 23 Causes of dementia

Degenerative
Alzheimer's disease
Frontotemporal dementias including Pick's disease
Parkinson's disease
Huntington's chorea

Vascular dementia
Cerebrovascular disease
Cerebral emboli

Demyelinating
Multiple sclerosis

Head trauma
One-off traumatic injury; repeated injury (e.g. boxing)

Space-occupying lesions
Tumour (secondary tumours are more common than primary)
Subarachnoid, subdural and other haemorrhages

Infections
Dementia resulting from HIV disease
Syphilis
Prion diseases
Creutzfeldt–Jakob disease

Physiological
Epilepsy
Normal pressure hydrocephalus (e.g. secondary to head trauma)

Anoxic damage
Cardiac or respiratory arrest
Cardiac failure
Carbon monoxide poisoning

Metabolic
Chronic vitamin deficiencies; metabolic disturbances; endocrinopathies
Liver or renal failure

Drugs and toxins
Alcohol-induced dementia
Substance misuse
Heavy metals

• *Carer abuse* must be considered in vulnerable patients. Dementing illness in an immobile patient is a tough challenge for any home carer. Overwork, isolation, lack of support and stress can combine to frustrate, even anger, carers. As with the abuse of children and all vulnerable adults, it can be physical, emotional, neglect or (rarely) sexual. Abuse can be subtle: Nancy might be giving Daniel alcohol to sedate him, making him less 'vocal' but making her life easier. However, alcohol has multiple negative health consequences (Table 18, p. 62). Here, there will be increased risks of drug interactions and falls

What will you do now?

His physical state is poor and he needs admission to a medical ward for review. There may be reversible organic causes of his current confusion and visual hallucinations that need to be identified and treated (Box 23). Subsequently, the degree of his cognitive decline and any persistent psychotic or affective features can be more confidently ascertained (on a psychiatric ward if necessary) before deciding whether or not psychotropic medication is indicated.

At this point in his history, Daniel is likely to have been extensively physically investigated in the past. Once any delirium is addressed and corrected (Table 20, p. 69), a dementia screen can be completed (Box 24).

Once on the medical ward Daniel's mental state fails to improve and no reversible causes for his confusion are identified. Other than psychomotor retardation, there are no other signs of depressive illness. He eats and sleeps well. A magnetic resonance imaging (MRI) brain scan shows generalized atrophy and a minor degree of small vessel disease. He is transferred to your psychiatric ward.

What treatment can be provided for Daniel?

Physical health needs to be maximized and risk factors

Box 24 Dementia screen

Bloods: full blood count, urea and electrolytes, glucose, liver function tests, calcium and phosphate, vitamin B_{12} and folate, thyroid function, syphilis serology
Scans: CT/MRI
If indicated: EEG, cerebrospinal fluid, metabolic screen, genetic and HIV test, ferritin, copper

for worsening confusion need to be kept under review (e.g. vascular disease and its antecedents should be treated).

Potential iatrogenic causes of confusion need to be avoided. Psychotropic medication should be prescribed with great care – if antidepressants are prescribed on an empirical basis, dosage should be cautious ('start low, go slow') and there should be a clear time-frame to assess any potential benefit.

KEY POINT

Antipsychotics should *not* be routinely prescribed for behavioural disturbance in dementia as they are of no proven benefit and their potential for side-effects is high – worsening both physical and mental states.

Drugs licensed for Alzheimer's dementia, acetylcholinesterase inhibitors (ACIs), are not currently approved for routine use in the UK given their limited benefits in delaying progression. This remains contentious. Box 25 summarizes Alzheimer's dementia, the most common cause of dementia.

KEY POINT

ACIs should form part of a comprehensive care package combining the best environment, reduction in comorbidities and social treatments.

The question of where he will live in future needs to be addressed. Clearly, he has not been coping at home. While in hospital he needs an occupational therapy review of his activities of daily living (ADLs) to look at his functional level. For example, can he wash himself, get to the shops to buy food, prepare and cook it safely himself?

Consider too how liable he is to falls as a result of his Parkinson's? Are there other areas of vulnerability in addition to forgetting to close or lock his front door? His GP, Nancy and his family will be able to provide you with more collateral information.

You manage to speak to his daughter Liz and she tells you she was first aware of Daniel becoming confused a year ago when Jill found him in the garden in his pyjamas one night. Since then, until her death, Jill locked all the doors at night. Liz tells you she and her brother are busy with their own families: there is no question of them looking after

---

Box 25 Alzheimer's dementia (AD)

1 AD occurs on its own or in combination in up to 70% of all dementia cases
2 Postmortem diagnosis of AD is established by cerebral atrophy with extracellular plaques (comprising amyloid load) and intracellular neurofibrillary tangles (filaments comprising microtubules of highly phosphorylated tau protein). Both correlate with the degree of cognitive impairment present before death. Tau protein in the hippocampus is believed to be the first pathological process in AD
3 Early features include word-finding problems, repetitions, circumlocutions (confabulation comes later) and memory loss for recent events (remote memory is preserved until the late stages of AD)
4 The clinical features of AD are:
   ◦ Global cognitive impairment (dementia)
   ◦ Functional decline: after early stages, ADLs are reduced
   ◦ Psychotic symptoms causing behavioural disturbances
5 Personality changes are common in the middle and late stages of AD:
   ◦ Flattening of affect
   ◦ Emotional lability

◦ Catastrophic reactions (sudden overwhelming despair)
◦ Disinhibited behaviour (swearing, sexualized behaviour, aggression)
6 AD is universally fatal, though the cause of death may be recorded as one of its complications: pneumonia, bone fractures due to falls, etc. Due to the age of these patients, other conditions may cause death before AD
7 The cholinergic hypothesis of AD links cognitive impairment with the degree of losses of cholinergic neurones. Inhibitors of acetylcholinesterase (donazepil, galantamine, and rivastigmine) raise levels of acetyl choline. Tacrine is also an ACI but it is not used due to toxic liver damage. The three drugs are expensive and have multiple side-effects, principally gastrointestinal symptoms of which patients may be unable to complain. They should only be used if they improve MMSE and objective quality of life markers
8 In addition to GPs, many physicians work in the long-term care of rising numbers of people with dementia: geriatricians, neurologists and psychiatrists of older adults. Planning of care should involve all professionals and the patient's family, with contingency planning and provision of practical carer support

---

Daniel. She has had to pay Nancy to keep her father safe for the past 3 months. She mentions she was never close to him ('He's always been very selfish') and wants to hear your plans for him.

KEY POINT

Prolonged hospital admission of people with dementia leads to loss of existing ADLs. Balance the need for investigation with long-term plans.

What do you tell her?

The option of home discharge seems remote here given his low MMSE, low level of functioning, absent family supports and poor mobility.

A case conference is an ideal setting to decide on the next best options: his GP and neurologist, occupational therapy, ward nurses and his family should attend. Does her father have a friend who might attend and act as an advocate for him? He may have left an advanced directive or appointed someone with power of attorney (other than his late wife) to determine his affairs. Daniel deserves a say in his destination too.

KEY POINT

The prevalence of dementia increases with age. The prevalence is 5% in people over 65 years, 20% over 80 years and 70% over 100 years.

CASE REVIEW

There are many lessons here:
• Following patients over time reveals other, frequently linked, disorders
• He was a 'difficult patient' at first interview, but in a different way to other cases; he had personality traits of narcissism and was anxious about his situation

• Being challenged out of our 'comfort zone' by a colleague or celebrity can be unpleasant
• The identification of a rare complication of a common disease and negotiation of its management. Pathological gambling has a prevalence of 3% in Parkinson's patients, as opposed to 1% in the general population. The incidence
Continued

is further increased (7%) amongst patients on dopamine agonists
• Neuropsychiatric complications occur in about 50% of cases of Parkinson's disease, reflecting both the direct impact of the disease process on the brain and the relatively common psychological side-effects of treatment: delirium, psychosis, dementia, depression and compulsive behaviours
• A holistic interdisciplinary approach to dementia (Box 25) in Daniel's case did not include input from family members. This was about existing family tensions, probably reflecting his difficult premorbid personality
• Social treatments in dementia are important. In patients with Alzheimer's dementia, these have been shown to have equal efficacy to ACIs in improving MMSE and quality of life scores. They can be more expensive to deliver (transport, occupational therapy and suitably trained staff, materials) but they have far fewer side-effects.

Reference

Folstein, M.F. *et al.* (1975) Mini-mental state: a practical method for grading the cognitive state of patients for the clinician. *Journal Psychiatric Research* **12**, 189–198.

Further reading

Douglas, S., James, I. & Ballard, C. (2004) Non-pharmacological interventions in dementia. *Advances in Psychiatric Treatment* **10**, 171–177.

Holden, M. & Kelly, C. (2002) Use of cholinesterase inhibitors in dementia. *Advances in Psychiatric Treatment* **8**, 89–96.

Schneider, L.S., Tariot, P.N., Dagerman, K.S., Davis, S.M., Hsiao, J.K., Ismail, M.S., *et al.* (2006) Effectiveness of atypical antipsychotic drugs in patients with Alzheimer's disease. *New England Journal of Medicine* **355**, 1525–1538.

Wong, S.H. & Steiger, M.J. (2007) Pathological gambling in Parkinson's disease. *BMJ* **334**, 810–811.

Case 18 Complete loss of memory in a fit middle-aged man

A middle-aged man has walked into an A&E department in London asking for help because he has lost his memory. He is well-dressed in suit and tie, speaks with a Manchester accent and appears dazed. He is unable to tell staff his name, date of birth or where he is from. He says he cannot remember anything before finding himself outside a nearby train station earlier today.

What are your first thoughts?

This is either an *organic* or *functional* disorder. You need to exclude physical causes and establish that he has not had an acute insult to his brain, commonly head injury, infection, stroke or epileptic seizure.

In a physically well man, this presentation is more likely to be functional in origin. Dense amnesia with complete loss of *all* autobiographical memory is unlikely to be brought about by an organic cause in the absence of gross brain pathology in an otherwise cognitively oriented patient.

He is physically examined by a junior doctor in A&E and nil of note is found. You are called in to give him a psychiatric examination.

What do you do at this point?

Physical pathology has not been excluded here. Given the consequences of missing organic illness, it would be wise to insist that physical investigations carried out include routine blood screen, urine drug screen, blood alcohol levels and imaging of his brain (computed tomography [CT] or magnetic resonance imaging [MRI]), and perhaps brain activity if indicated (electroencephalogram [EEG]). Discuss this case with senior colleagues in the A&E department and the on-call neurologist if necessary.

KEY POINT

When psychiatric patients lack capacity or insight, or where their disorder makes them vulnerable, you need to advocate for them. As a rule they are underinvestigated, and less likely to receive physical treatments. If you are unhappy with their medical care, raise your objections in the most productive way.

Investigations are normal except for a mildly abnormal liver function profile.

How will you approach the interview?

• Avoid direct aggressive or incredulous challenging of his loss of memory – this is unhelpful as it can increase the patient's anxiety and level of arousal, thus making memory retrieval more difficult

• Gently explore what he can remember, his last memories of his movements and whatever personal and psychiatric history he is able to tell you

• Systematically go through a mental state examination (MSE), paying particular attention to cognitive testing

He continues to draw a blank, saying he cannot remember anything before finding himself outside the train station. He then wandered around nearby streets and found the hospital after asking a 'nice young lady for directions to the hospital'. He apologizes, but says he is unable to give you any background history. MSE is normal other than memory deficits. He is orientated in time and place, although not in person; cognitive testing is otherwise normal.

What else could you check at this point?

• Establish whether he has anything on him that might give you some clues as to his identity or recent movements

• Double check he is not wearing any MedicAlert bracelet/chain with details of medical conditions such as epilepsy or diabetes

You find a train ticket for today from Leeds to London in a pocket, along with a wallet including a bank card with the name Mr R. Smith on it. He seems unsure whether this wallet is his but then confirms his name is Smith. He then suggests his first name might be Robert, he is married to someone called Margaret, and he thinks he might be a lawyer in Leicester. He sips thoughtfully on a cup of tea during your conversation, appearing a little perplexed but not overtly distressed or anxious. If anything, he appears surprisingly unconcerned.

List your differential diagnoses

• *Dissociative fugue:* a functional state of amnesia during which an individual makes a sudden unexpected journey to somewhere beyond their everyday range of travel. The individual is unable to recall their past and may demonstrate confusion about their identity. In some cases they may assume a new one, which may evolve if the state persists. Dissociation in essence represents a functional *narrowing* of consciousness. This contrasts with the *lowering* and fluctuation of consciousness seen in delirious states (Case 5)

> **KEY POINT**
>
> Fugue states are rare and represent a severe form of dissociative *disorder*. As a *symptom* in its mildest form, dissociation occurs when an individual feels temporarily distant or cut-off from their own emotional or physical state (*depersonalization*) and/or what is going on around them (*derealization*).

• If this is a dissociative fugue, the underlying predisposing and precipitating causes are complex and you need to be aware of psychiatric *comorbidity* (affective disorders, substance misuse and personality difficulties) that might complicate the presentation. His liver function tests may indicate alcohol misuse

• Differential diagnoses include *any organic cause* of impaired consciousness, hopefully excluded by this point (Box 26) as well as *psychiatric ones* such as psychosis, affective disorders and (as a last resort) factitious disorder

> **Box 26 Organic causes of dissociative amnesia**
>
> Toxic insults to the brain including drugs (illicit and prescribed) and alcohol
> Epilepsy – especially complex partial seizures
> Head injury
> Brain tumour
> Brain haemorrhage
> Cerebrovascular accident
> Migraine
> Hypoglycaemia

> **KEY POINT**
>
> The hallmark of dissociative disorders is **lack of normal integration** of an individual's memory, identity and active self-awareness, including that of their current mental processes, physical sensations and motor movements. Examples of dissociative physical pathology include non-epileptic seizures and functional paralysis of voluntary motor control (including speech).

How would you describe the type of memory deficit he appears to have?

We can categorize his memory deficit temporally and in relation to type of memory loss:

• He appears to have a dense *retrograde amnesia* (i.e. he is unable to recall information from before a point in time). With acute brain injuries such as head injuries, retrograde amnesia may be for a matter of minutes before the injury; with longer-term conditions (e.g. dementia) the memory loss may spread back for years before the onset of the condition

• There is no evidence of *anterograde amnesia* (i.e. he is able to form new memories) as shown by his recall for events since finding himself outside the station (the 'nice young lady'). You have confirmed this with his ability to recall new information in getting here (asking just once for directions) and on cognitive testing of his mental state. This contrasts with organic memory impairment caused by delirium or dementia for example, where there is profound disruption in the formation of new memories, as well as varying degrees of (often patchy) retrograde amnesia

• While in this altered state of consciousness Mr Smith has maintained the ability to function – hence managing to negotiate the practical requirements of his amnesia. His behaviour may well have appeared normal to others. This is because the type of memory usually affected in dissociative states is *explicit episodic memory* rather than *implicit procedural memory* (Box 27). As the latter has

---

Box 27　Classification of memory

Clinical presentation
Memory can be broadly divided into three functional components: **registration** of new information; **retention** of stored information and **recall** of that information. In organic amnesias (e.g. dementia) all three processes may be impaired. With functional amnesia the primary problem is recall.

Short- versus long-term memory
Sensory memory: perceptual information held for around a second in the sensory modality in which it was perceived (e.g. sound; touch).
Short-term memory: sensory information processed by the brain and held for up to 20 seconds. Information is held in the brain by temporary changes in neuronal synaptic activity. Short-term memory is also known as **working memory** and is tested by immediate recall in the cognitive assessment (Table 19, p. 68) whereby the patient repeats a list of numbers back to the examiner.
Long-term memory: memories that have been stored and linked with other categories of existing memories. This linkage requires the synthesis of new neuronal proteins and new synaptic connections to be formed. Long-term memory is tested on the mini-mental state by recall of three items of data after 5 minutes.

Implicit versus explicit memory
Explicit or *declarative* **memory** concerns memories of past events and facts that are consciously remembered. It is divided into **episodic** memory that is personal to an individual (e.g. their mother's name, what happened on Saturday, the voice of a friend), and **semantic** memory, relating to facts about the world (e.g. the meaning of the word *rose*; what a rose looks like; how a rose smells). Dissociative amnesias usually pertain only to episodic memory. Alzheimer's dementia (Box 24, p. 161) by contrast involves both episodic and semantic memory impairment.
Implicit or *procedural* **memory** is non-declarative and is that which is known without an individual actively having to remember it (e.g. complex psychomotor tasks such as how to drive a car, how to take a medical history). Implicit memory tends to be most impaired in subcortical dementias such as Huntington's disease and Parkinson's.

---

been unaffected, he has continued to know how to buy a train ticket for example, and to remain aware that when in this kind of difficulty and needing assistance he should present to A&E.

KEY POINT

During a fugue state, difficulties may also occur in forming and retaining new memories, given the altered state of consciousness.

Speculate about the causes and onset of Mr Smith's fugue state
Fugue states tend to be abrupt psychological reactions to trauma and overwhelmingly stressful circumstances (e.g. an exit event such as divorce, financial collapse, job loss), often a culmination of stressors occurring simultaneously.

Are you surprised by the fact he does not appear distressed?
No. Dissociation is a psychological defence mechanism. It is an unconscious process, classically referred to as *hysteria*, now described as conversion disorder. Its purpose is to protect the individual from an overwhelming uncomfortable affect that they are unable to manage. It is a state during which difficult or disavowed feelings (e.g. anger, guilt, disgust) are avoided rather than experienced.

In a fugue state, the individual also physically removes him/herself from the reality of the stressful situation.

KEY POINT

The term *belle indifference* describes the abnormal incongruous affect associated with conversion disorders. It is an emotionally bland response to a seemingly serious disability (e.g. paralysis of a limb) or predicament (e.g. inability to recall identity).

Whose help do you need to manage Mr Smith?
Approach the police for assistance. They may be able to help establish his identity if someone fitting his description has already been registered as a missing person.

The police have no record of anyone missing of that name or description. They suggest if the current situation continues it might be possible to identify him at a later stage through his bank details.

For the short-term at least, it may be wise to admit him to a psychiatric ward while his identity and the best course of action are established.

No regular medication is indicated at present (antipsychotics will not help here). He may possibly require p.r.n. (i.e. as required) medication such as hypnotics to sleep, or sedative medication (e.g. a benzodiazepine) if his mental state changes and he becomes acutely distressed. If either occurs it would be wise for him to be reviewed to ensure medication is indicated and supportive psychological measures have been tried first. Avoid pre-emptive prescribing on a p.r.n. basis.

On the ward he should initially be nursed on timed regular observations, with the plan that this may need to be increased if his mental state changes. When the amnesia lifts, he might become highly emotional, depressed or even suicidal, depending on the circumstances that precipitated the fugue, combined with any pre-existing mental health difficulties.

Mr Smith agrees to be admitted and sleeps well that night. He wakes up the next morning able to recall his wife's name is Marcia and their telephone number in Leeds. Marcia sounds exasperated when you speak to her. She says her husband's name is Richard, not Robert, and he has done this at least once before 4 years ago when he ended up spending 2 days on a psychiatric ward in Plymouth. The precipitant to this fugue appears to be her asking for a divorce following his multiple infidelities. She also comments that Richard is an accountant, not a lawyer, and currently he is under investigation for fraud. She flatly refuses to come down to London to see him.

What do you make of the fact that Richard gave inaccurate information to you earlier concerning his name, wife's name, home town and occupation?

His answers were striking for being approximations of the truth – similar but incorrect (e.g. recalling his wife's name as Margaret). This is termed *paralogia* and is a recognized dissociative phenomenon called *Ganser's syndrome* – the syndrome of approximate answers. It is consistent with the diagnosis of fugue.

What might you do now?

• Check he is not already known to mental health services in Leeds as they may be able to give you more information

• When practically possible, arrange transfer for Richard to a psychiatric ward local to his area. He is not yet sufficiently orientated for discharge and there would be concerns about his vulnerability if he left your ward to make his way back to Leeds

• The mainstay of his treatment (here or there) will be supportive, treating comorbid illness as necessary, and gently exploring his account of recent events

• Once under a team in his area, meetings with his family (parents, any siblings or friends, perhaps Marcia) will be central to his care

• It might be helpful to ask Marcia to speak to Richard on the telephone to jog his memory, bearing in mind she may be hostile and it could upset him

Marcia speaks to Richard on the telephone and he appears to become distressed. He refuses to discuss anything with the nurses afterwards but later approaches staff requesting to use the telephone, saying his memory has returned and he needs to speak to his brother Steve. Later, the nurses receive a call from Steve who sounds angry. He says Richard is 'faking it' and he should come back to Leeds and 'face the music'. He goes on to say it is Richard's fault his marriage is breaking up because he has no idea how to treat people and does not care about anyone but himself. He also intimates Richard is due to appear in court to answer fraud charges. Steve has asked you to call him as he wants to know what is going on. Your nursing colleagues comment that it sounds like Steve is right and they cannot believe anyone could just lose all their memory like that.

How might you respond to Steve's allegations?

• Call Steve and establish why he views Richard's presentation as consciously induced

• Take this opportunity to get collateral history to fill the gaps

What do you tell Steve at this point about Richard's presentation?

Nothing until you have obtained Richard's permission. Remember, you do not have the right to *disclose* a patient's confidential clinical information without their consent, assuming they have capacity to give consent. There is nothing here to suggest that Richard lacks capacity (Box 12, p. 82). Even if lacking capacity, you would need to consider carefully whether it was necessary and in Richard's best interests to disclose information to his brother at this point. Relationships certainly sound fractious as it is.

While you do not need Richard's permission to *obtain* information (as distinct from disclosure from his relatives), it is good practice to discuss with Richard your intention to do so (or the fact that you have done so) to maintain an open honest dialogue with Richard.

> **KEY POINT**
>
> Where family relationships are complex, remember your duties to your patient of care and confidentiality, unless there are threats to self or others.

Evaluate Steve's allegation that Richard is faking it

'Faking it' implies conscious deceit on Richard's behalf. If that is the case, he has not done a very good job of it. Actual details such as his retaining ID on his person and his relatively brief period of memory loss, terminated by his own recollection of his home telephone number, suggest he was not consciously seeking to gain from his behaviour.

Conscious fabrication of symptoms is often fantastic and detailed, with exaggerated symptoms, striking historical details and mechanistic behaviour that fits the patient's idea of what appropriate illness behaviour should be. Obvious clues would include physical complaints that do not fit known anatomical patterns (e.g. neurological symptoms that do not correspond with nervous distribution and functioning).

Fabrication of symptoms can be difficult to detect, relying on clinician acuity and experience, specifically the clinical intuition developed from seeing many patients with the actual disorder. Overall then, implicit rather than explicit memory forms the basis on which a clinician has an intuitive sense of how patients with particular disorders tend to present themselves, how they describe their symptoms, how they subsequently discuss them and the match (or mismatch) with their associated emotional state and behaviour. Experience also informs awareness of how these factors can differ depending on an individual's personality, age, gender and cultural background. We learn about disorders primarily through memorizing lists of signs and symptoms but, in reality, we grasp the overall clinical picture first and then go on to look for specific features of a presentation in keeping with suspected diagnosis or diagnoses.

If the issue of fabrication arises and one struggles to explain to colleagues why a presentation does or does not fit, it can be helpful to break-down the features of the presentation and ask common sense questions of whether they would be consistent with achieving the alleged external gains.

Behavioural motivations are complex. Even if an individual's behaviour has been previously deceptive, it does not exclude genuine disorders in future.

> **KEY POINT**
>
> Consciously induced symptoms – physical or mental – may represent either a **factitious disorder** (one form of which is referred to as Munchausen's syndrome) or **malingering**. Key to distinguishing between the two is the motivation behind the deceit. Factitious disorder is driven by *internal* motivations (e.g. to illicit care and concern from others or to gain a social role as a patient), with an identity and symptoms of interest to others. The motivation for malingering is *external* (e.g. to avoid a difficult situation such as criminal proceedings or financial gain through compensation).

What might you say to Steve at this point?

Avoid a debate about the degree to which conscious processes are at play, or whether Richard has brought his difficulties on himself. Dissociative processes are by their nature unconscious (Box 28), but that is not to say Richard's conscious behaviour has not contributed to his difficulties and even precipitated them in the immediate sense at least: it is not your role to make moral judgments either way.

You may wish to defuse the situation with Steve by acknowledging things are complicated, his family sounds under stress because of the situation, and making a fairly bland statement about mental health difficulties often being complex in their origins, without committing yourself to discuss of Richard's case.

What will be the focus of Richard's future treatment?

If his dissociative difficulties persist, the mainstay of his treatment will be psychodynamically informed psychotherapy (Table 45, p. 147). This will involve exploration

Box 28 Dissociative disorders and their clinical features (based on ICD-10)

Dissociative amnesia

Memory loss may be selective or densely localized to a period of time. The amnesia may be circumscribed for certain categories of information, such as all memories associated with a person, place or specific event (e.g. trauma). More rarely, amnesia is complete for identity and all historical information, and for a period of time there may be ongoing difficulties in forming new memories. Note the amnesia must not be explained by organic pathology and is too great to be caused by ordinary forgetfulness or fatigue.

Dissociative fugue

Amnesia for one's identity combined with seemingly purposeful travel. Organic fugue states also occur (e.g. post-seizures). At a population level the prevalence of dissociative fugue states is known to increase during times of social upheaval, such as war or natural disasters. If a new identity is assumed, it tends to be in keeping with the individual's baseline personality (as opposed to the new contrasting identities of dissociative identity disorder, see below).

Dissociative identity disorder

This is the new, agreed term for *multiple personality disorder*. It is a very rare condition, strongly associated with very severe childhood trauma, whereby an individual harbours two or more quasi-autonomous personality states. Each state has its own characteristic patterns of cognition, affective range and interpersonal behaviour. These characteristics are often in sharp contrast between different states, where they may be exaggerated versions of a social norm (e.g. one personality may be supremely confident, another extremely submissive). Painful or disavowed

emotional states (e.g. depressed, hopeless states or angry aggressive states) tend to be circumscribed within particular personalities. One personality state is operational at any one time, with the other personalities experienced as 'other' and referred to in the third person. Dissociative amnesia may occur for the other personality states, or events and experiences associated with them (i.e. memory may be state-dependent).

Derealization – depersonalization disorder

Derealization as a symptom is the sense of removal from one's surroundings; depersonalization is a sense of removal from one's body or part thereof. The emotional state tends to be one of detachment and feeling numb, although the sense of removal may in itself be experienced as unpleasant. There is no delusional elaboration of the experience. As symptoms, derealization and depersonalization often occur as part of a constellation of symptoms in other psychiatric disorders, such as depression. They commonly occur in association with other dissociative disorders. When they are the predominant feature, these disorders are diagnosed in their own right.

Dissociative trance disorder

Trance states are an altered state of consciousness associated with a loss of normal sense of personal identity; possession trance states entail the sense one's identity has been taken over by an external agency, such as a spirit or another person. This diagnosis is only made when this state occurs outside what is considered normal for the individual's religion and culture.

of his childhood: dissociation (to varying degrees) in response to stress is a faulty coping style he probably developed in response to trauma or unmanageable emotional experience as a child. The aim of therapy would be to help him integrate his sense of self and strengthen the continuity of his experience.

What is his prognosis?

Even if he makes a full and speedy recovery at the present time, you would advise him to consider some form of psychodynamic psychotherapy to address his vulnerabil-

ity to such episodes in future. Given his history he has a propensity to dissociation that is likely to recur when faced with future stress.

KEY POINT

Dissociative fugue usually resolves spontaneously after hours or days. Fugue states may be recurrent (as here), reflecting an individual's propensity to dissociate as a way of managing emotional difficulties.

CASE REVIEW

Covering A&E as a psychiatrist will never be boring: you cannot know who will walk through the door. Having insisted on a thorough evaluation for organic illness, your repeated examinations elicited dissociative fugue with features of **Ganser's syndrome**. This is more common in men and usually overlaps with other **dissociative symptoms** and syndromes, as in this case. More so than in other cases, his family pressurized you to intrude into his management – for understandable reasons. They asked one question: is he **faking**? The wise course is to avoid being the adjudicator of what is conscious and what is unconscious: restoring social function is the priority, and

from this stability, combined interventions work to prevent relapse. You followed the same principles, ensuring the patient did not lose face, as in Case 10.

You should avoid being drawn into long-standing family disputes. Not described here, prolonged hospital admissions may become a perpetuating factor in both dissociative disorders and factitious illness (internal motivation to be a 'patient'). In Richard's case, the safe option was hospital admission to clarify and support. If – and this is a big if – Richard engages in therapy, he should develop new ways of coping with future stressors.

Further reading

Owens, C. & Dein, S. (2006) Conversion disorder: the modern hysteria. *Advances in Psychiatric Treatment* **12**, 152–157.

Steinberg, M., Coons, P., Putnam, F.W., Loewenstein, R.J., Simeon, D. & Hollander, E. (2000) Dissociative disorders. In Sadock, B.J. & Sadock, V.A. (eds). *Kaplan & Sadock's Comprehensive Textbook of Psychiatry*, 7th edn. Lippincott Williams & Wilkins, Philadelphia.

Case 19 A 32-year-old woman puts her GP under pressure

Tara is a 32-year-old science graduate, off work for 4 years. For most of the past 2 years, she has attended your GP colleague, Dr Ward, on average twice weekly. Despite these visits, she also attends four A&E departments up to 12 times yearly, and has regular outpatients' appointments in three hospitals.

You are a consultant psychiatrist asked to see her to give your opinion about her psychiatric diagnosis, or possible psychological contributors to her presentations. Dr Ward has sent you a computerized list of her attendances with his practice for the 2 years she has been on his list (Tables 46 and 47). Dr Ward tells you he 'swapped' her case with another local GP 2 years ago – her attendances then were identical to her current pattern. He says he spends more time on her than all his psychiatric patients put together. He tried to swap her with colleagues but she is something of a local medical celebrity and no-one will agree to her transfer, even for 10 other 'heart sinkers'. He tells you that you are his last hope.

Where will you begin?

> **KEY POINT**
>
> Most experienced clinicians can cope with the consequences of excessive expectations in their patients ('No-one else understands, you are my last hope'). The same skills are required to deal with high expectations in a colleague.

She has been described as a 'heart sink patient': the doctor's heart sinks as she enters the room. Already, the sincere efforts of many physicians have failed to reduce – or may have increased – the demand for health care. All you can promise here is an assessment, and even if some psychological treatments might change illness behaviour, progress is not guaranteed, and this patient may refuse or undermine them.

Before you see her, you need to gather even more information than the summary supplied by her doctor (Tables 46 and 47):
• What is the physical evidence (X-ray, laboratory and direct evidence) that established each medical diagnosis? This means obtaining summary letters from the hospitals she attended, and information from her previous GP(s)
• What are her active medical conditions at this time?
• Does she have any new physical problems at this time?
• Did she have a psychiatric assessment before this one?

Assisted by Dr Ward and with the dogged determination of your secretary, you have gathered a comprehensive account of Tara's presentations. These are summarized in Table 48. You are now fairly confident that she has two definite medical conditions, asthma and eczema, and she is unlikely to have any other life-threatening pathology.

What are the likely psychiatric diagnoses here?

1 *Depressive disorders* are the most common cause of medically unexplained symptoms (MUS). Highly treatable, depression is both a cause of MUS and a comorbid condition that exacerbates somatic symptoms (e.g. lowers pain threshold). So common is depression in new onset MUS in adults (up to 70% of MUS cases) that some clinicians institute a trial of antidepressant treatment – although the introduction of psychological explanations to this patient group can be a challenge.

> **KEY POINT**
>
> MUS make up at least 20% of all GP visits.

171

Table 46 Summary of Tara's medical attendances, 2006.

Presentation	Diagnosis	Outcome
January 2006: first visit to the practice	*(from Dr Tony, previous GP)* Migraine Unstable bladder Recurrent UTIs Eczema Diverticulitis Asthma	Renewal of current prescription: mebeverine hydrochloride, omeprazole, ispaghula husk, lactulose, salbutamol (by inhaler), sumatriptan, codeine phosphate, oxybutynin, and topical ointments: liquid paraffin, sodium pidolate and diflucortolone valerate
February 2006: new onset abdominal pain	Premenstrual tension	Additional medication: NSAIDs, oil of evening primrose
March 2006: flu-like symptoms	Viral illness: no physical signs	Additional medication: 2 weeks' antibiotics
April 2006: urinary frequency	No UTI: four separate urine tests were clear of cells, glucose or protein	No action taken Tara complained about Dr Ward to the Practice Head
April 2006: relapse of migraine headaches	Extended after-hours consultation: no new history or exam findings	Long discussion about pain relief, stress avoidance and sumatriptan use. Anxious that latter medication not be changed
May 2006: shortness of breath	No physical signs: chest did not sound wheezy; peak flow was slightly reduced. Normal chest X-ray	Inhalers changed: addition of terbutaline by inhaler and home nebulizer
June 2006: attended for pregnancy test	Normal pregnancy test	No action taken. Tara complained that the receptionist was rude to her during her visit. Practice issues an apology to Tara
September 2006: discharged from GI clinic	Letter sought from Dr Ward to further her complaint against her (former) GI consultant	Tara reassured that if her abdominal symptoms returned, she would be referred to another GI specialist
October 2006: acute diarrhoea	No diagnosis made	Referred to another GI specialist
October 2006: numbness both hands	Mild tremor, felt to be anxiety related. No neurological signs	Referred to Practice GP colleague with a special interest in neurology. MRI brain scan normal. No treatment prescribed
November 2006: weakness of left arm, difficulty writing	Clear differences between subjective complaints and objective findings (all normal). Writing is normal until she becomes tired	Telephone call to her most recent neurologist: she says she cannot see her because of a conflict of interest. She is banned from their clinic following the alleged theft of her notes. By return, Tara is suing their department
December 2006: recurrence of migraines	Repeated visits, 'crying with pain of headaches'. No physical signs	Increase of dose of sumatriptan per GP. Not referred to neurology

GI, gastrointestinal; MRI, magnetic resonance imaging; NSAID, non-steroidal anti-inflammatory drug; UTI, urinary tract infection.

Table 47 Summary of Tara's medical attendances, 2007.

Presentation	Diagnosis	Outcome
January 2007: tiredness	Associated insomnia, loss of pleasure with some anxiety features. Possibility of depressive illness	Prescribed SSRI medication 'to reduce her stress': paroxetine
February 2007: 'drug allergy' to paroxetine	Complaining she is over alert, cannot concentrate, nausea and tremor. Symptoms of her migraine and diverticulitis are worse since paroxetine	Tara took paroxetine on five occasions in total, spread out over 2 weeks. Decision that paroxetine may have contributed to her symptoms but she is not allergic to it. Discontinued. Counselling refused
March 2007: Tara is 'devastated' when her benefits are questioned	The 'benefits doctor' has written to state she has no medical reason preventing her from working	Letter written to the benefits doctor, by Dr Ward listing her six medical conditions of January 2006 (Table 46), with copy to Tara. Although she is satisfied with the outcome, she makes a complaint against the benefits doctor
April 2007: chest pain	Pain is sharp but radiates down both arms. Tara cannot be sure about cardiac family history: her father left when she was 4	Referral to A&E reveals normal ECG and enzymes ×3. Cardiologist recalls Tara from previous post (in another hospital): 2004 coronary angiogram was '100% normal'. Discharged
May 2007: palpitations and syncope	Night-time painful palpitations. Has passed out on three occasions	Refuses referral to previous cardiologist. 24-hour ambulatory ECG is normal. Decision taken *not* to refer for further investigations
September 2007: urinary symptoms	Recurrence of stress and urge incontinence: normal exam and urinalysis	Urgent gynaecological re-referral (same unit had investigated pelvic pain in 2003): pelvic exam and urodynamics normal. Discharged
October 2007: urinary symptoms	Symptoms of urinary frequency. Normal urine	No antibiotic prescribed. Threatens complaint to General Medical Council
October 2007: upper abdominal discomfort	No physical findings. Full blood count and occult blood screens normal	No referral made. Subsequently presented to A&E and was admitted for emergency gastroscopy. Normal
October 2007: skin burning and blotchy	Examined on four separate occasions: no evidence of any lesion other than dry skin as a result of eczema	No new medications or ointments prescribed. Decision to discontinue topical steroid led to an argument – Tara escorted from GP surgery
November 2007: blurred vision	States she cannot read except when objects are very close to her. No physical findings on visual acuity and fields testing	No referral made. Dr Ward informs driving licence authority of visual symptoms and driving is suspended. Tara makes complaint about him to the General Medical Council
December 2007: collapses while waiting for appointment	Examined as normal by practice partner but referred to A&E urgently	A&E discharges her that day. She begins a letter-writing campaign against that hospital and the GP practice

ECG, electrocardiogram; SSRI, selective serotonin reuptake inhibitor.

Table 48 Summary of Tara's medical investigations over past 11 years.

Disorder (latest tests)	Investigations	Likelihood of physical basis (%)	Feedback for the patient
Coronary heart disease (2004)	Exam, ECG, enzymes and coronary angiography normal	0%	You do not have coronary heart disease
UTIs (2007)	Two urine tests showed equivocal evidence of infection in 2001; over 30 normal urine tests	If urinalysis is normal at this time: 0%	At this time, you do not have a urine infection
Unstable bladder (2007)	Exam + investigations of urinary flow within normal limits	0%	There is no structural problem with your bladder
Pelvic disease (2004)	Exam + investigations normal	<5%	At this time, it is unlikely you have a problem with your reproductive system
Premenstrual tension (2006)	Historical diagnosis, exam (above) normal	50% Difficult to prove or disprove diagnosis	You may have premenstrual tension
Eczema (2007)	Physical examinations: no lesions documented since 2002	>50% She may have thinned her skin with topical steroids (diflucortolone) **Attends dermatologist**	You may have a tendency to dry skin
GI ulceration (2005)	Normal endoscopies ×3, barium swallows ×5, pH studies ×2	<5%	It is unlikely you have a stomach ulcer
Diverticulitis (2004)	Normal endoscopies ×4, barium enema ×1	<10%	It is unlikely you have any pouches (diverticula) in your lower bowel
Migraine (2006)	Diagnosed on history but do not conform to typical migrainous episodes. Over 11 years, five normal CT/MRI scans	5% likelihood that these are migraine headaches; history confirms tension headaches, not migraine	Your headaches are not migraine but the pain is real, and likely to be related to muscle tension
Epilepsy, brain lesion (any cause) (2005)	No abnormal findings on exam, scans, EEG	<1%	There are no structural or electrical abnormalities in your brain
Eye disease (2002)	No abnormal findings	<1%	Your eyes are normal
Asthma (2007)	In 2005, a chest physician carried out extensive tests and proved reversible airways obstruction	80% **Attends chest physician**	It is likely that you have asthma, but it is a mild form

ECG, electrocardiogram; EEG, electroencephalogram; UTI, urinary tract infection.

2 Somatic symptoms are a recognized feature of *schizophrenia* but are typically bizarre in nature: delusions that body parts have been replaced, items inserted into the body or outside forces have caused physical symptoms. Delusional disorder may present in the arena of physical health. This is not health anxiety (an overvalued idea) but has acquired delusional intensity. In older people, one classic component of psychotic depression is a nihilistic delusion that part of the body is dead, rotting or missing – Cotard's delusion.

3 This presentation is likely to be associated with a comorbid *anxiety disorder*, although unlikely to be caused by one; panic disorder can be misdiagnosed as asthma, and both headaches and urinary frequency can be part of generalized anxiety disorder (Table 11, p. 38). You would need to establish both cognitive and somatic features of anxiety to establish an anxiety disorder here. **Health anxiety** is a useful clinical term that describes a patient's disproportionate preoccupation with illness and its investigation that leads to impairments in social func-tioning. It is far less pejorative a term than the previous term – hypochondriacal anxiety.

4 *Somatoform disorders* (Table 49) can be conceptu-alized as the combination of mood and/or anxiety symptoms in the presence of (trait) health anxiety. These patients have lots of symptoms *and* a conviction that they have a physical illness. One example of these – rare, but a distinct category – is somatization disorder (Briquet's syndrome). This patient meets all three ICD-10 criteria:

Table 49 Somatoform disorders (as listed in ICD-10).

Name	Description	Clinical examples
Somatization disorder	As Tables 46–48, 50	Case 19
Undifferentiated somatoform disorder	Falls short of criteria for somatization disorder	Undifferentiated psychosomatic disorder
Hypochondriacal disorder	Persistent belief that there is at least one physical illness/deformity despite evidence to the contrary	Body dysmorphic disorder Non-delusional dysmorphophobia Hypochondriasis Nosophobia
Somatoform autonomic dysfunction	Predominant symptoms refer to autonomic functions: typically excess arousal or fleeting autonomic activation	Cardiac neurosis (Da Costa's syndrome) Gastric neurosis Irritable bowel syndrome Functional diarrhoea Psychogenic urinary frequency
Persistent somatoform pain disorder	Persistent pain that cannot be explained by physical disorder or physiological processes	Somatoform pain disorder Psychogenic backache Psychogenic headache Functional anorectal pain
Other somatoform disorders	Symptoms limited to specific parts of the body or organs, but with no tissue damage	Globus hystericus Psychogenic torticollis Psychogenic pruritus (Teeth grinding, thumb-sucking, hair-pulling and nail-biting are classified elsewhere in ICD)
Somatoform disorder, unspecified	Somatoform disorder that does not fit into any of the categories above	N/A

PART 2: CASES

• At least 2 years' multiple and variable physical symptoms for which no adequate physical explanation has been found

• Persistent refusal to accept the advice or reassurance of several doctors that there is no physical explanation for the symptoms, and

• Some degree of impairment of social and family functioning attributable to the symptoms

> **KEY POINT**
>
> Current diagnostic classifications use the broad term 'somatoform disorders' ('-form' meaning similar to) to describe presentations where physical symptoms are not fully explained by organic pathology.

5 *Alcohol and/or substance misuse* are unlikely to be causative of this presentation, but either/both may have become a perpetuating factor during several years off work through boredom, as a displacement activity or as a remedy for pain and other unacceptable symptoms.

6 *Conversion disorder* is part of the differential here but usually presents acutely and with dramatic symptoms specific to a particular system, typically neurological (Table 50). It is classically known as hysteria (Case 18).

7 Voluntary symptom production is always a diagnosis of exclusion. A *malingering* patient has an identifiable advantage in continuing to feign symptoms

Table 50 Comparison of conversion (dissociative) and somatization disorders.

Factors	Conversion disorder*	Somatization disorder (SD)
Age and gender	Equal sex ratio in childhood, but female excess thereafter	Excess of women over men; most cases present in early adulthood
Systems	Mostly, neurology: paralysis, numbness, tremor, abnormal movements/gait of limbs; non-epileptic seizures; blindness; unusual visual symptoms	DSM-IV requires pain in at least four systems to diagnose SD. Patients have usually attended at least four specialist services (Tables 46–48)
First presentation	Dramatic symptoms (sudden loss of a major function): a minority show apparent indifference to the seriousness of their symptoms ('la belle indifference') and are not curious about medical causes	Insidious, subacute onset; present to many doctors before SD is suspected. Presentation is forceful, but not dramatic: they show great concern about the symptoms, requesting immediate explanations
Precipitant	Life events usually precede presentation; for many patients, the symptoms rescue the patient from a difficult adverse event	No identifiable precipitant of individual presentations. A pattern may develop where there is an identifiable illness model (see text)
Outcome	Usually good. Of patients whose symptoms resolve, one-quarter will relapse: stressful events commonly herald their return	Tend to run a chronic course, where one set of symptoms is replaced by another – frequently from another system (Tables 46–48)
Interactions with health care staff	Reassured by 'normal' test results. Unlikely to complain against physicians who acknowledge their difficulties	Not reassured/disbelieving of/angered by 'normal' test results. Frequently pursue complaints (as in Case 19)
General medical interventions	Respond to interventions that do not provoke a 'loss of face': physiotherapy for limb symptoms, speech and language therapy for conversion aphonia, etc.	Symptoms frequently become more severe with medical treatments; blaming of health staff (for delays in treatment, wrong treatment, poor techniques etc.)
Psychiatric interventions	Usually accept links between their anxiety and symptoms; do not resist antidepressant treatment	May accept links between their anxiety and symptoms; tend to resist antidepressant treatment

*American classifications list conversion disorder as a somatoform disorder, but it is not listed as a somatoform disorder by ICD-10 (Table 49).

(Case 18, p. 168). Most A&E staff will have encountered the patient who fakes renal colic to gain a narcotic such that these are now rarely prescribed to unknown patients. The second form of voluntary symptom production, *factitious illness*, is rare and difficult to diagnose. These patients are highly inventive and go to extraordinary lengths to feign abnormal physical investigations (heat up thermometers to fake a fever, adulterate urine samples, mix microbes into specimens) or inflict abnormal states on themselves (insulin to achieve hypoglycaemia, laxative-induced hypokalaemia, self-poisoning to mislead investigations not to self-harm, or self-inflicted skin lesions; 'dermatitis artefacta').

> **KEY POINT**
>
> Although patients who fake illness (voluntary symptom production) *behave psychiatrically*, many have no underlying psychiatric condition. Remember, they can feign psychiatric symptoms too.

| *From discussions with Dr Ward, it appears that somatization disorder is her diagnosis.*

With what you now know about her, comment on the presentation patterns as set out in Tables 46 and 47, and identify the points at which psychological interventions were attempted

- *April 2006:* extended consultation carried out acknowledging her difficulties
- *January 2007:* antidepressants prescribed, although the patient explanation was for 'stress' rather than an antidepressant
- *February 2007:* counselling was offered but refused
- *At other times:* despite his anxieties and her protests, Tara has established a therapeutic relationship with her GP Dr Ward. The problem with it is that it has not reduced her need for more medical interventions

How might her behaviour have influenced her medical care?

- Negotiation of increases in existing medication (May and December 2006) and new medications (February 2006 and January 2007). Alongside these, she frequently

requested more medication, and in only one instance (paroxetine) did she strive to have a medication discontinued

- Devaluing medical advice/doctor shopping: September 2006, second gastrointestinal opinion sought; November 2006, rejects normal findings of her GP and his specialist partner; May 2007, refuses to attend previous cardiologist with new symptoms; October and December 2007, calls to A&E despite the 'all clear' from her GP; and her public campaign attacking local health services
- Seven separate complaints about health care staff: April 2006, June 2006, November 2006, legal action; March 2007, October 2007, threatens 'more serious' complaint; November 2007 and December 2007, letter campaign
- One documented episode where she was overtly aggressive to staff (October 2007) was when a medication was removed rather than added to her prescription
- Her alleged theft of her medical notes (for unknown reasons)

| *Because of their complexity, patients with somatization disorder are frequently the subject of multidisciplinary case conferences. Two doctors are essential to this case discussion: her GP and her chest physician. Both (or a representative) should attend to balance the consensus that her symptoms are somatoform.*

> **KEY POINT**
>
> In treating somatoform disorders, you need to establish your credibility with the patient. Make clear you will not ignore life-threatening conditions, but will shift emphasis from the physical to the psychological.

| *Given her limitless consumption of health services, there may be specialist nurses, physiotherapists, occupational therapists, home visitors and others involved in her care: they should always be invited. Think too about the timing of participation of her family.*

In addition to presenting your findings and differential diagnosis, you are asked to comment on her recent escalation (Tables 46–48). Where did Dr Ward go right (and wrong) in the past 2 years?

He has a duty of care to his patient and (even with hindsight) was right to take every new symptom seriously. Had he ignored her symptoms or refused to carry out examinations and investigations, we would not now have reached the consensus represented in Table 48.

Unless you have worked as a GP, you cannot imagine how hard it is to say no to requests for unnecessary antibiotics (e.g. March 2006) or excessive medications (May 2006). By October 2006, he resisted prescribing new treatments where pathology was unproven, bravely so during the following October when she had made multiple complaints against him and others.

It is also clear that having showed flexibility in referring Tara to 'new' specialists, her requests continued to escalate. He has referred for a psychiatric opinion at the end of a series of comprehensive negative findings in cardiac, gynaecological, neurological and gastrointestinal systems.

The only criticism that could be made of her care is her acquisition of 'special patient' status. If the receptionist was rude to her, then the practice was right to apologize. However, if the rudeness was Tara's, this could have been handled differently – although many would argue Tara would have tried to attend another GP practice without this face-saving apology.

When, in October 2007, her behaviour became unacceptable, she was 'escorted from the surgery'. She may have resented this – and it may have provoked more complaints – but it did not undermine the therapeutic relationship with her GP.

> *Tara is having a good run at the moment. She organizes the local parish tennis tournament every year during the summer. With local sponsorship, she achieved funding for a recent indoor tennis tournament that 'kept me busy' and was 'a great success'. She consents to a conventional psychiatric interview, and agrees that you can share your findings with Dr Ward and the respiratory team.*

How will you approach her psychiatric assessment?

1 Begin with exploration of her account of the medical ailments described thus far. Use open questions to establish her current attitudes to each system (Table 48). You will be asked by her and you will be tempted to comment on the 'realities' of her ailments. *It is best not to do so at this stage.* The feedback comments (Table 48) should be introduced gradually, one by one in different attendances, **after** she has built up some confidence in you and the process. They are quoted, system by system, to share with every health professional, lest Tara uses one professional's explanation to challenge another's.

2 Screen for psychiatric symptoms as comorbidity or possible perpetuators of her symptoms (see differential diagnosis above). You might begin by explaining that these questions are part of your assessment of every patient, and ask her to be patient as many questions will not apply to her. This is not to reinforce her status as a 'special patient' but to foresee objections or anger that her problems are 'all in the mind'. Try to establish her understanding of the contribution psychological processes (stress, having a low mood, health beliefs) could make to each of these systems.

3 You are likely to find events in her personal and family history relevant to her presentation (see next section). Equally, it would be unlikely if she did not have abnormal personality traits. Take your time in establishing these factors as they will be a major influence on your treatment plan.

KEY POINT

The added cost to the US health care system of somatization is over \$250 billion each year. This does not include self-prescription, costs of alternative therapies, disability payments or work days lost.

---

4 Social supports: you already know a great deal about her. When she is busy (as a tennis organizer every summer), she does not need to see her doctors. Are there networks that support her then but not at other times? To whom does she talk when symptoms become intolerable? Apart from friends, is there a family network? Has she fallen out with anyone? Who lives at home with her? Is she in a relationship now? How are relationships for her in general? Explore her request for a pregnancy test (June 2006) with sensitivity: did she plan or wish for pregnancy?

> *Tara is the elder of two children, with a normal birth history and milestones. She has one younger brother (now 26). Tara*

PART 2: CASES

never met her father, and her early years were spent with her mother's parents while her mother returned to her acting career. After her grandmother's sudden death (Tara was 4), she lived for short periods with her aunt and then friends of her mother's 'who liked kids or had some of their own'. She moved house frequently, even after her stepfather 'moved in on the scene'. Her stepfather was strict and left when his son (her brother) was 7. She remembers getting 'stuck with' her younger brother quite a bit during his early years, and still keeps in touch despite their 'on–off' relationship. Her mother lives 40 miles away, but has chronic fatigue syndrome, diagnosed 5 years ago. They seldom meet as a result of their illnesses. She loved school and university, where she did well, and says if she has a fault it is that she 'idolizes her friends'. She is the one who keeps in touch with school and college friends. She has three close friends (two women and an ex-boyfriend) in whom she confides. Her last relationship was with her 'ex' and it ended 4 years ago.

Tara asks you if she could have the same disease as her mother.

Set out your understanding of chronic fatigue syndrome

Diagnostic guidelines are set out as Box 29. From details of Tara's history so far, it is highly unlikely she has this. Details of her mother's symptoms and how she copes with these are relevant to Tara and her future management.

KEY POINT

A key part of history taking in people who somatize is to examine their experience of physical and other illnesses in people who were close to them.

Tara recounts the medical experiences of her wider family. Her grandmother had rheumatoid arthritis. She never complained about her health, and no-one knew why she died at only 62. Her mother developed brittle diabetes when she was 6 but, by Tara's account, it took some time before she accepted the diagnosis or got 'proper medical help'. Her brother is the 'fittest man on the planet' but Tara remembers her mother taking him repeatedly to the doctor to find the diabetes he does not have. Her 'ex' is a tennis

Box 29 Chronic fatigue syndrome: guidelines for diagnosis (Fukuda et al. 1994)

Definition
Fatigue > 6 months: verified, and backed up by history, *mandatory* MSE, physical exam and investigations. The fatigue must cause substantial reductions in the patient's activities.

Verification of fatigue
Treadmill and other exercise tests; CFS instruments have been described (see references).

Excluded by:
medical conditions that explain fatigue (e.g. those causing depression in Table 14, p. 47, severe obesity and malignancies); depression with psychotic or melancholic features; other psychiatric disorders: bipolar illness, psychosis, dementia, eating disorders and recent (2 years) alcohol/substance misuse.

Conditions that do not adequately explain CFS (i.e these do not exclude a CFS diagnosis)
Physical and psychiatric conditions for which there are no objective tests – depression that is nether psychotic nor melancholic, anxiety disorders including somatoform disorders, neurasthenia, fibromyalgia and multiple chemical sensitivity disorder. Some tests cannot exclude CFS: weak antinuclear antibody, treated Lyme's disease, infectious mononucleosis (positive monospot test) and syphilis.

Investigations
Full blood count, erythrocyte sediment rate, alanine aminotransferase, alkaline phosphatase, total protein, albumin, globulin, calcium, phosphorous, glucose, urea, electrolytes, creatinine, thyroid stimulating hormone and urinalysis.

Additional tests are based on abnormalities and positive physical findings.

coach and 'probably only sees the doctor to check he has not caught a sexually transmitted disease'.

Speculate about how Tara's attachment style, past losses and relationships might impact on her psychiatric diagnosis of somatization disorder
Attachment style

Preoccupied attachment style resulting from inconsistent carers. She has a strong internal model of herself: she achieves her goals, people like her and she deserves to get the best medical care.

Losses

The key loss here is her grandmother. She lost her mother (to acting) some years before. As her domestic circumstances approached normality, a step-father then a brother emerged: her 'only child' status was removed. Despite evidence that her illnesses have a psychological basis, she has lost her health. She may have hoped for a pregnancy in June 2006.

Relationships

Parentification describes how a child becomes parent to mother or father, perhaps because of parental illness and frequently as a result of alcoholism in a parent. In the context of her insecure attachment, her relationships are one-sided. Because she lacks control over these, she invests much energy in trying to control relationships with health professionals. Ex-boyfriend and brother are described in terms of their apparent lack of need for medical care, and her description of her grandmother (who needed but failed to get 'proper medical help') is also relevant.

> Tara's mother has a diagnosis of chronic fatigue syndrome (CFS).

What is CFS, and is this relevant to Tara's condition?

Of people with a diagnosis of CFS (including many self-diagnoses), only a proportion meet the criteria (Box 29). You need to be clear if her mother has CFS. It is more prevalent than somatization disorder, with which it has considerable overlap:

- There could be yet undefined shared genetic aetiologies
- They may share the same attachment style (see above)
- Environmental contributions include learned responses to illness, modelling the sick role or attitudes to medical interventions (Table 51, p. 198)
- Effective CFS treatments are cognitive–behavioural therapy (CBT) and antidepressants: these also help patients with somatization disorder, but in both disorders, people resist psychological explanations

---

> **KEY POINT**
>
> CFS is a subjective complaint (more than 6 months of fatigue that is not caused by exertion and not relieved by rest) which must be evaluated clinically (Box 29). It cannot be a self-diagnosis.

How would you manage Tara over the next 2 years?

Tara needs a lead clinician for psychological symptoms and a second lead clinician for physical ones. Her GP is the key bridge between the two:

- Agree that there will be one prescriber: he/she prescribes only with the agreement of all three physicians
- All assessments and decisions must be clearly communicated to everyone, including Tara
- The strongest predictor of good outcome here is the quality of therapeutic relationship between Tara and her psychiatrist
- With Tara, begin with the areas on which you can agree. Try to prioritize systems where the case for missed organic pathology is weak and there is good evidence for the contribution of stress (Table 48). Decide which systems to 'shut down' first
- Messages must be consistent: examples quoted in the fourth column of Table 48
- CBT: re-education and alternative explanations comprise the C, and the B examines activities, illness behaviours, etc (Table 4, p. 13).
- Symptomatic treatment of depression and anxiety if these arise
- Resilience therapy: supportive interventions identifying positive coping skills, in Tara's case her tennis tournaments are a model for other activities
- Family therapy and/or psychodynamic psychotherapy may be required

> **KEY POINT**
>
> Managing people with MUS and somatization disorder involves complex long-term negotiations. Your aim is to withdraw two elements: existing medical attendances and current medications. Use the model of drug dependency: reduce one thing at a time, and reduce it by predictable, small increments – with a contingency plan.

PART 2: CASES

CASE REVIEW

Somatoform disorders, typified by somatization disorder, have much in common with other severe enduring mental illnesses:

- Complex aetiologies
- Multiple psychiatric comorbidities
- Chronic illness with multiple relapses and remissions
- Major losses of social functioning
- Poor treatment response
- Multiple health service utilizations

Somatoform disorders are common but because the vast majority of medical student and postgraduate training is devoted to the identification and treatment of 'real' illnesses, doctors feel frustration when managing these patients. In addition, demonstrable physical disorders frequently coexist with somatoform (functional) ones. This adds our anxiety to our patients'. In this case, her GP's meticulous documentation allowed you to see the overall picture in Tara's history. This is far more difficult if you are one investigating doctor examining one system. The case also covered CFS, making clear its parallels with other somatoform disorders. High service utilization is driven by strong beliefs in patients who go to great lengths to fight their corner. If the cycles of symptom → investigations → no/unsuccessful treatments → more dissatisfaction → new symptom can be broken, even intensive psychiatric follow-up with individual psychotherapy is substantially cheaper *and safer* than the alternatives.

Reference

Fukuda, K., Straus, S.E., Hickle, I., Sharpe, M.C., Dobbins, J.G., Komaroff, A. & the International Chronic Fatigue Study Group (1994) Chronic fatigue syndrome: a comprehensive approach to its definition and study. *Annals of Internal Medicine* **121**, 953–959.

Further reading

White, P.D. (2002) Commentary on 'Physical or mental? A perspective on chronic fatigue syndrome'. *Advances in Psychiatric Treatment* **8**, 363–365.

Case 20   The 21-year-old critical medical student

The Dean of Medicine at your university asks you to see Declan, a 21-year-old third year medical student. Declan came to his attention the first time 1 month ago when his then consultant wrote to the Dean. During his psychiatry attachment, he started to question patients' diagnoses. This would not have been a problem but for the manner with which he did this – in front of vulnerable patients and, on three occasions, shouting and making accusations against the professionals involved. When his consultant tried to speak with Declan about this, he told her to 'rev up and f*** off'. He did not settle into his attachment for the previous month and, prior to these confrontations, he had regularly interrupted ward meetings (where everyone sat to discuss cases) by standing up and walking around the room. He said this was as a result of back pain.

Declan has signed consent for you to interview him and send a written report to the Dean, with copies to his GP.

How might you begin the interview?

• Remind him that he has waived confidentiality and that you are seeing him for the purposes of a report to the Dean. This will require detailed questioning – with collateral history – not unlike a court report (Table 33, p. 114)

• Has he had any psychiatric assessments before this one?

• How does he see his difficulties in the light of the allegations against him?

• Does he have any psychological symptoms?

What are the possibilities here?

• *Organic illness* is always a possibility. Back pain is unusual in someone so young, and a primary or secondary tumour could have caused confusion (Table 20, p. 69), mood (Table 14, p. 47) or psychotic (Table 16, p. 53) symptoms. You need to decide if he requires further medical evaluation

• As with other cases, do not let his background distract you from investigating *alcohol and/or substance misuse*

• He has crossed a line in behaving so inappropriately towards vulnerable patients, with verbal abuse to his consultant. That this is 'new' raises concerns about functional *mood* or *psychotic* symptoms

• A primary *anxiety disorder* (Table 11, p. 38) seems unlikely. He might be restless (Fig. 2, p. 37) but he has behaved in an excessive manner – unusual even for severe disorders such as post-traumatic stress disorder (PTSD; Table 32, p. 108)

• There may be evidence of *personality disorder* (PD) here, specifically dissocial PD (Box 19, p. 149). Does Declan have features suggesting psychopathy (Box 18, p. 148)? He might have paranoid traits that were activated by discussions on the ward rounds or by specific psychiatric patients

• The possibility remains that Declan has been *unjustly accused* of these charges as punishment for challenging a (malevolent) consultant psychiatrist. The Dean should have verified he had a case to answer based on more than one account

• Less likely is ~~voluntary symptom production~~. He could be malingering to get time off his studies or 'special consideration' at exam time. Your assessment of him presents another opportunity for direct gain in escaping a disciplinary hearing or achieving mitigation in front of the Dean. Factitious psychiatric illness (without a clear direct gain) is reported as being more common in medical and other health professionals

Declan arrives 20 minutes' late, dressed in a suit but wearing trainers with one lace missing and a crumpled dirty shirt. His hair is long and uncombed. He appears restless but stays seated. His eyes wander around the room and eye contact is only fleeting. At the start of the interview, Declan makes a brief reply then falls silent: 'There's nothing about me or my personality you can tell me that I do not already know. And what you don't hear from me, you'll make up anyway. You, Dr Hooper (the consultant who contacted the Dean) and Professor Brown (the Dean) are three sides of the same coin. Just greedy stenocrats. That is it, the end.'

With that, he terminated the interview. Will you?

No. You can continue to observe him for a limited mental state examination (MSE):

• *Appearance and behaviour:* as summarized above. There are signs of anxiety. He looked anxious as he left
• *Speech:* thought disorder ('three sides of the same coin') and neologism (use of the term 'stenocrats' – was he distracted by seeing you writing?)
• *Mood:* subjectively unknown, objectively anxious affect that failed to calm during the interview. Just before he walked out (10 minutes after his comments), his eyes watered. He could be depressed
• *Suicidality:* not yet established
• *Thoughts:* possibility of paranoid delusions. He describes three doctors as 'greedy', and may have additional ideas about this
• *Perception:* no abnormalities could be elicited based on truncated interview
• *Cognition:* untested
• *Insight:* unknown. Unlikely to be good

Declan's cousin has left his phone number with your secretary. You had intended to speak with him after your assessment, but call him immediately in the light of your new concerns. He grew up with Declan – he knows him well, and shared a house with him for 2 years until they fell out 2 months ago. At that point, Declan said he wanted to buy a derelict house to fix it up for them and for others. 'There was no talking to him about it – he was going to do it, even if the bank would not lend the money.' Since then, they have not been in contact and he knows nothing about recent events: Declan tells his parents nothing. The last he heard of Declan, he was sleeping at the hospital in rooms usually given to relatives who stay over.

Do you have any further questions for this informant?

You can now fill in the rest of his history: medical and family history, and his premorbid personality. You might also get the details of the people best placed now to describe recent events to support or refute your working diagnosis.

Declan was always 'one of a kind'. By the time he knew him well (about 15 years ago), he would approach complete strangers to tell them about himself. He made up wild stories which he insisted were true 'until the very end'. 'Very popular with the ladies', Declan 'is the life and soul of every party, but when the party's over, you don't want to be there': he hates being on his own and will phone anyone to keep himself going. His cousin could not name one family event in the past 10 years that did not become 'all about Declan'. The only quiet time for him was a few months some years ago when their cousin died in a car accident. He took her death 'the hardest of everyone', and went in on himself. There is also a family history of mental illness: your informant's mother has been on haloperidol 20 years. The rest of his birth, medical and other history are unremarkable. He enjoys a drink, but he has never used illegal drugs.

Does your new understanding of his personality explain the presentation?

No. Even if Declan has a histrionic personality disorder (Box 30), this could not explain his recent behaviour – on the wards or during your assessment. If anything, someone with histrionic traits might have enjoyed a long interview. The fact that he achieved a place in medical school and stayed below the radar for so long indicates he is able to keep his personality in check and achieve his goals.

There has been a clear change of behaviour, beginning with his ambitions to buy a house but now characterized by his falling out with a succession of people. His previous personality could be *contributing* to this presentation – but it is unlikely to be the sole cause.

We are left with the first three diagnostic headings listed above. All raise the possibility of risks to him (physical illness, effects of intoxication/withdrawal, suicide, exploitation by others) if they remain undiagnosed, and psychosis adds the more remote possibility that Declan might pose a risk to other people.

> **Box 30 Features of histrionic personality disorder (ICD-10)**
>
> Histrionic PD shows features of:
> - Self-dramatization, exaggerated expression of emotions
> - Feelings that are easily hurt
> - Shallow and labile affectivity
> - Impulsive seeking out of exciting situations, the appreciation of others or striving to be the centre of attention
> - Inappropriate seductiveness in appearance or behaviour
> - Easily influenced by others (suggestibility)
> - Over-concern with physical attractiveness
> - Others may feel manipulated by their behaviour
>   Histrionic personality disorder is wrongly stereotyped as being a caricature of excessive femininity (it occurs in men too). Its name is less than perfect, but it has replaced highly stigmatizing terms such as 'oral hysterics', 'good hysterics' and 'psychoinfantile personality'. Additional confusion arises in that American classification (DSM-IV) includes a category of hysterical PD, but ICD-10 does not. While people with this latter diagnosis tend to share some of the traits above, they have better impulse control and are less exhibitionistic.

> **KEY POINT**
>
> Just as we do not accept our patients' accounts of their own personality as the definitive one, be cautious in accepting the views of one informant. They may be too close or not familiar enough with the patient, could have their own agenda (relationship problems, individual issues) or be just plain wrong. Record details for later reflection.

Declan is outside in the car park as you leave to go home. There are other people around and he does not appear surprised to see you. His jacket is torn and he has a bundle of A4 pages, perhaps 100. He wants to show you 'the evidence'. He spreads the pages on the ground, making several points at once: about his studies, his family, his investments and his plans for the future. The notes indicate disturbed thinking and are mostly indecipherable. He wants to show you a mathematical formula for his 'ready reckoner', but when he cannot find it, he throws the papers down and runs away.   irritable

Will you physically restrain him?

No. A physical confrontation *on your own* (short of a declaration he is going to end his life *right now*) is not justified. If you were based in an A&E department or a psychiatric ward, gentle restraint by suitably trained personnel could be justified – at least until you are more certain of what is happening for him.

Will you await further contact from him?

No. You now have good presumptive evidence of *hypomania or mania* (Table 13, p. 45).

You do not know *why* his mood is elevated. In order of likeliness, its causes are functional, substance-induced or organic – but he requires urgent physical examination, investigations that include urine drug screen, and assessment of risk.

There is a past depressive episode (his cousin's death) and a family history of psychosis (aunt).

Discuss his case with the on-call psychiatry team. He may present elsewhere this evening. Copy any correspondence to the sector team for his area.

> **KEY POINT**
>
> Boundaries are important to define in all situations. It was reasonable to talk to him in the car park – once your safety was considered – until you knew what was happening. Your original brief was to provide a report about him, but events turned this into a psychiatric emergency.

Overnight, Declan presented to A&E but he did not accept any treatment. He did agree to come to your office the next morning. You are able to complete an MSE.

Set out the degrees of elevated mood that are possible here. Which does he have?

1 *Hypomania* is the mildest form of elevated mood. Many features are there (Table 13, p. 45) but, by definition, hypomania shows neither delusions nor hallucinations. It can be diagnosed after only a few days and causes '**considerable**' disruption of work or social activity. Declan has progressed well beyond this stage of elevated mood.

2 *Mania* implies '**complete**' disruption of work or social activity. It must last 1 week or more. By this point, the patient cannot control the associated behaviours and lacks insight that a psychiatric condition is causing them.

3 *Mania with psychotic features*, the most severe form of bipolar disorder, is his diagnosis. The vast majority of patients require admission. Extreme irritability or hostility may dominate, and it can be difficult to differentiate from a first episode of schizophrenia. Declan has grandiose and paranoid delusions and his pages of 'evidence' indicate thought disorder.

> Declan needs hospital and will come in voluntarily, but not to the hospital he has been attached to as a student. Your clinical director tells you that we cannot afford to fund a bed for him in another facility.

What will you do?

You cannot admit him to the ward where he has been as a student as he already knows details of the patients there that could compromise them and him. With mood elevation or any disinhibition, he may be unable to keep confidential matters to himself. It might even be dangerous for him to be admitted there if patients resent the 'them and us' attitudes of staff.

It is unlikely that there is another ward in the same hospital that could manage him – the nature of most facilities is to mix patients for therapy interventions and at mealtimes. It would be wrong to put him in that hospital against his will. He has already given consent to an admission, and made a reasonable request of you.

Telephone other colleagues in neighbouring hospitals. This sort of situation arises frequently and even the most hard-hit services show flexibility.

If all else fails, you must insist to your managers that funding is found to treat Declan in a safe and secure environment.

> You are allowed to admit Declan to a hospital 15 miles away that has no links with the university. The only condition is that you are the responsible consultant for his care: you agree. It is Friday, and a plan for the weekend is needed.

Will you prescribe? If so, what will you prescribe?

Observation of his mental state can continue on the ward, but you know enough to justify the prescription of a benzodiazepine.

In the short term, you should use an antipsychotic (AP) as adjunct (Box 11, p. 77; Table 8, p. 18): this way you do not have to choose a highly sedating AP

and, when he settles, he can go home on this AP but *not* the benzodiazepine. Better sleep with the tranquillizing effects of this combination will improve insight and help maintain his current resolve to stay on the ward.

It is the weekend, and extra doses can be given – provided he is reviewed by senior staff.

Will you prescribe a mood stabilizer?

Yes, but not now. We need to see his response to first line agents. Starting three medications at the same time is bad practice.

> At Monday's ward round, Declan is unrecognizable. He is pale and quiet, and has been crying for almost 24 hours. He says he has hit 'rock bottom', his food tastes like paper and he believes he will never leave hospital.

What might have happened?

- There could have been an *incident on the ward* that upset him: check this out
- Try to conceptualize each patient's *reaction to illness* (and confinement) as unique: we can guess the significance of rheumatoid arthritis in a pianist, but how might a young medical student deal with a potentially lifelong psychiatric disorder?
- He could have *gained insight with full recollection* of his behaviours. Did he have any calls or visitors that might have precipitated this reaction?
- Check his medication chart: was he given *excessive doses of AP*? Most typical APs, and many atypicals, induce dysphoria at higher doses
- If this episode is short-lived (moments or hours), it may be an adjustment to medication and circumstances, and described as a *microdepression*
- *Mixed bipolar affective disorder* is defined as the presence of both sets of mood symptoms (low and elevated mood; Table 13, p. 45), prominent for 2 weeks or more
- You have not yet seen a clean urine drug screen here. Declan could be coming down from the effects of amphetamines or other *substances*
- As a diagnosis of exclusion, Declan could be 'playing up' mild dysphoria for a multitude of reasons (e.g. reducing AP dose). He has a high *degree of knowledge* of the disorder and the system (as a medical student) and he might have *histrionic traits*. This is not a judgement you should make lightly

> **KEY POINT**
>
> Mixed affective state is a common presentation of bipolar disorder. Rapid cycling disorder is four episodes in 1 year of *any of*: mania, hypomania, mixed affective state or depression. Its most common cause is antidepressants.

His dose of AP is maintained at a therapeutic dose and other sedation reduced gradually: he is observed taking these. He sleeps well and he is reported as enjoying his food. A visit from his mother was 'a great success' and she left word she wants to know his discharge date. Urine drug screen is negative. Two days later, he is just as high and irritated as when he presented.

Outline your management

• He has bipolar type I disorder (Box 31) and will require a mood stabilizer (Table 9, p. 19). Each of the three drugs are effective in acute mania in over 50% of patients. Careful discussion about which agent is important. He will need medication as prophylaxis following discharge.

> **KEY POINT**
>
> Because of their potential toxicity (Table 9, p. 19) and narrow therapeutic ranges, mood stabilizers are the most hazardous of all psychoactive drugs.

• Check his physical health and review investigations for a physical cause of his elevated mood (Table 14, p. 47)
• Maximize management and ward environment (Box 11, p. 77)

> **Box 31 Classification of bipolar disorder (DSM-IV)**
>
> • Only a minority of patients with bipolar disorder experience mania
> • Bipolar type II disorder has episodes of hypomania (but not mania) and episodes of major depression (the DSM-IV equivalent of moderate/severe depressive illness)
> • Bipolar type I disorder is classic 'manic depression' (now an obsolete term) with episodes of mania and periods of major depression. The manic episodes do not need to have psychotic features to achieve this diagnosis

• Monitor his mood and any suicidal ideation at several points each day
• Cognitive–behavioural therapy (CBT) techniques are useful in symptom reduction and have been shown to prevent future relapses. CBT is an effective way to prevent and manage depression. You already know enough about the volatility of Declan's mood to make you very reluctant to prescribe an antidepressant should he become depressed in the future
• Even at this early stage, psychoeducation (to counter what *he thinks* he knows) will help with concordance and engagement
• Ward activities: Declan progressed from being a busy student to mania and is now doing little to occupy himself on the ward. Enlist the help of occupational therapy to programme activities. Practical projects would keep his day structured: where to live on discharge, managing his debts (it is likely he has been overspending), or building bridges with friends and family
• Future activities may be an issue. This is not the time to write a response to the Dean about his prior behaviour. Once he has responded to treatment, you can write a report to the Dean with his consent. He should arrange a meeting with the Dean, accompanied by a friend or family member

> **KEY POINT**
>
> Acute mania is unpredictable. With rapid changes in mood, suicidality varies considerably.

One month later, Declan has had 10 days' leave without incident. He approved your report to the Dean and Declan's apology has been accepted in full by Dr Hooper. The Dean will meet him next week to discuss a return to his studies. He is taking a mood stabilizer to excellent effect and agrees to remain on an AP for the next 6 months. At the discharge planning meeting, you explain to him that you cannot continue to be his psychiatrist and will be referring him to another team. Declan says that will not be necessary. His mother is a GP and wants to take things from here.

What needs to happen?

• His mother cannot be his doctor
• Declan needs formal follow-up, preferably by an Early Intervention Psychosis team as he is likely to relapse. We do not expect to find cognitive impairment but, if his functioning is lower than previously, formal testing would help decide future plans

Box 32 Early warning signs 'prodrome' of relapse in bipolar disorder (Watkins 2003):

Common prodromes of depression:
- Reduced interest in people or activities
- Feeling sad or depressed
- Disturbed sleep
- Tiredness
- Low motivation
- Increased worry
- Poor concentration

Common prodromes of mania:
- Reduced sleep/need for sleep
- Increased goal-directed activity
- Irritability
- More optimism
- Increased sociability/talking more
- Racing thoughts
- Distractibility

- He needs to agree safeguards to monitor his mental state with the university. In this episode, no patients were harmed (including Declan), but he may not be as fortunate next time
- His psychiatric illness should be notified to the medical licensing authority – with a clear relapse prevention plan (Box 32)

Reference

Watkins, E. (2003) Combining cognitive therapy with medication in bipolar disorder. *Advances in Psychiatric Treatment* **9**, 110–116.

CASE REVIEW

So far we have seen a spectrum of depressive illness (Cases 2, 7 and 12; Fig. 6, p. 146) and many other cases have presented with low mood and unhappiness, but short of the criteria for depression (Table 13, p. 45). Here, mania was characterized by irritability not infectious good humour. This feature is hard to tolerate by patients (suicidal acts are increased) and by those around them, in this case a consultant psychiatrist and you.

Declan's case was not complicated by alcohol or substance misuse – often used as the means of calming down or sleeping, but making mania worse and masking symptoms. Despite his degree of social impairment, he took 2 months to present: people with bipolar disorder can take years before the diagnosis is made. Unusually, he accepted admission: people with bipolar disorder are the most challenging Mental Health Act assessments. His treatment journey is only beginning here, and further episodes of high and low mood are likely.

Further reading

Frangou, S. (2005) Advancing the psychological treatment of bipolar disorder. *Advances in Psychiatric Treatment* **11**, 28–37.

Morriss, R. (2004) Early warning symptom intervention for patients with bipolar affective disorder. *Advances in Psychiatric Treatment* **10**, 18–26.

Smith, D.J. & Ghaemi, S.N. (2006) Hypomania in clinical practice. *Advances in Psychiatric Treatment* **12**, 110–120.

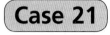 **A 24-year-old legal secretary with depressed mood and suicidal thoughts**

Vicki is referred to your community mental health team by her GP, Dr Edwards, who requests an urgent assessment. Vicki has been under pressure at work and has talked about feeling suicidal, saying voices in her head are telling her to take an overdose.

What are the key questions to ask Dr Edwards?

How quickly does Vicki need to be seen: *is she acutely suicidal?* Clarify whether Vicki needs to go to A&E now for assessment, or whether this can wait to be carried out by your community team over the next few days.

What diagnostic possibilities occur to you with this referral information?

Use the diagnostic hierarchy (Fig. 1, p. 7):
• *Organic illness:* unlikely in someone aged 24, with this presentation
• *Substances:* drugs would be a common cause of acute mental instability
• *Psychosis:* she is complaining of voices in her head
• *Affective:* suicidality is her presenting symptom
• *Anxiety disorders:* is this a reaction to an adverse work event?
• *Personality:* does she have long-standing difficulties exacerbated by stress?

Dr Edwards is extremely concerned about Vicki's suicide risk. He requests you see her today. She is refusing to go to A&E, saying she has been there before and the staff do not care. After some persuasion you agree, cancelling an important meeting to see her. She does not attend and you cannot contact her to find out if she is safe.

How might you feel at this point?

You are likely to be irritated; you have missed an important meeting to see Vicki and you are now left with the anxiety of whether she is safe. Without having even met her, you are caught up in concerns about her safety.

The next morning you speak to one of Dr Edwards' colleagues. He tells you Vicki called Dr Edwards on his mobile at midnight in a distressed state. This GP states with irritation that Vicki is 'attention-seeking' again. He also mentions she demands to see Dr Edwards 'practically every day' and refuses to see anyone else, saying they are all 'useless'. Dr Edwards is going on paternity leave in a month; Vicki is aware of this.

Describe Vicki's relationships with health care professionals

Vicki seems able to elicit sharply contrasting reactions from staff. She appears overly attached to Dr Edwards while completely rejecting his colleagues.

Vicki called Dr Edwards on his personal mobile at midnight. Is Dr Edwards having difficulties maintaining his boundaries with her?

Vicki has a long history of chronic depression, which has not responded to antidepressants. She was prescribed antipsychotics at times during the past 2 years because she had complained of hearing voices. She saw a practice counsellor but became more suicidal when this ended recently. Over the past year, she has presented to A&E twice after small overdoses but each time has self-discharged.

Does 'chronic depressive illness' sound like the right diagnosis here?

It is too early to define this as you have not yet met the patient (Fig. 6, p. 146). It sounds like depression but this is unlikely to be the whole story.

KEY POINT

Use of the term 'depression' must distinguish between depression as a disorder, as a discrete symptom and as a 'catch-all' term used by patients (and staff) to convey a host of uncomfortable emotional states, more accurately described by other terms such as emptiness, loneliness or boredom.

Reconsider differential diagnoses

• An *organic disorder* remains unlikely, although *substance misuse* could be complicating her presentation
• *Psychotic illness* is also less likely, as she describes hearing voices on occasion but is well known to the GP and there are no other features of psychosis
• An acute stress reaction or *adjustment disorder* are still possible (Table 26, p. 93), perhaps in addition to other more long-standing difficulties. Several stressors are happening around the same time: work pressure, the end of therapy and the imminent loss of *her* GP
• A *personality disorder with borderline traits* would explain chronic problems with mood instability, recurrent suicidality and quasi-psychotic symptoms, as well as the tensions evident in her professional relationships

> Vicki attends for assessment. She is articulate, funny and engaging, even flirtatious. She describes anxiety, depression and chronic insomnia, as well as some symptoms of bulimia. She tells you about two boyfriends who have been physically abusive to her and complains that her boss bullies her at work. She becomes tearful telling you about a recent sexual encounter with a stranger that was initially consensual but during which she felt out of control and frightened. This happened just after her counselling ended and she has been off work since. With little prompting she goes on to describe what sounds like an emotionally impoverished upbringing with a violent, sexually abusive father and a disinterested critical mother. You find there is much to admire in how she has coped overall. Vicki tells you you are a wonderful listener, better than her counsellor.

What is your reaction to Vicki at this point?

This information may enable you to feel empathy (p. 9) for her and thus help you to understand how she might feel so desperate and suicidal at times. If so, you are likely to feel a strong sense of wanting to help her.

You may feel flattered by her praise, although it is at others' expense. This may draw you further into wanting to help, elevating you to an idealized position of being 'that one special person' who can help where others have failed.

You might also start to feel anxious about how extensive her problems are and how you are going to complete your assessment in the short time left.

> You have two patients waiting. Vicki catches you trying subtly to look at your watch. Her manner changes abruptly to one of quiet hostility. After an awkward silence, she apologizes for taking too much of your time, when you must have other people worse off than her to see. She mutters something about the voices being right saying she is stupid because she was stupid enough to think you would care. She adds Dr Edwards is only doctor she has ever met who cares.

What do you think has just happened in the interview between you both?

• She appears unusually sensitive to the social cue (looking at your watch) indicating there is a limit to the time you can give her
• You are likely to feel defensive when negatively compared with Dr Edwards
• Her reaction appears disproportionate, suggesting she might have experienced this as a rejection. Her seemingly abrupt emotional withdrawal from you was to protect herself from experiencing further rejection
• Her comments would be commonly described as 'passive aggression'. While the other person's outward behaviour is not aggressive, and indeed may be the opposite (meek, submissive), you are under attack in an unspoken way and are likely to feel irritated (perhaps intensely and seemingly irrationally so) in response. *It is your own emotional response that alerts you this is occurring*

How might you manage the rest of this interview?

You need to manage both the interview's content and process:
• Do not respond defensively or with irritation. It tells you something about how she feels about herself and her relationships with other people. By this point, you can see why she has evoked such contrasting reactions from different doctors

---

KEY POINT

Do not act out your emotional reactions to patients: use them. Your own emotions are a tool to understanding the internal worlds of others (i.e. how they are feeling at that moment, how they tend to relate to other people and how others are likely to relate to them).

• Openly acknowledge time is limited, and that this is difficult as there are important areas you have not had time to cover together
• Orientate her to what she can expect now in terms of time and what she can expect after today (e.g. an appointment to continue the assessment next week)
• Decide what your priorities are and what you need to know before she leaves the room today – everything else can wait

What do you need to establish today?

1 Current problem list, rather than an exact diagnosis
2 Level of current risk to self
3 Management plan for the short term (e.g. reviewing medication, how often she will see you, date of next appointment and what she will do if she feels suicidal again to keep herself safe)

• Clarify her risk history and explore other possible forms of self-harm (e.g. has she burnt or cut herself, or restricted food?). Ask how she views her sexual behaviour – is this for her a way of harming herself via the exploitation of others?
• What are its triggers? How serious is the harm caused? How often does it happen and when was the last time?
• Does she have active thoughts of self-harm at present?
• What strategies has she found useful in the past for managing her feelings without harming herself?

You establish Vicki is not acutely suicidal but if she becomes so she will come to your team base to see the duty worker, or out of hours she will present to A&E. She also seems interested in the idea of telephoning the Samaritans for support. You agree to meet in a week to continue the assessment. She asks if you could prescribe her another antidepressant today. From her history you confirm she has had extensive treatment with medication with no benefit.

> **KEY POINT**
>
> It is common to be asked something important at the last possible moment of a consultation: the 'door knob question'. The patient may have been anxiously avoiding bringing it up or hoping to elicit a reply quickly without negotiation. Acknowledge you may have to frustrate your patient by not providing an immediate response because the topic demands more time for discussion.

Do you start another antidepressant today?

This is a difficult clinical judgement. Although a diagnosis of depression by this point clearly does not explain either the nature or extent of all her difficulties, arguably prescribing is a simple way to help her feel cared for, thereby increasing the chance she will engage with your service (i.e. there may be some short-term placebo benefit).

By contrast, if you withhold a prescription she may assume you do not see her problems as sufficiently serious. She may feel rejected by that and it may contribute to her feeling more worthless and suicidal again.

If you rush into prescribing for her, however, you establish a precedent of responding to her distress by reaching for a prescription. Furthermore, premature prescribing will be positively unhelpful if it maintains a biological focus for her difficulties when you need to be engaging her in exploring a psychological one.

Whether or not you decide an empirical trial of medication is justified, the important point is to clarify previous responses to antidepressants and make the patient an active participant in this decision. This is a longer discussion (not for today) that will be a valuable gateway to discussing the more difficult reality that there may not be a simple medication solution to their difficulties.

> **KEY POINT**
>
> Patients often hope that their difficulties are caused by an illness that medication will cure. If you perpetuate unrealistic hopes around medication, you may be successful in providing temporary reassurance that pleases the patient but risks disappointment later on.

You see Vicki for further assessment. You are confident that her primary diagnosis is borderline personality disorder (BPD) and she does not have an affective or psychotic illness at the present time. The voices she hears are in keeping with dissociative symptoms under stress. You explain what BPD means (Box 33) and she is able to recognize that its features apply to her.

> ### Box 33 Features of borderline personality disorder (ICD-10)
>
> The **general criteria** for personality disorders must be met (Box 13, p. 89), i.e. the individual must have enduring patterns of *cognition, inner experience, behaviour* and *ways of relating to others* that cause distress.
>
> **Borderline** personality disorder (in ICD-10, *Emotionally unstable personality disorder, borderline type*) shows features of:
> - Unstable mood
> - Liable to outbursts
> - Impulsive behaviour
> - Disturbed sense of self
> - Chronic feelings of emptiness
> - Involvement in intense, unstable relationships
> - Excessive efforts to avoid abandonment
> - Recurrent threats or acts of self-harm

> ### KEY POINT
>
> *Hearing voices* does not always mean psychotic illness. Voices can also occur as a dissociative symptom and are a common phenomenon in BPD. The critical voices the patient carries with them can be understood as persistent fragments of childhood abuse. Antipsychotics will only help by sedating the patient.

You agree with Vicki to refer her for cognitive–analytic therapy. She leaves in a positive mood, expressing her gratitude for your help. Three days later you hear Vicki has been admitted to psychiatric hospital. Dr Edwards went on paternity leave sooner than expected. His colleague then refused to see Vicki as an emergency. She subsequently traced Dr Edward's home address via the General Medical Council (GMC) register, turned up on his doorstep, having freshly cut her arms and accused him of being 'an uncaring bastard'. His wife called the police, but Vicki ran off and took an overdose soon after. The GP practice will remove Vicki from their list.

What can be learnt from this?

The bubble of 'perfect care' provided by Dr Edwards has burst. Vicki felt rejected and was unable to manage those feelings, while Dr Edwards and his family will have been frightened by her behaviour and the strength of her emotions. The end result for is her actual rejection by Dr Edwards and his practice.

> ### KEY POINT
>
> People with BPD may seek fulfilment of a fantasy of 'perfect care' or perfect closeness with others ('emotional fusion'), as opposed to the reality of abuse, lack of care and rejection they have actually experienced. When others cannot fulfil this fantasy, as ultimately no-one can, further help-seeking behaviour may paradoxically elicit a rejecting response from others, unable to cope with the emotional demands this need places on them.

With hindsight, some form of crisis around her GP's paternity leave was highly likely. It could have been anticipated and planned for by acknowledging and discussing the problem with staff and Vicki herself.

Also, with hindsight, Dr Edward's boundaries were poorly defined. Vicki had his personal mobile number and phoned him outside office hours without sanction. Difficult conversations about this early on save much more difficult ones later. These discussions probably did not happen because of 'splitting' occurring between the professionals involved; staff experienced different aspects of Vicki's personality, hence their contrasting responses.

Staff splitting mirrors the patient's lack of internal integration. In BPD, the experience of others tends to be polarized. They are experienced as either good or bad, caring or abusive, rather than the more complex human reality: someone who cares can also disappoint sometimes. Children in nurturing relationships learn to integrate both good and bad aspects of their care givers and thus themselves. Having lacked that opportunity, patients with BPD tend either to idealize or denigrate others as one extreme or the other, and equally 'split off' or dissociate from the bad aspects of themselves. If staff are initially idealized, disappointment is inevitable, as Dr Edwards now knows.

When staff splits occur, there is a tendency to fail to recognize the bigger picture of what is happening and what that says about the patient's internal world. Individual staff may either naively pride themselves on their special relationship with the patient or become defensive about the patient's dismissal of them. Splitting therefore perpetuates the patient's pathological dynamics, and the lack of team integration mirrors this (Box 34).

Box 34 Treatment for borderline personality difficulties (BPD): general approach

Treatment is essentially psychological. Medication is indicated for any identified intercurrent mental illness (e.g. depression). Symptomatic prescription is on an empirical basis: the prescribing process itself may evoke unhelpful interpersonal dynamics and medication risks subsequent dependence that may distract from a more useful psychological focus.

Given the nature of their difficulties, patients with BPD may quickly establish a treatment relationship but it is often difficult for them to maintain one. Treatment relationships inevitably invoke their habitual relationship patterns. Patterns involving *idealization* (and/or denigration) of the health professional often emerge, with the patient seeking care, experiencing painful rejection as a result of the limitations of that care, and subsequently finding it difficult to manage their feelings safely as a result.

The following guiding principles (adapted from Gabbard 1994) anticipate and help contain these difficulties:

- *Establish a stable treatment framework:* be consistent. Let the patient know what they can expect. Set limits and stick to the boundaries of what can be provided (e.g. start and end appointments on time) and give the patient advanced warning of when their care will be disrupted (e.g. by your holidays)
- *Give the patient feedback:* be honest. Help them reflect on their behaviour and the feelings that they experience and invoke in others, including you
- *Contain the patient's anger:* do not get defensive. Use empathy where appropriate to help them reflect on why they are angry
- *Confront self-destructive behaviours:* do not ignore them. Explore the consequences of their self-harm, substance misuse, unsafe sex, etc.
- *Establish the links between feelings and actions:* connect them. Patients with BPD often struggle to understand their own behaviour. Their self-destructive behaviours are (maladaptive) ways of managing and avoiding difficult feelings. Help them identify the feelings so they can recognize what is happening and thereby learn to manage it differently
- *Remain aware of countertransference:* monitor your reactions. Reflect on the emotional response the patient invokes in you, otherwise you will simply act out on it, and perpetuate the patient's unhelpful relationship patterns

KEY POINT

In working with a patient with BPD, supportive and non-defensive communication amongst staff is vital to avoid splitting. Open and honest communication with a BPD patient is also essential, with a clear structure to their care so they know what they can expect and what its limitations are. Time set aside for open team discussion of difficulties arising with these patients is time well spent.

Finally, doctors should keep home addresses out of the GMC's public register.

Months later, Vicki sees a television programme on famous people with bipolar disorder and becomes convinced this is her diagnosis. Around this time she becomes depressed while addressing past abuse in psychotherapy. Her psychotherapist cancels a session because of illness and shortly after Vicki is admitted to hospital acutely suicidal, following a weekend of heavy alcohol use. The hospital psychiatrist agrees with Vicki she has bipolar disorder and starts her on medication. She sees you again after discharge and is angry with you for not doing so before. She also mentions that the psychiatrist advised her she should stop psychotherapy if it makes her suicidal.

What will you advise Vicki to do about the medication and therapy?

Clinical presentations change. It is entirely possible medication is now indicated. Anyone with a diagnosis of BPD is more vulnerable to other mental disorders, especially substance misuse (Box 33).

Even if you disagree with an alternative diagnosis, avoid unhelpful splitting between you and the hospital psychiatrist. Be wary of taking Vicki's account of their views at face value; discuss her directly with them. If Vicki believes her new medication is helpful, you would be unwise to stop it at this point anyway.

KEY POINT

It can sometimes be difficult to distinguish between the mood instability of bipolar disorder and that of BPD. In terms of predisposing risk factors, abusive childhood experiences are more common in both. A careful history of affective symptoms is key to deciding how the mood instability is most helpfully conceptualized.

Box 35 Borderline personality disorder: specific psychological treatments

There is no one right approach. The theoretical language and tools used by therapies differ, but generally the goal is for the patient to learn to manage their emotional experience and develop a more coherent, rounded view of themselves and others.

Cognitive–analytic therapy (CAT) is a time limited therapy (for BPD usually 24 sessions) that combines elements of CBT with psychodynamic psychotherapy. The therapist guides the patient in making links between their presenting problems and their habitual (maladaptive) patterns of managing their emotions and relating to themselves and others. These patterns are also actively explored as they occur in the treatment relationship itself. Central to this process are:

1 The therapist making these links explicit in a *reformulation letter* to the patient early in therapy that puts their current difficulties in the context of how they evolved in their formative relationships, and
2 The joint creation of a *diagrammatic reformulation*, which maps out the patient's repertoire of reciprocal relationship patterns (known as 'reciprocal roles') and links them to the problematic procedures they use to manage the difficult feelings that result (e.g. using alcohol to reduce anxiety)
3 The end of therapy is marked by the exchange of *goodbye letters* between therapist and patient, which aim to integrate both positive and negative aspects of the experience, making explicit what has and has not changed for the patient, what they may find difficult when the therapy ends, and how they might continue to grow in experiencing more reality-based and less damaging ways of relating in the future (www.acat.org. uk).

Dynamic psychotherapy: there are various schools of dynamic therapy that aim to address the patient's core deficiencies and work through their difficulties as they arise in the treatment relationship over a longer period of treatment (often years). The therapist tends to take on a more active and challenging (although not confrontational) role in the sessions (see Box 34), different from classic (silent therapist) psychoanalysis.

Cognitive therapy: schema-based cognitive therapy has developed as a goal-directed and problem-solving approach that seeks to identify the long-standing dysfunctional core beliefs that the patient has regarding themselves, others

and the world. While there is much overlap with CAT, this is a longer-term therapy (weekly sessions for up to 2 years) that has less of a psychodynamic focus. There is more emphasis placed on establishing and maintaining a treatment alliance (Young *et al*. 2003).

Dialectical behaviour therapy (DBT): a structured therapy that combines individual therapy with group sessions every week, with the individual's therapist available (including evenings and weekends) for telephone counselling between sessions to help manage crises. There is a treatment hierarchy of goals, namely:

1 To stop life-threatening and self-harming behaviours
2 To stop treatment-interfering behaviours (e.g. missing sessions), and
3 To stop crisis-generating behaviours (e.g. substance misuse).

Group work teaches patients to develop new skills for regulating their emotions and managing them in a safe way, to tolerate distress and to develop mindfulness, i.e. the ability to reflect on one's own and others' emotional experience (Linehan 1993). DBT is suitable for clients too disturbed for only once-weekly psychotherapy and for whom focused work on stopping self-harm needs to occur as a priority. A successful course of DBT might be sufficient. Alternatively, a patient who has completed DBT may need more in-depth therapy such as schema-based CBT or CAT.

Therapeutic community treatment: combines psychodynamically informed individual therapy with group therapy in the *milieu* of a day hospital or residential setting. Here the patients and staff experience themselves as part of a community, with the opportunity to work through the difficulties that arise in relation to others in that context. Group therapy is based on the principle that key to our experience of ourselves is our active experience of ourselves in relation to others. When problematic interpersonal dynamics occur, individuals learn to recognize and understand their emotional experience better through a process of *mentalization*. This entails developing one's capacity to reflect on one's own and others' mental states. Through their interventions and open reflections with patients, staff provide a model for this process. The support and feedback (or 'reality checks') the patients give each other is also integral to this experience (Bateman & Fonagy 2004).

Explain that you are the treating doctor in the long term and will have opportunities to review medication and diagnosis regularly.

Focus instead on a more useful discussion that tries to help her understand why she became suicidal again. Identify her use of alcohol as a maladaptive coping mechanism for managing (i.e. avoiding) difficult emotional experience. Explain how alcohol is a depressant, which in turn would have made her more depressed in addition to other psychological problems (Table 18, p. 62).

Suggest Vicki returns to her therapist to discuss continuing therapy. If it would be helpful, offer to become involved in this discussion.

This crisis may offer a valuable opportunity for positive change. Reassure Vicki it is not unusual for people to become more depressed when they confront painful realities that much of their maladaptive behaviour functions to help them avoid.

This might be a good time to consider principles of her management in the long term (Box 34).

KEY POINT

Like everyone, doctors and psychotherapists disappoint (e.g. they go on leave or change jobs). For patients with BPD this can be intensely upsetting as past painful feelings are evoked – activating fear of abandonment. Where possible pre-empt with the patient when this might occur. What matters is that unlike in their formative damaging relationships, in a therapeutic relationship the patient has an opportunity to have their feelings recognized and understood.

What types of psychotherapy are suitable for Vicki and other patients with BPD?

Generic counselling frequently makes these patients worse, as it did here at the start of this presentation. Psychological treatments need to be specialized and based within a coherent theoretical framework that directly addresses the patient's difficulties. Most require many years training, and ongoing regular supervision of the therapist (Box 35).

CASE REVIEW

Vicki has long-standing traits of BPD originating from childhood abuse and neglect. Having previously managed to function as a legal secretary, she decompensated and became more disturbed when several stressors happened around the same time. Once engaged in treatment, pathological dynamics arose with staff; these reflected her underlying difficulties.

There is no curative medication or single psychological treatment solution for BPD. However, positive change can occur over time through providing consistent and honest treatment relationships that support the patient, while challenging their habitual unhelpful and painful ways of relating to, and thinking about, others and themselves (Box 34). In doing so, the patient can be helped to develop their capacity to understand and manage their emotional experience more effectively.

Although we have represented psychopathic traits in a man (Case 16) and borderline traits in a woman in this case, do not assume that these disorders are always gender-specific. Mixtures of both traits can also occur in one person.

References

Bateman A. & Fonagy P. (2004) *Psychotherapy for Borderline Personality Disorder: Mentalization Based Treatment*. Oxford University Press.

Gabbard, G. (1994) *Psychodynamic Psychiatry in Clinical Practice*. American Psychiatric Press, Washington DC.

Linehan, M. (1993) *Cognitive Behavioural Therapy for Borderline Personality Disorder*. Guilford Press, New York.

Young, J.E., Klosko, J.S. &Weishaar, M.E. (2003) *Schema Therapy: A Practitioner's Guide*. Guilford Press, New York.

Further reading

Ryle, A. (1997) *Cognitive Analytic Therapy and Borderline Personality Disorder*. Wiley, Chichester.

Ryle, A. & Kerr, I.B. (2002) *Introducing Cognitive Analytic Therapy*. Wiley, Chichester.

Case 22 A 41-year-old woman with epilepsy develops a different pattern of fits

Sally has a clinical diagnosis of generalized epilepsy. She had childhood petit mal (absence) seizures that resolved after 4 years' treatment, but developed tonic–clonic seizures last year. Despite being on medication, she continues to have 2–5 generalized fits each month, confirmed by electroencephalogram (EEG) as recently as 3 months ago. This restricts her from driving, and adds additional pressures to her life as a working mother of two children. She is reviewed by the neurology trainee who detected new 'counting rituals'. Her partner says 'she goes off on one' once, sometimes three times, every week. She gets angry

when he tries to stop her pointing at things and counting. The trainee prescribes her 20 mg fluoxetine for obsessive-compulsive disorder and contacts you after 4 months' treatment – the counting episodes are more frequent.

Was the trainee mistaken in prescribing fluoxetine for Sally?

Yes. Obsessive-compulsive disorder (OCD) is a difficult diagnosis to make at one assessment and by people who do not see enough cases (Box 36). Sally may have rituals but this does not mean OCD. The fact that they are epi-

---

Box 36 Obsessive-compulsive disorder (OCD): ICD-10 criteria and phenomenology

OCD is diagnosed on the basis of obsessional thoughts or compulsive acts. Either or both must be present on most days for at least 2 successive weeks. OCD is a lifelong condition, manifesting by early adolescence and continuing through adult life. It may have active periods where the person has comorbid depression, anxiety or panic disorder (all very common in acutely unwell OCD patients) or is under stress. To diagnose OCD, it must cause distress or interfere with normal activities.

Obsessional thoughts must have the following properties:
- Recognized as the individual's own thoughts
- At least one thought (initially every obsessive thought) is resisted, but without success
- The thought of carrying out the act (ritual) must not in itself be pleasurable
- Thoughts/images/impulses are repetitive and unpleasant

Both the thoughts and the rituals are stereotyped. The same thoughts occur over and over: in many cases they are worrying (that they have left the gas on, that germs will kill someone), obscene (sexual content, blasphemy) or senseless (numerical sequences, patterns). The rituals too are stereotyped: a monotonous task that as if by magic will rid the patient of the original obsession. The individual will repetitively check the gas, clean to excess, say specific sentences to atone for some obscenity or blasphemy, count

to self or aloud (both are acts), rearrange items, etc. The rituals are a symbolic attempt to avert a bad outcome: the individual *knows* they will not prevent anything, but cannot resist carrying them out. From a behavioural standpoint, as the rituals are practiced, the acts reinforce any original unpleasant thoughts, and these will recur *more* frequently.

The *unpleasant* nature of either thoughts or acts has been described as egodystonic and ego-alien. The terms are synonymous, meaning that although the person knows they originate from within themselves (they are not delusions of thought interference or made acts of somatic passivity delusions), their content is out of keeping with their beliefs and personality. Common examples are obscene words in a prudish individual or blasphemy in a religious person.

If someone does not meet these criteria, they may have an anakastic (obsessional) personality disorder:
- Preoccupation with rules, details, schedules
- Traits of inflexibility and perfectionism
- Excessive conscientiousness, pedantry
- Insistent, unwelcome thoughts (not meeting criteria above)

In anakastic PD, thoughts and behaviours are egosyntonic; they are not experienced as unpleasant (e.g. the accountant taking pleasure in keeping meticulous bookkeeping).

---

sodic rather than occurring *on most days* (Box 36), and that something else is happening to her consciousness (she 'goes off on one'), make OCD less likely here.

OCD is unlikely to present for the first time in people over 20 years. Even if she has the disorder, in the context of new onset epilepsy 1 year ago, there could be an organic illness (possibly a cerebral lesion) explaining both.

People with OCD *resist* their thoughts and behaviours (Box 36), at least initially. Any anger they feel is self-directed for thinking and doing pointless things. Sally gets angry with others, raising the possibility of delusional thinking or an automatism (see below) rather than a compulsion.

A trainee neurologist may have missed epileptic symptoms.

Putting a patient with poorly controlled, generalized (or other) epilepsy on selective serotonin reuptake inhibitor (SSRI) medication lowers their seizure threshold, and could have induced seizures.

If she has OCD (i.e. the trainee is right for the wrong reasons), about 70% of OCD patients present with comorbid depression. This needs to be treated vigorously (Table 15, p. 49), with careful monitoring of suicide risk. Doses of up to 60 mg fluoxetine are required to treat OCD symptoms.

> ### KEY POINT
>
> In clinical medicine, being right for the wrong reasons can be just as dangerous being wrong.

A consultant neurologist reviews her, stops her fluoxetine and discusses her case with you. Sally has new episodes where she hears the voice of her dead mother, her arms and legs jerk vigorously, and this terminates with extreme sadness. Towards the end of these episodes, she counts softly to herself.

What additional information and investigations will you suggest?

• Are there other symptoms to support that the episodes are seizures (aura, urinary incontinence)? Partial seizures have manifestations that are localized to one region of the cerebral cortex, and complex partial seizures have localized features *plus* impaired consciousness. Does the neurologist think the episodes are likely to be epilepsy?

• Is there any temporal relationship between these new episodes and her generalized fits?
  ○ ictal: episodes occur *during* fits
  ○ postictal: they occur *afterwards*
  ○ interictal: they occur *in between*

• She is relatively young, but are their vascular risk factors (smoking, high lipids, family history of premature heart disease) or antecedents of cancer (smoking, weight loss)?

• What are the doses and levels of anti-epileptic drugs (AEDs)? Concordance?

• Does she have other neurological symptoms? Abnormal neurological signs? Other physical findings?

• Was her magnetic resonance imaging (MRI) scan normal? She will have had extensive investigations *last year*, but these may not have been repeated in the past 4 months

• Did 24-hour EEG record one of her new episodes?

• Results of blood tests: general and metabolic screen. Postictal prolactin levels are usually elevated, although not always

• Previous psychiatric assessments, family history of psychiatric illness and date/details of her mother's death (normal bereavement; Box 16, p. 119).

> ### KEY POINT
>
> Postictal psychoses are organic psychoses occurring after a seizure. There is usually a lucid interval before the onset of psychotic symptoms that last hours, rarely days, and resolve spontaneously. Treatment is aimed at reducing the epileptic seizures. Antipsychotics lower seizure threshold, making epilepsy worse.

All physical investigations are normal. She did not have an episode during 24-hour EEG, but further testing with video EEG has been booked. Her consultant tells you that she is a 'reliable witness' and finds her accounts consistent and plausible, but cannot decide whether this is 'real' or 'psychiatric'. It is hard to define it, but there is 'something different about her'. Additional details of her childhood epilepsy are that they were simple absences with 'blanking' for 4–5 seconds, but became complex absences, lasting minutes, with increases in muscle tone during episodes. She 'grew out of them' by age 14 and had no recurrence. You review her.

What is your differential diagnosis?

1 *Organic illness:* single pathology (neurological conditions of Table 20, p. 69) could have caused new epilepsy or an extension of previous seizure pathways. The same pathological lesion(s) could also have caused organic personality change. Many other conditions mimic seizures (e.g. complicated migraine, transient ischaemic attacks, episodic hypoglycaemia). It is important that further testing takes place, with regular neurological review.

2 *Substance and/or alcohol misuse* (Tables 18 and 42, p. 62 and p. 138): Sally does not have to misuse alcohol for it to interfere with the plasma levels of her AEDs. At the very least, carry out a urinary drug screen randomly, and after an episode.

3 *Psychosis:* ictal, postictal or interictal. Many other disorders must be considered as causes of her voices before making a diagnosis of functional psychosis, but details thus far suggest bizarre, out of character behaviour, and other symptoms must be explored (Box 9, p. 54).

4 *Depression:* very common and can present with somatic symptoms or behaviours. Sally has new counting 'rituals' and a depressive episode could have brought out previously latent obsessional traits (Box 36).

> **KEY POINT**
>
> Each of a history of psychosis and depression are associated with three times the incidence of epilepsy. People with epilepsy have up to 10 times the incidence of psychosis.

5 Sally could have an *anxiety disorder* (Table 11, p. 38), including panic disorder. This latter diagnosis is supported by the symptom of extreme dysphoria after the episode terminates, but neither voices nor rituals are recognized features (Case 1). With her recent diagnosis of epilepsy, Sally could have developed *health anxiety* – a conviction that something is definitely wrong with her, despite normal investigations.

6 These may be *non-epileptic seizures* (NES).

> **KEY POINT**
>
> The highest incidence of NES is in patients who have a confirmed diagnosis of epilepsy: 30% of people with epilepsy have NES.

7 She may be exhibiting *abnormal illness behaviour* (Table 51). This is her third experience of fits with her second experience 1 year ago. She is a busy professional, and 41 is a transition age. Has she completed her family? Is she frustrated by the side-effects or the teratogenic potential of her AEDs (Table 9, p. 19)? Illness behaviour has cognitive, perceptual and behavioural components (see her symptoms above).

8 While she may not meet the criteria for *personality disorder* as a diagnosis in itself, she may have traits that mediate responses to illness (Table 52). The possibility arises that the distress of new generalized epilepsy has activated previously controlled obsessional traits in this patient (Box 36). However, the presence of rituals excludes anakastic personality as a possible diagnosis.

9 *Factitious disorder/malingering:* there is no current evidence to support either, but they are a possibility when all others are excluded.

You interview Sally and are satisfied she does not have an affective or anxiety disorder. She has never misused illegal drugs, and drinks less than 5 units weekly: urine drug screens are negative. As best you can tell, her responses to her generalized epilepsy and recent episodes are within normal limits (Table 51). She has adapted positively to changes imposed upon her. She takes carbamazepine and plasma levels are in the therapeutic range. Her personality does not display any maladaptive behaviour (Table 52), but collateral history is unavailable. Simon is minding their two young children (aged 6 and 2 years). Assume there are three possible explanations for her episodes:

Complex partial seizures (CPS)
Interictal psychosis (IIP)
Non-epileptic seizures (NES)

> **KEY POINT**
>
> CPS are the most common seizure disorder in adults. Over half are associated with psychiatric disorders.

How will you decide between these three options?

Each option is considered under four headings: description of individual episodes, other details from the history, description of the aftermath of episodes, and investigations.

Table 51 Schema to conceptualize reactions to illness.

Responses to illness	Factor	Example
Normal illness behaviour	Resilience	A patient, after a myocardial infarction or psychotic episode, decides to work less and exercise more
	Normal stages of grief (Box 16, p. 120)	Brief adjustment disorder in a diabetic or depressed patient who later accepts diagnosis and treatment
Abnormal illness behaviour	Inadequate response to symptoms	• Denial of symptoms or illness • Delayed help seeking • Treatment non-concordance • Defaulting from follow-up
	Excessive response to symptoms	• Hypervigilance leading to excessive health care utilization • Self-medication: alcohol, over-the-counter, prescribed and illegal drugs • Anxiety syndromes (Table 11, p. 38) • Health anxiety, somatization (see Case 19)

All three parameters below contribute to abnormal illness behaviour

Responses to illness	Factor	Example
Individual factors	Attachment disorders	See Case 19
	Personality traits, personality disorder	See Table 52
	Coping styles	Overgeneralization, catastrophization: a patient, after a myocardial infarction is convinced (despite normal tests) that he will have another myocardial infarction or die if he takes any exercise at all
Cultural norms (including person's subculture)	Disclosure to doctors*	• People from Afro-Caribbean families are more likely to contact the police not health services for a psychotic family member
	*Factors preventing disclosure may rest within the doctors	• Although disputed, patients from the Indian subcontinent are said to somatize to excess: they complain more of physical symptoms even if they have psychological disorders • Doctors are less likely to diagnose psychological symptoms in minority ethnic groups
	Spirituality	Many cultures believe that the Devil plays a part in mental disorders: as spirits, possession, punishment (Case 2)
Other social factors	The sick role	This is a socially agreed notion of how sick people should behave and the benefits that accrue to them. It can be over played
	Stigma	Has negative effects on recognition, presentation, diagnosis, treatment, reintegration and outcomes of all mental disorders and some physical (e.g. HIV)
	Socioeconomic group/income	Patients are stereotyped (e.g. wealthy people are less likely to have domestic violence identified despite its equal prevalence); some treatments are given in a disproportionate way: higher income groups more likely to be offered psychotherapy

Table 52 How different personality traits react to illness differently. After Querques and Stern (2004).

Personality type	Traits	Reactions to physical or psychological illness	Recommended management strategies
Anxious avoidant (Case 4)	Feelings of tension, inferiority; avoidance and restrictions in lifestyle	May be overwhelmed by illness; will have multiple questions but might be too anxious to ask them of professionals	Supply reassurance; ask directly about concerns and tactfully about anxieties; discuss any procedures clearly
Paranoid (Table 24, p. 89)	Suspicious, tenacious personal rights' awareness, grudges, misconstrue neutral actions	See illness as an external assault; suspicious of medical interventions – that something is being hidden from them	Acknowledge effects of illness; information about causes and procedures; disclosure of side-effects in advance of treatment
Schizotypal (p. 57)	Eccentric, odd behaviours; ideas and experiences that fall short of psychosis	Similar to paranoid personalities but communicate their concerns poorly (odd speech and mannerisms) if at all	As paranoid traits; allow self-isolation; extra efforts to communicate with person: similar to autism and LD (Box 22)
Dependent (Table 31, p. 105)	Excessive need to be taken care of: submissive and clinging behaviours	Cycles of ↑ anxiety and ↑ demands on staff; perceived abandonment by family and professionals	Clear information by one nominated staff member; state your care is comprehensive and that all options have been considered
Dissocial (Box 19, p. 149)	Callous unconcern for others, low frustration, high guilt thresholds; disregard social norms; frequent lying and rule breaking	May appear unconcerned but use their illness as opportunity for other goals; see medical advice as applying to others, not them; capacity for destructive acts	Tailor medical advice to self-preservation rather than feelings; address concordance frequently; limit set if anger/inappropriate or destructive behaviour
Narcissistic (Case 17)	Strive to appear independent and smart; grandiose when under duress, may lack empathy	Illness may challenge sense of self and self-esteem; unlikely to request and will resist help	Encourage efforts to 'beat' the illness; accommodate excessive/intrusive participation in decision-making
Histrionic (Box 30, p. 184)	Exaggerated emotions but shallow affect; excitement seeking and suggestible	Illness interpreted as threat to self or sexuality; premature trust of medical staff may disappear; tendency to dramatize	Acknowledge patient's grace under pressure; 'less is more' in explaining causes and proposed treatments
Borderline (Case 21)	Emotional instability; fear of abandonment; self-damage from impulsive behaviours; extremes in relationships	Dramatic presentations but may abscond; misinterpret staff action/words: anger; dissonance between staff's and patient's different realities	Education of non-psychiatric staff is essential about what to expect; agreed consistent information, with limit setting; avoid splitting (see Case 21)
Obsessive (Box 33, p. 191)	Place high value on detail, proper protocols and order; minimize pain as 'normal'	Illness threatens self-control; need for certainty increases anxiety further; unlikely to complain of problems early	Provide more detailed information at all times, including written; show tolerance to 'pedantic' questions; encourage self-efficacy

LD, learning disorder.

What aspects of the episodes will help you make one diagnosis over another?

• *The nature of the precipitant:* an emotional trigger suggests NES, sometimes suggestion alone by the clinician will bring on an episode. Flashing lights can provoke seizures in many forms of epilepsy, including CPS: 'television epilepsy'. Psychotic symptoms do not have a precipitant or a warning/aura.

• Onset of NES is gradual, and they last longer (>3 minutes) than CPS. Psychotic symptoms tend to endure longer than both.

• An *aura* is a simple partial seizure. It is highly individualized as what people can remember up until the time their consciousness is impaired (when the seizure generalizes). People with CPS may experience foreboding, visual symptoms (colour changes, macropsia/micropsia, visual hallucinations), epigastric aura (bizarre gastrointestinal symptoms), déjà vu, jamais vu and hallucinations in any modality (smells, tactile sensations, voices).

> **KEY POINT**
>
> Temporal lobe epilepsy (TLE) is a CPS with a temporal lobe focus. People with TLE are often misdiagnosed as 'psychiatric'.

• We expect *more drama* during NES (e.g. speaking, shouting, crying, complex emotional expressions, laboured breathing). These are highly unusual activities in epileptic seizures: during tonic–clonic seizures, a patient breathes normally but cannot speak or emote in any way.

• During any NES, the patient is *responsive* to specific commands: 'Lift your head for this pillow. Move your legs up. Hold your arm still while I take this blood sample.' Unlike a generalized seizure, the person's conscious and unconscious instincts for self-preservation remain intact.

• You will need to witness a variety of epileptic fits to contrast their *motor features* with NES: the latter may show head bobbing, pelvic thrusting, limb thrashing, asymmetry of movements, and (in some cases) are a poor impersonation of what lay people might imagine epilepsy to be.

• *Urinary incontinence* can occur in many generalized seizures. It is unlikely to occur in NES, but anything can happen if someone wants to convince others and themselves that they have epilepsy.

• Sustaining *injury* is said to favour a diagnosis of CPE over NES. It is unethical to 'put this to the test' when supporting someone during a seizure, but you should observe, and ask about injury as part of your history-taking.

List the points in her history (not presenting complaints) that will help you decide

Primary epilepsy is supported by the presence of learning disability (LD; Box 21, p. 152) or a family history of epilepsy. Common causes of secondary epilepsy are:

• Head trauma, more so if penetrating head injury
• Any brain haemorrhage
• Cerebral and systemic infection: febrile convulsions are associated with TLE
• Metabolic disorders, drug and alcohol effects
• Vascular disease and cancer (in adults over 40 years) may present with any type of epilepsy

Psychosis is suggested by:

• Low birth weight: in this instance, obstetric complications favour CPS via LD
• Previous or family history of psychosis
• Cannabis and amphetamine use
• Good response to antipsychotic drugs: these raise the seizure threshold and would increase the frequency of CPS

NES are more likely to have:

• Medically unexplained symptoms (especially neurological)
• Unusual features of previous epileptic seizures. Sally presented with classic childhood absence seizures, but these (unusually) developed a different and atypical pattern. Were there familial or other environmental factors occurring at this time that might give alternate explanations for this change?
• A history of childhood sexual abuse
• Apparent indifference to the consequences and risks of fits
• Persistent seizures despite adequate trials of AEDs by a neurologist

What aspects of the aftermath will help you choose one option over another?

• People with CPS are confused after the event
• People with NES are lucid with clear recollections of everything about their episode
• Functional psychotic symptoms occur in clear consciousness and symptoms persist for some time

=CPS ej TLE

- An automatism is a state of clouding of consciousness at the end of a seizure where posture and muscle tone are normal. The person *appears* well (although careful observation reveals vacant expression), but performs simple or complex actions and is unaware of these. Simple behaviours include lip smacking, head nodding, or tapping; more complex includes counting things, sitting up and lying down (in a repetitive stereotyped way), monotonous speech (same phrase over and over), even writing (this will be meaningless). Once the pattern of an automatism is established, it rarely changes over time
- People with NES might mimic automatisms – but just as they are rousable during their 'fit', they could be distracted during strange post-episode behaviour. Never confront a true automatism

---

KEY POINT

It is dangerous to interrupt a true automatism: people may become violent if prevented form carrying out stereotypical actions. Supportive nursing is essential in postictal patients – including people who have just had electroconvulsive therapy (ECT).

- Epileptic *fugue* states have been described. The patient can wander for hours, but rarely days. Their behaviour is similar to that described in Case 18, and clinical/EEG evidence differentiates this from psychogenic fugue
- *Twilight state* describes unusual postictal behaviours where consciousness continues to be impaired. It includes automatism and fugue, but in its minor form, a twilight state might be dream-like absent-minded behaviour where the person can speak with subtle impairments (e.g. vague, stock answers, perseverations) after a seizure

Which investigations might help you decide?

All physical examinations, blood tests and functional brain investigations are normal in psychosis and people with NES. In CPS:

① • upgoing plantar reflexes
② • Prolactin may be elevated after a seizure
③ • EEG during CPS will show focal then generalized hyperactive waves
- If her counting ritual is part of a postictal twilight state, EEG during this period will indicate impaired consciousness

You receive conclusive video EEG evidence that Sally's episodes are NES. Her neurologist appears surprised because 'she seemed like a very nice person – even if she had daft symptoms, she didn't strike me as a faker'. He heard of a similar case some years ago; when a man was confronted with the diagnosis of NES, he committed suicide. Your advice about best management here is sought.

How might you reassure your colleague?

Suicide is a rare outcome in NES patients. You need to reassure him that there may have been individual factors in the previous case, or provocative aspects of the confrontation that led to his suicide. You will manage all risks, including suicide, by regular review (Cases 7 and 8).

He may have black and white views of neurology/psychiatry: nice people get epilepsy, but 'bad' or 'mad' people get 'fake' fits. Unhelpfully, NES used to be called *pseudo-epilepsy*. Try to win the argument that Sally is probably unaware that she is doing this, and needs support managing the stressors that maintain her episodes.

There is unlikely to be a single cause of her NES, but her neurological condition is the main contributing factor. One explanation might be Sally's frustration that her generalized epilepsy has not been sorted: she is a working mother who cannot now drive. These new episodes could be an indirect request (of her neurologist) for effective treatment of her original problem.

Drawing on other clinical cases in this book, how will you manage Sally's NES?

Her safety is the main priority and procedures need to be in place to prevent any injury from either generalized seizures or NES:

- In many presentations (Cases 3, 6, 7, 13, 17, 19 and 20), you managed patients who did not concede they were experiencing mental health difficulties. In each case, perseverance and demonstrating to them that you were acting in their best interests won them over
- Vague non-organic symptoms (Case 10) were managed by a multidisciplinary team, without loss of face for the patient (p. 106)
- Unpredictable dissociative symptoms (Case 18) were managed by consistent non-judgemental interventions. In Sally's case this is unexplored, but Richard's family had a major role in the evolution of symptoms. The best chance of reductions in the frequency of these episodes is to enlist the help of her partner, family and friends

• You were able to begin the long process of separating physical illness from functional illness in a logical non-confrontational way (Case 19), supported by liaison with other physicians. Alongside your therapeutic relationship with Sally, and your alliances with her social networks, the key relationship here is with her neurologist

• Although not currently present, psychiatric comorbidity is likely to occur in Sally's case. You can manage any anxiety (Cases 1, 4 and 10), depression (Cases 2, 7, 8 and 10), substance misuse (Cases 4 and 14) and new physical/psychological symptoms (Cases 10, 18 and 19)

Sally agrees to joint outpatient care between neurology and psychiatry. She accepts your explanation that she has two related diagnoses: (i) generalized epilepsy – partially responsive to carbamazepine medication; and (ii) stress-related episodes (agitation, voices and counting). This second diagnosis is "not epilepsy but acts like it". Your role is to support her with additional measures to reduce their frequency. She has no anxiety or mood symptoms, and no suicidality.

Are there any other risks here and how might you address them?

Yes. She has two children whose care she shares with her partner. You need to ensure that she is not left as their sole carer. She is unlikely to harm them through generalized or NES, but she will be incapacitated by both, and contingency needs to be in place for her young children. She has already accepted limitations on her driving and should agree to placing their safety first.

As a final point, and this is a highly contentious area, the possibility of voluntary symptom production remains. There are documented cases when parents with extreme variants of factitious illness (the rare but fanciful *Munchausen's syndrome*) were confronted about their symptoms, they subsequently manufactured symptoms in their children. So great is the legal reaction to this diagnosis, that the term *Munchausen's syndrome by proxy* never appears in a patient's case notes. If you have any concerns, raise them.

CASE REVIEW

We saved the hardest case for last. The interface between psychotic symptoms and epilepsy is a highly complex area. Sally's case was made more complicated by a misdiagnosis of OCD (see Case 2 where 'obsessions' turned out to be a diagnosis of depression). Personality impacts on any diagnosis of illness. Any of the previous 21 cases would have presented differently if the person had other traits or mixtures of them (Table 52).

Sally's symptoms could be seen as a reaction to generalized epilepsy. Differential diagnosis represented the main section of her case: this can take weeks to establish, and features would require careful documentation by everyone involved in her care. Many cases end without 'conclusive' proof of NES over other epilepsy variants, and patients are followed up by neurologists and psychiatrists. In this uncertain context, evidence about prevalence and prognosis of NES is currently inadequate to speculate about Sally's outcome. However, with what you now know about psychiatric disorders and their management, we expect her to do very well under your care.

Reference

Querques, J. & Stern, T.A. (2004) Approaches to Consultation Psychiatry: Assessment Strategies. In: Stern, T.A. et al. (eds) *Handbook of General Hospital Psychiatry*, 5th edn. Mosby, Philadelphia.

Further reading

Davidson, S.E. (2002) Principles of managing patients with personality disorders. *Advances in Psychiatric Treatment* **9**, 1–9.

Nicholson, S.E., Mayberg, H.S., Pennell, P.B. & Nemeroff, C.B. (2006) Persistent auditory hallucinations that are unresponsive to antipsychotic drugs. *American Journal of Psychiatry* **163**, 1153–1159.

MCQs

For each situation, choose the single option you feel is most correct.

1 *Concerning post-traumatic stress disorder (PTSD):*

a. The onset of symptoms is usually immediate after trauma
b. There is wide variation in inherent vulnerability to develop PTSD after any given trauma
c. The diagnosis can be made after any event described as 'traumatic' by the patient
d. The development of the disorder can usually be prevented by professional debriefing after a trauma by trained counsellors
e. Antipsychotic medication is an effective treatment for flashbacks

2 *Dissociation is:*

a. An acute organic confusional state
b. Synonymous with the defence mechanism of denial
c. A functional (i.e. psychological) narrowing of consciousness
d. A chronic decreased level of consciousness resulting from organic brain compromise
e. Splitting of reality leading to delusional beliefs

3 *Depressive illness is usually:*

a. An illness of late middle age
b. A one-off episode
c. Recurrent
d. Independent of current life events
e. Treated by psychiatrists in secondary care

4 *Concerning the typical onset and progression of obsessive-compulsive disorder (OCD):*

a. Symptoms manifest during adolescence, continue through adulthood, and may vary in intensity depending on life events and psychiatric comorbidity
b. Symptoms manifest during adolescence and continue through adulthood, usually with a chronic but stable clinical picture
c. Symptoms tend not to manifest until early middle age and may be episodic in nature
d. Symptoms may manifest during infancy as repetitive stereotyped play
e. Symptoms usually have a sudden onset in early adulthood and tend to be episodic in nature

5 *The first line treatment for panic disorder is:*

a. Psychodynamic psychotherapy
b. Benzodiazepines
c. Anticonvulsant mood stabilizers
d. Group therapy
e. Cognitive–behavioural therapy (CBT)

6 *Patients with factitious disorder:*

a. Have psychosomatic symptoms resulting from health anxiety
b. Fabricate symptoms for external gain (e.g. avoiding criminal proceedings)
c. Fabricate symptoms for internal gain (e.g. eliciting care from others)
d. Respond well to selective serotonin reuptake inhibitor (SSRI) antidepressants
e. Were formerly diagnosed with 'hysteria'

7 In a man over 40 years the most likely cause of new onset unexplained physical symptoms is:

a. Multiple sclerosis
b. Depression
c. Alcohol abuse
d. Nihilistic delusions in schizophrenia
e. An early onset dementia

8 A diagnosis of schizophrenia:

a. Requires a history of auditory hallucinations
b. May follow a previous diagnosis of drug-induced psychosis
c. Can be made 2 weeks after the onset of symptoms
d. Requires a history of paranoid delusional beliefs
e. Is excluded when symptoms of a mood disorder are present

9 The symptom of 'hearing voices':

a. Has high specificity for schizophrenia
b. Is usually a psychiatric emergency
c. Can occur with borderline personality disorders and dissociative states
d. Is rare in dementia
e. Always indicates psychiatric disorder

10 Non-epileptic fits occur most commonly in people who have:

a. Epilepsy
b. A learning disability
c. Somatization disorder
d. PTSD
e. Severe depression with psychotic features

11 Medication failure in psychosis is most often caused by:

a. Drug interactions
b. Patients not taking the tablets as prescribed
c. Prescribed dose being too low
d. Prescribed dose being too high
e. Slow metabolism of the liver's cytochrome p450 enzyme system

12 Antidepressant treatment:

a. Is a first line treatment for mild depression
b. Has a more than 70% response rate to the first agent
c. Is contraindicated in dementia
d. Is commonly associated with sexual side-effects
e. Increases the risk of diabetes

13 Personality disorders can be:

a. Excluded if a diagnosis of anxiety or depression is made
b. Diagnosed in childhood
c. Comorbid with other mental disorders
d. Diagnosed after a brief assessment
e. Cured with medication

14 Mood instability and recurrent thoughts of self-harm characterize which of the following personality disorders?

a. Borderline
b. Narcissistic
c. Anxious-avoidant
d. Paranoid
e. Histrionic

15 Alcohol withdrawal symptoms usually peak around how many hours after the last drink?

a. 5 hours
b. 24 hours
c. 16 hours
d. 48 hours
e. 72 hours

16 A manic episode in bipolar disorder:

a. Can be prevented by antidepressant stabilization
b. Is by definition always characterized by elated mood
c. Is commonly precipitated by antidepressants
d. Is rarely followed by a depressive episode
e. May rarely be associated with delusional beliefs

17 *The assessment of capacity is:*

a. Situation-specific
b. A one-off assessment applicable to all future decisions
c. Only relevant to decisions involving medical care
d. Only applies to patients with dementia
e. Performed by formal testing of IQ

18 *In people with a learning disability:*

a. Rates of epilepsy are decreased
b. Criminal behaviour is more common
c. Medication for mental illness should be avoided
d. Mood disorders usually occur only with an IQ above 60
e. The prevalence of mental disorders is increased

19 *Considering antipsychotic medication:*

a. Weight loss is a common side-effect
b. Prolactin levels are decreased
c. Clozapine may cause neutropenia
d. It raises the seizure threshold
e. Olanzapine is known to cause a photosensitive rash

20 *Panic attacks terminate within:*

a. 5 minutes
b. 12 hours
c. 60 minutes
d. 30 minutes
e. 24 hours

21 *Up to what proportion of people relapse after their first psychotic episode?*

a. 1/4
b. 2/3
c. 4/5
d. 1/5
e. 1/10

22 *After recovery from a first psychotic episode patients should be advised to take medication for a minimum of:*

a. 5 years
b. 1 year
c. 10 years
d. 6 months
e. 1 month

23 *The recommended safe alcohol limits per week are:*

a. 21 units for women and 30 for men
b. 7 units for women and 10 for men
c. 20 units for both men and women
d. 10 units for both men and women
e. 16 units for women and 21 for men

24 *The most common reported side-effect of electroconvulsive therapy (ECT) is:*

a. Hypersalivation
b. Memory loss
c. Status epilepticus
d. Limb trauma
e. Tongue biting

25 *Which of the following is associated with a better prognosis in schizophrenia?*

a. Male gender
b. No affective component
c. Family history of psychosis
d. Low premorbid IQ
e. Older age of onset

26 *What proportion of cases of delirium are caused by prescribed medication?*

a. <1%
b. >80%
c. 10%
d. 40%
e. 5%

PART 3: SELF-ASSESSMENT

27 *Which of the following is not a risk factor for postnatal depression?*

a. Age – very young or over 30
b. Low socioeconomic group
c. Past history of depression
d. Low normal IQ
e. Immigration in the past 5 years

28 *Concerning mood stabilizers and side-effects:*

a. Lithium has few side-effects and a wide therapeutic range
b. Valproate levels correlate closely with efficacy
c. Ataxia, dysarthria and diplopia are recognized uncommon side-effects of carbamazepine
d. Carbamazepine reduces liver metabolism of oral contraceptives
e. Valproate is associated with thirst, polyuria and hypothyroidism

29 *Concerning medically unexplained symptoms:*

a. Somatization disorder entails at least 1 month of multiple unexplained symptoms
b. Depression is rarely a contributory cause
c. They represent around 20% of all GP consultations
d. Somatization disorder is synonymous with chronic fatigue
e. Somatization disorder is synonymous with conversion disorder

30 *With OCD:*

a. The disorder usually occurs in people with premorbid anakastic (obsessional) personalites
b. The individual takes pleasure or pride in their obsessional preoccupations and compulsive behaviour
c. The patient may have delusional beliefs about the origins of their obsessions or compulsive behaviour
d. The content of obessional thoughts and the associated rituals tends to vary from day to day
e. Obessional thoughts, images and associated rituals are experienced as repetitive and unpleasant

EMQs

1 Diagnostic differentials

a. 'The Queen has stolen my identity. I've heard the police talking about it' 5

b. 'I am the Queen!' 9 ✗ 11

c. 'My mood has always been up and down. Sometimes I just feel nothing and that's when I don't care anymore and overdose' 7

d. 'I felt sick with panic all day about having to meet people at the wedding' 10

e. 'I don't feel anything. I deserve to die' 8

f. 'I just feel really anxious all the time, it's making me physically ill' 3

Which is your first diagnostic differential on hearing the above presenting complaints?

1. Bipolar disorder
2. Moderate depression
3. Generalized anxiety disorder
4. Panic disorder
5. Schizophrenia
6. Phobia
7. Borderline personality disorder
8. Severe depression
9. Dissociative identity disorder
10. Social anxiety disorder
11. Delusional disorder
12. Chronic fatigue syndrome

2 Diagnoses

a. Delusional disorder 7

b. Paranoid schizophrenia 8

c. Bipolar disorder, manic episode 6

d. Severe depression, psychotic episode 4

e. Delirium 1

Select the mental state examination (MSE) finding that would be most consistent with the above diagnoses

1. Fleeting delusional beliefs and visual hallucinations
2. Orientation in place and time but not person

3. Repetitive handwashing because of fear of contracting disease
4. Hearing critical voices calling one offensive names
5. Fixed beliefs about widespread corruption in public life
6. Mood objectively characterized by extreme irritability c
7. False fixed belief about partner's infidelity in a high functioning male
8. Hearing critical voices discussing one's actions b
9. Non-epileptic seizures
10. Difficulty with recall of long-term but not short-term memory

3 Substances

a. Amphetamines 5

b. Benzodiazepines 7

c. Opiates 1

d. Antipsychotics 2

e. Cocaine 7

Match the substance to the picture of withdrawal states

1. No recognized withdrawal state
2. Up to 5 days of dysphoria, anxiety and insomnia; no physiological withdrawal
3. Acute psychosis characterized by visual and auditory hallucinations
4. 5–10 days of anxiety, dysphoria with severe cramps, sweating, rhinitis, lacrimation
5. 2–5 days of mood elevation, tactile hallucinations, fluctuating blood pressure
6. Up to 7 days of potentially severe dysphoria, anxiety and insomnia; no physiological withdrawal
7. Potentially weeks of irritability, anxiety, depression; nausea, tremor (seizures if severe neurological rebound), tachycardia
8. 24–48 hours of fluctuating concentration, hypersomnia, respiratory depression

4 A woman survives a car crash

a. Her car hits a lamp-post narrowly avoiding a child on the pavement. Afterwards she is in a dazed and confused state, which resolves over the following few hours.

b. Her fellow passenger is killed. Several hours later she finds herself outside her old school, unable to account for the lost time or how she got there following the crash.

c. She is accused of reckless driving by the driver of the other car. He sustains a neck injury and proceeds with a legal claim. She is tense and irritable for weeks after the incident, ruminating about what happened and the injustice of the claim. She is signed off work sick with stress for 2 weeks and asks her GP to write a report for the court about her injuries.

d. A pedestrian is killed in the crash. Initially she feels numb and then after a week she starts to have nightmares where she sees the man dead on the road. She is sleeping poorly and has lost her appetite. She feels unable to get back into a car and she becomes increasingly tense and irritable. She starts to avoid leaving the house where possible, choosing to work from home.

e. Her fellow passenger, her husband, sustains severe injuries from the crash and requires extensive surgery. He blames her for the crash as she had been drinking and their relationship suffers. Over the following months she becomes withdrawn, starts to refuse to leave the house and sleeps excessively. She says God has told her she should have died in the accident as she deserved to. She was arrested and charged after the crash but fails to attend court.

Which of the following primary diagnoses would best fit the presentations?

1. Adjustment disorder
2. Moderate depressive episode
3. Post-traumatic stress disorder
4. Dissociative fugue state
5. Acute stress reaction
6. Factitious disorder
7. Severe depressive episode with psychotic symptoms
8. Malingering
9. Chronic fatigue syndrome
10. Bipolar affective disorder, depressive relapse
11. Agoraphobia
12. Acute psychotic episode

5 A mother complains her child is difficult

a. A 13-year-old who has refused to attend school since the start of the new term. She spends days in the local shopping centre with friends.

b. A 6-year-old boy who frequently gets into trouble at school and home for his clumsy impulsive conduct. He is restless and over-talkative in class and his reading and writing are behind the other pupils.

c. A 10-year-old boy with marked personality change and the onset of temper tantrums after sustaining a head injury while skiing.

d. A 12-year-old who has failed to attend secondary school since she briefly attended at the start of her first term. She becomes intensely distressed when her mother tries to insist she goes. She spends most of the day in her bedroom watching TV.

e. A 14-year-old girl who has lost a significant amount of weight following a sexual assault by an uncle. She is spending most of the day in bed sleeping, is refusing to go to school and is having tearful outbursts against her mother.

f. A 6-year-old girl with an 'imaginary friend' who she talks to when she is alone and says she can hear talking to her. The mother is concerned as her daughter refuses to accept her father walked out of the family home 6 months ago and is not expected to return. She continues to insist her imaginary friend has told her 'Daddy is coming home soon.'

g. An 8-year-old who has had angry outbursts at home since the birth of his little sister. He has hit and scratched his mother when she has tried to discipline him. His school reports are unremarkable.

Which of the following primary diagnoses would best fit the presentations?

1. Autistic spectrum disorder
2. Attention deficit hyperactivity disorder
3. No diagnosis
4. Oppositional defiant disorder
5. Organic brain pathology
6. School refusal
7. Early onset schizophrenia
8. Conduct disorder
9. Depressive disorder
10. Moderate learning disability
11. Anorexia nervosa
12. Anxious-avoidant personality disorder

6 Scenarios

a. A 55-year-old man with no history of psychiatric or physical problems complains to his GP of heaviness in his head and difficulty breathing. He becomes tearful when his wife complains he is trying to manipulate her into not leaving him.

b. A 30-year-old man with cerebral palsy who self-catheterizes is admitted to a urology ward from A&E with a history of nausea, high temperatures, seizures and proteinuria. While on the ward he has what appears to be a prolonged generalized seizure, unresponsive to rectal diazepam, while he exhibits no signs of hypoxia. He is later observed by nurses to be surreptitiously introducing some kind of powder into his catheter bag.

c. A 22-year-old man presents at A&E with a small bruise on his leg which he says has been caused by his neighbours putting poison in his water supply.

d. A 34-year-old woman describes to her GP a 3-month history of excessive but unrefreshing sleep, generalized joint pains and profound physical exhaustion arising hours after even brief exercise. She denies any psychological difficulties.

e. A 40-year-old woman falls into debt through seeking repeated private medical opinions and complementary therapies for a range of physical complaints that date back around 5 years including whole-body numbness, abdominal bloating and a pain that travels around her head to her feet.

f. A 21-year-old woman presents to A&E with sudden onset paralysis of her left arm.

g. An 18-year-old man in police custody is brought to A&E after telling police he has taken a large paracetamol overdose in the morning before his arrest. Blood tests show no paracetamol detected.

h. A 52-year-old woman self-presents to a private dermatologist preoccupied and distressed by the belief that she has a parasitic infestation under the skin of her forehead and temples. She has refused to accept the reassurances of her GP, who suggested the cause might be 'stress-related'. The GP found her mental state examination otherwise unremarkable.

Match the most likely primary diagnosis from the list below to the above scenarios after nil has been found on examination and investigation to explain the presentation:

1. Chronic fatigue syndrome
2. Somatization disorder
3. Depressive disorder
4. Dissociative conversion disorder
5. Factitious disorder
6. Psychotic disorder
7. Health anxiety
8. Malingering
9. Delusional disorder

7 'Doesn't that medication cause . . .?'

a. 'Sodium valproate causes hair loss'
b. 'Antipsychotics prevent you from getting pregnant'
c. 'Carbamazepine gives you a rash'
d. 'I don't want to get fat. Doesn't olanzapine cause weight gain?'
e. 'I have epilepsy. Don't all antipsychotics and antidepressants increase my risk of seizures?'
f. 'Haloperidol causes hair loss'
g. 'People get addicted to antidepressants'
h. 'Antipsychotics make you tired'

Which response would you give when a patient tells you they have heard the above about medication:

1. That is not a recognized side-effect of this medication
2. That is a common side-effect
3. Yes, they all do
4. That is a recognized side-effect but rare
5. That is only thought to happen with the SSRI paroxetine
6. Some can but not all, and it may depend on dose

8 Statements in a mental state examination

a. 'He is putting thoughts into my head'
b. 'I am his best friend'
c. 'I can hear him talking about me with his Cabinet'
d. 'He was talking about me on the TV news'
e. 'I can hear him telling me I'm his best friend'
f. 'He has tapped my phone because he wants to steal my ideas about government'
g. 'I keep seeing him on the bus'
h. 'He keeps making my legs shake'

How would you categorize the above statements regarding the Prime Minister in a MSE, taking it as read none reflect reality:

1. Thought content: persecutory delusional belief
2. Thought content: delusion of thought insertion

3. Thought content: delusion of somatic passivity
4. Perception: visual illusion
5. Thought content: thought echo
6. Thought content: grandiose delusion
7. Perception: second person auditory hallucinations
8. Perception: third person auditory hallucinations
9. Thought content: delusion of reference

5. Neuropsychiatric assessment
6. Child case conference
7. Medical examination, with white cell count and creatine kinase levels
8. Forensic psychiatry referral
9. Music therapist
10. Urinary drug screen
11. Physician and anaesthetist to assess suitability for ECT

---

9 Clinical presentations

a. A 29-year-old man with a past diagnosis of personality disorder refuses to see you, his psychiatrist. He says if he is made to see you, he will make sure you will 'live to regret it'. You have never seen him and members of your team say he will agree to see someone else.

b. A 69-year-old woman is mute on the ward. She is cooperating with all requests made of her but acting in a suspicious manner. No staff member has broken through her silence. Her GP says she was cognitively intact and appeared well – with normal bloods and brain scan – when he saw her last week.

c. A 22-year-old motorcyclist has sustained a severe head injury, but his IQ remains in the normal range. He insists on going home against medical advice to be with his partner and 4-year-old daughter.

d. A 42-year-old woman was admitted 3 months ago to treat her severe depressive episode with psychosis. She stopped eating and drinking this week and today's urea and electrolytes are within normal limits.

e. A 28-year-old man has been sectioned to a medium secure ward during his first episode of psychosis following a violent assault on another patient. He told the nurses the medications have completely slowed him down and stop his arms and legs from working. He presents as drowsy.

f. A 54-year-old woman with moderate learning disability has returned to hospital following breakdown of her placement. The learning disability team has investigated her fully. She was aggressive to people by day and is said to howl like a dog at night-time.

---

10 Personality traits

a. Feelings of tension, apprehension, inferiority, insecurity
b. Tendency to bear grudges, misconstrue neutral actions as malign; tenacious sense of personal rights
c. Eccentric, odd behaviours; ideas and experiences that fall short of psychosis
d. Callous; low threshold for frustration; disregard for social norms; dishonest
e. Excessive need to be taken care of; submissive and clinging behaviours
f. Exaggerated emotions but shallow affect; excitement seeking and suggestible
g. Mood instability; fear of abandonment; recurrent acts of self-harm; impulsive behaviours
h. Perfectionist; excessively conscientious; preoccupation with details; rigid

Match the traits above to the personality type:
1. Paranoid
2. Dependent
3. Borderline
4. Anxious (avoidant)
5. Dissocial
6. Narcissistic
7. Schizotypal
8. Histrionic
9. Obsessive (anakastic)

Match the specialist assessment with the clinical presentation:
1. Psychology: measurement of IQ
2. Psychology: assessment for suitability for psychodynamic group therapy
3. Occupational therapy assessment of activities of daily living
4. Behavioural therapy assessment

SAQs

1 *A 57-year-old man with no psychiatric history has become aggressive on a medical admissions unit following a myocardial infarction 24 hours earlier. He is crawling on the floor of the ward and appears to be hallucinating, shouting at invisible rats.*

a. What is the most likely diagnosis?
b. You are asked by the medical registrar on call to arrange his transfer to a psychiatric unit. How do you respond?
c. What needs to be prioritized in his management?
d. What do you advise the nurses?
e. The man is settled back into bed by the nurses but he tells them he does not want to stay because 'This is the worst hotel I've ever stayed in'. He is persuaded to stay until the morning but staff are concerned about his capacity to decide to accept or refuse treatment. What are the criteria for assessing capacity?

2 *An 82-year-old woman is brought to her GP by her daughter who is concerned about her mother's gradually worsening memory. She says her mother keeps repeating herself and forgetting things. Physical examination is unremarkable.*

a. What is the most likely diagnosis?
b. What type of memory tends to be affected first?
c. How might you systematically assess this patient's cognition?
d. What other features do you need to look for in her history and on mental state examination?
e. Are there any medication cures for this disorder?
f. What are the key neuropathological findings on postmortem with this disorder?

3 *A 21-year-old medical student presents to her GP complaining that her periods have stopped. She denies any other difficulties, physical or emotional, although she admits to being under pressure with exams. Her medical and psychiatric history is otherwise unremarkable. She appears underweight. Her BMI is calculated as 18.*

a. What is BMI?
b. What is the normal range of BMI?
c. On further questioning she admits she has felt fat as long as she can remember. Following the break-up of her relationship she started to become increasingly preoccupied with reducing and controlling her weight. Recently, she has started to eat only one meal a day and she fills up with water otherwise. What are the diagnostic criteria for anorexia nervosa?
d. After establishing her pattern of diet restriction, what other methods of weight control do you need to explore?
e. What other related behaviour do you need to enquire about?
f. What is the key blood test?
g. What are the long-term complications of anorexia nervosa?
h. What is the prognosis of anorexia nervosa?
i. She insists she does not have 'a real problem' with her weight and is against considering whether she might need more specialist psychological help of any kind. What should you do at this point, her first presentation?

4 *A 20-year-old man is brought into A&E by his flatmates having taken an overdose. He reports taking 10 paracetamol, 7 diazepam tablets (5 mg) and 20 tablets of citalopram as a suicide attempt.*

a. What is your first priority in assessment?
b. What investigations do you need to do?
c. What is your advice to nursing staff?
d. He tells his nurse in A&E that he just wants to be dead. How do you assess the degree of his suicidal intent?

5 *A 57-year-old headteacher presents to A&E with an upper gastrointestinal bleed from a peptic ulcer. She was admitted 2 months previously with acute pancreatitis, at which point an enlarged liver and blood results consistent with harmful use of alcohol (raised liver enzymes and mean cell volume) were noted. She strongly denied drinking and self-discharged before having a psychiatric review. When alcohol was brought up again on this admission she burst into tears and threatened to make a formal complaint 'if I'm accused of that again'.*

a. What three broad categories, or areas, do you need to remember to cover in a history when considering the impact of harmful alcohol use?
b. What are the features of alcohol dependence?
c. She reluctantly agrees to a psychiatric review because her husband insists he is not taking her home until she sees someone 'and gets some help'. He says he wants to see you with her because otherwise 'she'll just hide everything'. Before you see her, how do you plan to approach the interview?
d. What might you suggest as a management plan to address her drinking?

6 *A 28-year-old Polish woman, who is a committed Catholic, has a stillbirth of a much-wanted baby. Over the course of the following week she stays off work, shuts herself away in the bedroom at home, avoids her partner and, much to his concern, refuses to see their local priest when he visits.*

a. What are the usual stages of adjusting to loss?
b. After 2 months she is back at work but continuing to struggle with the aftermath of what has happened. She continues to wonder whether she did not take enough care over her diet during the pregnancy, or whether she was working too hard. She has problems with poor sleep and is often tearful. What is the most likely diagnosis?
c. Two years later she has a complicated pregnancy, giving birth to an underweight baby after a prolonged labour. She subsequently has little sleep for the first 48 hours and, despite her excellent English, she has difficulty grasping the midwife's instructions about breastfeeding. She becomes tearful when her baby seemingly rejects her breast and she has to use formula milk. How common is it for women to develop transient emotional difficulties after birth?
d. Her symptoms of low mood and poor sleep (even when the baby is resting) persist over the following weeks and she discloses to her health visitor she is finding it hard to bond with or feel affection towards her baby girl. She also admits she wanted a boy because she knew that is what her husband wanted. How common is postnatal depression?
e. From the above information, what predisposing factors to depression might you formulate as potentially significant in her case?

7 *A 42-year-old man with a past history of generalized anxiety disorder and social phobia presents to A&E with shortness of breath, chest pain and tingling and cramps in his hands. He is reviewed medically and his blood gases show a respiratory alkalosis resulting from his ongoing hyperventilation. A panic attack is diagnosed after physical causes are ruled out.*

a. How do you differentiate pathological anxiety from anxiety as a normal (even self-protective) emotional reaction?
b. How do you manage his ongoing panic attack?
c. What are the features of panic disorder?
d. What treatments are available for panic disorder?

8 *A 15-year-old boy is brought to his GP by his mother. For several years he has insisted on checking all the light switches and power points at home before leaving the house or going to bed and he becomes agitated when his family have tried to prevent him from doing so. Recently, he has started to take up to 30 minutes to brush his teeth morning and night, much to the consternation of the family who have only one bathroom. He admits he is making his gums bleed.*

a. What is the likely diagnosis?
b. What are the features of this disorder
c. Is this an unusual age for presentation?
d. Which other disorder is commonly comorbid with this disorder?
e. How do you differentiate this diagnosis from a personality disorder presentation?

9 *A 39-year-old woman with an extensive history of overdoses and cutting her arms presents to A&E after burning her arm on a kettle. She recently had counselling for alcohol misuse but discontinued treatment because she alleged her counsellor 'hates me'. She tells staff she needs to be admitted to hospital because she feels suicidal and she can hear the voice of her dead twin telling her to kill herself.*

a. What is the most likely diagnosis?
b. What are the features of this disorder?
c. How do you understand her presenting symptom of her dead twin telling her to kill herself?
d. Do you think hospital admission to a psychiatric ward is likely to be helpful?
e. What are the types of psychological treatment for this disorder?

10 *A 20-year-old woman is brought into A&E after a member of the public called the police to report seeing her walking naked in a supermarket car park. She has told the police they cannot arrest her because she is the Virgin Mary and she has a message of peace and love for the world that she has heard directly from the voice of God. In A&E she is sitting calmly, greeting those who see her with a brief prayer.*

a. What are your differential diagnoses?
b. What do you need to ensure happens before she is seen psychiatrically?
c. What are the organic causes of an elevated (manic or hypomanic) mood state?
d. Physically she appears well. She denies any drug or alcohol use and there is no clear evidence of the same. How will you conduct your interview?
e. She tells you she was naked because she rejects the capitalist system and all its hypocrisies. She laughs when you ask her about voices and if she believes she is the Virgin Mary. She tells you, 'That's for me to know'. She confirms she believes she has special powers of healing of some kind but says these are secret. Although she does not agree she is unwell, she offers to see her GP in the near future and calmly requests that she be allowed to go home and get some sleep because she has not slept for 3 days. What is her most likely diagnosis at this point?
f. Will you let her go home provided she promises to see her GP the next day?
g. You make contact with her brother who confirms that she has a diagnosis of bipolar disorder and has been under stress recently. He also thinks she has been smoking cannabis in recent weeks and comments that she often stops taking her medication. What are common prodromal symptoms of a manic episode?

MCQs Answers

1. b. Evidence shows if anything 'debriefing' in the immediate aftermath of trauma worsens prognosis.
2. c.
3. c.
4. a.
5. e.
6. c.
7. b.
8. b. ICD-10 requires symptoms for at least 1 month before a diagnosis of schizophrenia is made; DSM-IV requires 6 months.
9. c.
10. a.
11. b.
12. d. Between 50% and 60% respond to the first antidepressant.
13. c.

14. a.
15. d.
16. c.
17. a.
18. e.
19. c.
20. d.
21. b.
22. b.
23. e.
24. b.
25. e.
26. d.
27. d.
28. c.
29. c.
30. e.

EMQs Answers

1
a. 5
b. 1
c. 7
d. 10
e. 8
f. 3

2
a. 7
b. 8
c. 6
d. 4
e. 1

In contrast to schizophrenia, in a delusional disorder the delusional beliefs are circumscribed to one topic and they are not bizarre or completely improbable. They are also not associated with any other features of schizophrenia such as thought disorder or hearing voices. In delirium, delusions and hallucinations are fleeting. In mania, the predominant affect is often one of extreme irritability rather than elation.

3
a. 2
b. 7
c. 4
d. 1
e. 6

Remember to differentiate between intoxication and withdrawal (Case 14).

4
a. 5
b. 4
c. 1
d. 3
e. 7

Factitious disorder and malingering both relate to symptoms that have been consciously induced by the individual (although the motivations between the two differ). In none of these scenarios was that the case, although court proceedings complicated two of the presentations.

5
a. 8
b. 2
c. 5
d. 6
e. 9
f. 3
g. 4

Personality disorders are not diagnosed in childhood. Schizophrenia can be but it is very rare, and not diagnosed at this age. The 6-year-old's imaginary friend is a normal experience for a child; here this experience helps protect the child from the reality of her father's departure, which she is too young to comprehend or accept. See Case 9 for further discussion of these diagnoses.

6
a. 3
b. 5
c. 6
d. 1
e. 2
f. 4
g. 8
h. 9

This form of delusional disorder is often referred to as 'primary delusional parasitosis' and it is notoriously difficult to treat. Another example of a delusional disorder is so-called Othello syndrome (i.e. a delusional belief about a partner's infidelity). The classic case of this is in males with alcohol misuse problems.

7

a. 2. In a minority of patients. Loss occurs gradually as the patient notices more hair on their brush, pillow or in the shower, etc. Hair tends to grow back as curly.

b. 6. They differ in propensity to elevate prolactin and not all will prevent pregnancy.

c. 4. It occurs in 3% of people taking carbamazepine.

d. 2. Some people do not put on weight at all but for those that do, the weight gain can be considerable. The mechanism is likely to be insulin resistance; there is not a clear dose relationship.

e. 3. All antidepressants and antipsychotics vary in their propensity to do so. It is a relatively common problem with clozapine for example, where anti-epileptic medication may be started as prophylaxis if higher doses of clozapine are needed.

f. 1.

g. 1. Antidepressants may certainly cause significant *withdrawal* symptoms if they are stopped abruptly (Table 7, p. 17). However, addiction is a term that also incorporates the key features of *increased tolerance and craving* (Table 41, p. 137) in relation to a substance, neither of which occurs with antidepressants.

h. 6. By contrast, amisulpride and aripiprazole may be alerting in about 5% of people.

8

a. 2
b. 6
c. 8
d. 9
e. 7
f. 1
g. 4
h. 3

9

a. 8. You should not ignore a direct threat to you and he is willing for assessment by others.

b. 9. She is not confused and a recent screen showed normal results.

c. 3. There are no current grounds to convene a child case conference.

d. 11. Three months' antidepressant treatment has failed. Do not wait to consider ECT until she deteriorates medically.

e. 7. Details are suggestive of neuroleptics malignant syndrome.

f. 4. This patient's IQ is known, she has been closely followed up by the learning disability team. Her behaviour is the problem and needs to be evaluated.

10

a. 4
b. 1
c. 7
d. 5
e. 2
f. 8
g. 3
h. 9

SAQs Answers

1

a. Delirium.

b. Transfer to a psychiatric ward is not appropriate here and would put him at risk. Delirium is a medical emergency. This man's brain has been acutely compromised and you need to establish why. Hypoxic damage resulting from the myocardial infarction is one likely cause but you need to consider ongoing possible causes – physical and iatrogenic – that may be contributing to the problem and need to be addressed. In addition, always remember to consider alcohol withdrawal, which can present up to around 72 hours after someone's last drink.

c. Establish any potentially reversible causes of his delirium (Case 5).

d. Advise the nurses how he needs to be managed in the ward environment (Box 10, p. 70). Advise on medication management as a last resort if his behaviour is unmanageable once the above have been addressed and appropriate nursing measures instituted. One treatment goal is to promote sleep by night.

e. To establish capacity you must demonstrate his ability to *understand*, *retain* and *weigh up* the information given to him about a specific topic to make a decision and he must be able to *communicate* that decision (Table 21, p. 70; Box 12, p. 82).

2

a. Alzheimer's dementia – the most common histopathological type.

b. The most recent long-term memories. Short-term memory function (i.e. 'working memory' of what has just occurred) is relatively preserved until later in the disease process (Box 27, p. 166).

c. Test orientation; attention and concentration; short-term and long-term memory; plus specific tests of frontal, parietal and temporal lobe function (pp. 6 and 68).

d. The presence or absence of other features associated with dementia: abnormal behaviours (e.g. disinhibition associated with frontal lobe decline); affective disturbance, mood symptoms as a cause of recent decline or as comorbidity; psychotic symptoms (e.g. auditory hallucinations); personality change. Social history: her level of current functioning and current social circumstances – how and to what degree is her cognitive decline affecting her ability to live independently? How is she managing in her current accommodation? Does she need other support in place?

e. No. Acetylcholinesterase inhibitors may delay progression but are not recommended for routine use in the NHS (see p. 161 for discussion of treatment).

f. Cerebral atrophy with *extracellular plaques* and *intracellular neurofibrillary tangles* (Box 25, p. 162).

3

a. Body Mass Index: weight (kg) divided by height (m)².

b. Between 18.5 and 25

c. 1 Weight loss with a BMI of 17.5 or less (i.e. weight at least 15% below expected weight for height)
2 Weight loss is self-induced
3 Distorted self-perception of being too fat with morbid dread of fatness
4 Widespread endocrine disorder involving hypothalamic–pituitary–gonadal axis: leads to amenorrhoea in women, loss of sex drive in men

d. Self-induced vomiting; laxative, diuretic and appetite suppressant abuse; excessive exercise.

e. Does she have episodes of bingeing on food? Given her BMI, if she does this it is likely to be associated with vomiting.

f. U&Es: if she is repeatedly vomiting potassium, levels are particularly important given the risk of hypokalaemia.

g. The list is long. Complications include metabolic, endocrine, cardiovascular, gastrointestinal, renal, neurological, musculoskeletal and haematological (Table 40, p. 133).

h. In people who meet the diagnostic criteria for anorexia nervosa, about one-third of people fully recover, one-third have partial recovery and the remaining one-third have a chronic and unremitting course. The mortality for the disorder is 18%.

i. Her physical presentation is not life-threatening and her BMI is not at 'danger level' so there is no question of enforcing any treatment on her against her will. However, it is an ideal opportunity to try and start to address the issue before further weight loss and associated physical damage occurs. Take baseline measurements of pulse, BP, BMI and routine blood screen and then arrange to see her again in the near future. Explain you think it important to monitor her weight, and to continue this discussion about her eating that has only just started at this her first presentation with a weight-related problem (endocrine changes). Avoid trying to dictate a plan to her, as eating disorders often involve difficult dynamics for the patient around control. Rather, try and engage her in thinking about how her weight might be a problem. A shared concern you can agree on to start with is her amenorrhoea. It can be helpful here to be mindful of the 'stages of change' concept drawn from motivational interviewing techniques used within the field of substance misuse (Table 43, p. 140). For a variety of 'addictive' or problematic behavioural patterns people go through different stages in the path to recovery, including precontemplation (where this patient is), contemplation, determination, action, maintenance and relapse. You need to target your interventions to where the person is currently in relation to the problem. Here you are only at the first precontemplative stage of trying to raise awareness, so a rush to 'action' before she is ready for it may overwhelm her and lead her to disengage from treatment entirely.

4

a. To ensure he is medically stable.

b. He needs routine observations to be carried out and a physical examination, with blood tests including paracetamol levels. Even if paracetamol ingestion is not reported, levels should be performed routinely

in case the antidote *N*-acetylcysteine (Parvolex) is required. Here, he may have taken 20 g of the drug. Obviously, a suicidal patient may not always give an accurate account of what they have ingested. Remember also to establish if he has harmed himself in any other way that might require acute treatment (e.g. by cutting or burning himself).

c. He needs to stay in the department until a psychiatric review has been performed. He should have a named nurse to monitor him and a private room needs to be made available for the psychiatric assessment (Case 7).

d. Establish:

1 Context of the suicide attempt: degree and examples of preparation, perceived lethality of method used, influence of substances (e.g. alcohol)

2 Mental state at the time of the attempt (e.g. pervasive death wish, suicidal intent)

3 Mental state now (Table 27, p. 94)

5

a. Substance misuse damage crosses three main domains:

1 *Physical health*: gastrointestinal (the starting point here), neurological, cardiac, respiratory, haematological, metabolic and trauma (e.g. any history of head injury while intoxicated)

2 *Mental health*: alcohol dependence; alcohol misuse as both cause and consequence of affective disturbance; psychotic symptoms; cognitive damage; intoxication as habitual maladaptive coping style within vulnerable personality structure

3 *Social*: employment difficulties; forensic history (e.g. drink driving offences); history of aggression to others or victim of aggression (e.g. sexual violence) when intoxicated and vulnerable (Table 18, p. 62)

b. Alcohol dependence describes a constellation of cognitive, behavioural and physiological features, namely a strong compulsion to drink; neglect of other activities and obligations; difficulty controlling use; narrowing of drinking repertoire; increased tolerance; presence of a withdrawal state; persistent use despite harm (in medical, psychiatric and social domains as above)

c. It sounds as if she is probably terrified of her alcohol problem being exposed. Start by considering why. This does not sound like denial as a psychological defence mechanism. Although denying it to others, it does not sound as if she is denying it to herself in the sense of unconsciously refusing to allow that fact into her consciousness. By contrast, her level of arousal suggests she is well aware of and concerned about the possible repercussions of this problem being out in the open. The most obvious external factor to consider is her status as a headteacher, and whether she fears her position might be compromised by her seeking help. Her drinking may also be her only (albeit maladaptive) way of coping with stress, whether work-related or otherwise. She may be unable to countenance the idea of managing without it.

See her alone. She is more likely to disclose information to you if she can avoid losing face, and she has already had to do so by agreeing to see you. There will be time to talk to her husband later. You need to avoid jumping into the middle of a disagreement that sounds as if it is already well established. You might start the interview by acknowledging her reluctance to see you and thank her for doing so. Before you launch into the provocative topic of why she thinks other people are worried, try and establish some rapport by asking her how she is feeling physically after the surgery. Rather than force her into naming the problem of alcohol out loud before she is ready to, make the observation that she appears very stressed, exploring why and whether you can link this to how she copes with that stress (e.g. by using alcohol). If she remains reluctant to talk to you, generate a hypothesis as to why this might be the case and share this with her, as a speculation you invite her to comment on (e.g. 'I'm wondering if you are concerned about discussing alcohol because of potential repercussions at work'). Remember 'push where it moves' (p. 10) and focus on what you need to establish from this interview:

1 The nature of her alcohol use (e.g. alcohol dependence)
2 Any comorbid mental disorder
3 Past psychiatric, risk and treatment history
4 Current MSE
5 What support or intervention she might accept at this point

d. 1 *Short-term:* if she is alcohol-dependent, having been admitted to hospital she risks entering an alcohol withdrawal state and then developing delirium tremens, so ensure she is on a reducing regime of benzodiazepines while she remains on the ward. If she has not yet withdrawn from alcohol but she is now about to go home, do not advise her to stop drinking abruptly without a plan for a medically supervised (to some degree at least) withdrawal. Advise her to stop driving (see 'L is for legal', p. 25) until her next review.

2 *Medium-term:* feed back your assessment to her GP. By starting with a focus on monitoring her physical health, it may be possible for her GP to engage her over time in addressing her drinking from a psychological standpoint. Referral via her GP to an alcohol counsellor would be ideal. They can thoroughly assess the nature of her drinking problem and devise a management plan (see below) that takes account of the severity of the problem and what kind of help she would find acceptable. If she has a severe problem with dependence and/or her physical health is fragile, withdrawal is likely to be complex and she could even require inpatient detoxification and rehabilitation on a specialist unit.

3 *Long-term:* in addition to one-to-one counselling, group therapy can be helpful. Self-help groups such as Alcoholics Anonymous can be a great support, but this approach does not suit everyone. It may be important to involve her husband in her treatment at some point, possibly through couples' therapy, as ultimately her drinking – the causes and consequences – will be a problem that involves them both.

6

a. • Shock
• Denial
• Numbness
• Anger
• Disengagement
• Searching
• Bargaining
• Acceptance (Box 16, p. 120)

Remember these stages are not necessarily sequential. Here for example her loss might represent a spiritual crisis: her prayers for a healthy baby have been unanswered, leaving her angry and disillusioned with her faith. Prayer – in a religious sense or as an ill-defined call to 'another power' of some kind – can sometimes be understood as bargaining or a promised exchange of a certain behaviour or sacrifice for a desired outcome (e.g. 'If only my child can live, I promise to be a better person').

b. Adjustment disorder (Table 26, p. 93). Remember not to rush to diagnose depressive disorders when symptoms occur in the period of adjustment to a significant life event.

c. Around half to two-thirds of women experience brief periods of labile mood and poor concentration ('baby blues') after birth. This is not a psychiatric disorder as such.

d. Postnatal depression (PND) occurs after around 10% of live births.

e. Structure your answer as follows:

1 *Factors relating to the mother:* as an immigrant she may well be disconnected from her social support network of family and friends. This can be particularly important as a first-time mother. She also has a history of stillbirth: this birth may reactivate feelings related to that loss. This was, in some sense, a 'replacement child' but her arrival is tinged with sadness as both parents wanted a boy.

2 *Pregnancy and birth-related factors:* complicated pregnancy and difficult labour. Also note her disappointment about breastfeeding. This can be profoundly disappointing if a woman places pressure on herself, or feels under pressure from others, to be the 'perfect mother'. This may relate in part to personality style (not known here).

3 *Factors relating to the child:* the baby has been unwell and is not the hoped-for boy. Connected to that may be underlying relationship difficulties with her husband, potentially exacerbated if the baby disappoints as a hoped-for solution (an impossible role that is an enormous burden to inherit, again not known here).

7

a. Pathological anxiety is:

1 Disproportionate to circumstance

2 Prolonged

3 Severe enough to interfere with normal functioning

b. 1 Reassure him that he was having a panic attack and the doctors have ruled out a heart attack – probably his main concern – or any other physical pathology

2 Explain to him that his fast breathing is actually causing the tingling and cramps in his hands, so you need to help him slow his breathing down

3 Talk him through the steps of the slow breathing technique (Box 4, p. 12).

c. Recurrent unpredictable episodes of sudden onset severe anxiety symptoms, which occur in various (sometimes similar) situations.

d. *Short-term:* (i) Learn breathing and relaxation techniques (via self-help books, leaflets, websites; e.g. Royal College of Psychiatrists, www.rcpsych.ac.uk); and (ii) address lifestyle factors that may exacerbate anxiety (Case 1)

Medium term: CBT. Medication may be needed as an adjunct but is not curative (p. 40)

Long-term: psychotherapy would seek to address the psychodynamic origins of anxiety disorders

8

a. Obsessive compulsive disorder (OCD).

b. Recurrent, stereotyped obsessions (thoughts, ideas, images) and/or compulsions (acts) that have the following characteristics:

• They are repetitive and unpleasant

• They cause the individual distress and/or interfere with functioning

• The individual attempts to resist them, at least initially

• They are not experienced as pleasurable

• Obsessions are recognized as the individual's own thoughts (thus differentiating them from the psychotic symptom of thought insertion; Box 36, p. 195)

c. No, it usually presents in adolescence.

d. Up to 70% of patients with OCD have comorbid *depression* during its exacerbations.

Remember to screen for symptoms of other anxiety disorders (generalized; phobias; panic), which are also common amongst people with OCD. Not surprisingly, low mood and other manifestations of anxiety tend to worsen in tandem with periods of more disabling OCD. In turn, CBT and SSRI medications are effective treatments for OCD as well as depression and other anxiety disorders.

e. OCD is pathological. The individual is disturbed by the obsessions and compulsions and they interfere with their life, often by the time absorbed in unnecessary rituals but sometimes – as in this case – by causing physical injury and disruption of relationships with others, also unable to cope with the demands and limitations the rituals place on them.

Anakastic (obsessional) personality disorder is not experienced as pathological by the individual as such. The traits of this disorder (preoccupation with rules;

inflexibility and perfectionism; excessive conscientiousness) are inherent to the individual's character. While these traits may lead the individual into difficulties or conflict with others, equally in some contexts, they may help them flourish (tax inspector, surgeon).

9

a. Borderline personality disorder (BPD).

b. BPD consists of the *general features of personality disorder*. These are enduring patterns of *cognition, inner experience, behaviour* and *ways of relating to others* that cause distress plus *specific features of borderline personality* disorder:
- Unstable mood
- Liable to outbursts
- Impulsive behaviour
- Disturbed sense of self
- Chronic feelings of emptiness
- Involvement in intense unstable relationships
- Excessive efforts to avoid abandonment
- Recurrent threats or acts of self-harm

c. The voice she reports is likely to be <u>dissociative</u> in nature, in keeping with her fragmented borderline personality structure, rather than a feature of psychotic illness such as schizophrenia. It is common for such voices to have an identity that <u>carries personal meaning</u>, here that of her dead twin; the content often <u>reflects the internalized criticisms</u> from abusive adult carers in childhood.
Remember do not rush to a diagnosis of psychotic illness when presented with a seemingly psychotic symptom. All symptoms need to be understood in the wider context of a patient's presentation, history and MSE.

d. It is not likely to be helpful as such. In exceptional circumstances, however, it may be necessary to contain an acute exacerbation of suicidal feelings and intent. Acute wards do not offer structured periods of psychological treatment for long-term personality difficulties, and dynamics with other patients and staff often sharply evoke the difficult dynamics around care and rejection (e.g. discharge may be experienced as the latter) that are painfully difficult for the individual to manage.
Here the challenge is to ensure this patient knows her distress is recognized and taken seriously, and from that to support and develop her capacity to manage her intense feelings safely, hopefully without recourse to hospital admission. If she gets the message from busy staff – implicitly or explicitly – that she is not thought to be 'really suicidal' on account of her numerous presentations before, it will distress and probably infuriate her. Ultimately, it will *increase* her risk if she feels she has no option but to behave in an even more destructive way to get the care she feels she needs. Remember that she *does* pose a serious long-term risk of completed suicide – 1% of people who present with deliberate self-harm kill themselves within the year, intentionally or otherwise, with acute intoxication often blurring the boundaries around intent.
Whatever the treatment context, whenever assessing a BPD patient's immediate and longer-term treatment needs, remember the general principles of working with patients with these difficulties (Box 34, p. 192).

e. • Cognitive analytical therapy (CAT)
- Dynamic psychotherapy
- Cognitive therapy
- Dialectical behavioural therapy (DBT)
- Therapeutic community treatment

DBT and therapeutic community treatments tend to be preferred for more disturbed patients, whose difficulties are difficult to address and safely contain within one-to-one weekly individual sessions with a therapist.

10

a. Three main categories of disorder would explain this presentation:
1 Organic psychiatric disorder: physical illness or acute intoxication
2 Bipolar affective disorder – manic presentation
3 Schizophrenia

b. Physical examination, blood tests if possible, urine drug screen.

c. • *Alcohol and substance misuse:* intoxication and withdrawal
- *Iatrogenic:* antidepressants may precipitate mania/hypomania, steriods
- *Neurological* (e.g. multiple sclerosis, trauma, HIV)
- *Infectious disease:* encephalitis
- *Immunological:* systemic lupus erythematosus
- *Endocrine:* hyperthyroidism
- *Other rare causes:* cancer, deficiency states

If you remember a mnemonic for causes of delirium (e.g. 'I watch death'; Table 20, p. 69) it will serve you as a broad systematic checklist for all possible medical causes of any seemingly psychiatric presentation (Table 14, p. 47).

d. • Her behaviour may be unpredictable so while you want to conduct the interview with some privacy, you need to remain near the support of other staff

• You would be well advised to see her with a nursing colleague present, given she has a history suggestive of sexual disinhibition

• Given the concerning nature of her presentation, you know that you are going to need to get some collateral information. Before seeing her you could gather information about her past psychiatric history (if any) from her GP, and early on in your interview you may wish to ask her if there is anyone she could call who would be able to come into A&E to support her, and help you understand what has been happening

e. Bipolar disorder: manic episode. Manic/hypomanic presentations are often characterized by excessive energy, hyperactivity and pressure of speech. Mania may also present with benign calm euphoric states such as seen here.

Key clues here to differentiating her presentation from schizophrenia is her self-report of a biological symptom of mood disorder (markedly disturbed sleep) alongside her objectively elevated affect and the mood-congruent nature of her grandiose delusional beliefs and previously reported hallucination. There is also no evidence of any other symptoms of schizophrenia (it is worth reminding

yourself here of the diagnostic criteria for schizophrenia; Box 9, p. 54).

f. No, not yet. You do not yet have enough information to make a full assessment (including risk assessment) and the history of her behaviour today makes it clear she was in a very vulnerable state earlier. She appears to currently lack insight and the capacity to make sound judgements about her behaviour or treatment. Overall then, it is too early to have any confidence that she is well enough to go home alone, even with the support of others.

Remember you make a management plan based not only on someone's minute-to-minute presentation in front of you, but on the history available to you, which you ignore at your peril. It is common for people in manic/hypomanic states to have labile mood and vary in their presentation and self-report, as is the case here.

g. • Reduced need for sleep

• Increased goal-directed activity

• Irritability

• Growing optimism; making of expansive, increasingly unrealistic plans

• Thoughts faster, experienced as clearer, but gradually concentration decreases, distractibility increases

• Increasingly sociable, talkative and decreased inhibition

• Increased libido

• Increasingly talkative

Index of cases by diagnosis

Index